Emergency Nursing

made

Incredibly Easy!®

Emergency Nursing

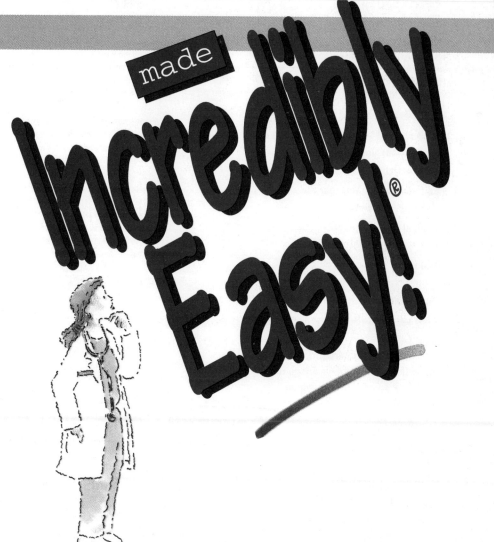

made
Incredibly
Easy!®

 Lippincott Williams & Wilkins
a Wolters Kluwer business
Philadelphia · Baltimore · New York · London
Buenos Aires · Hong Kong · Sydney · Tokyo

Staff

Executive Publisher
Judith A. Schilling McCann, RN, MSN

Editorial Director
David Moreau

Clinical Director
Joan M. Robinson, RN, MSN

Senior Art Director
Arlene Putterman

Art Director
Mary Ludwicki

Senior Managing Editor
Tracy S. Diehl

Editorial Project Manager
Gabrielle Mosquera

Clinical Project Manager
Beverly Ann Tscheschlog, RN, BS

Editor
Brenna H. Mayer

Clinical Editor
Maryann Foley, RN, BSN

Copy Editors
Kimberly Bilotta (supervisor), Jane Bradford,
Scotti Cohn, Amy Furman, Shana Harrington,
Dorothy P. Terry, Pamela Wingrod

Designer
Lynn Foulk

Illustrator
Bot Roda

Digital Composition Services
Diane Paluba (manager), Joyce Rossi Biletz

Associate Manufacturing Manager
Beth J. Welsh

Editorial Assistants
Megan L. Aldinger, Karen J. Kirk, Linda K. Ruhf

Design Assistant
Georg W. Purvis IV

Indexer
Karen C. Comerford

ENIE010706—021106

Library of Congress Cataloging-in-Publication Data
Emergency nursing made incredibly easy.
    p. ; cm.
    Includes bibliographical references and index.
    1. Emergency nursing. I. Lippincott Williams & Wilkins.
    [DNLM: 1. Emergency Nursing—methods. 2. Emergencies—nursing. 3. Emergency Treatment—nursing. WY 154 E5239 2007]

RT120.E4E44 2007
610.73'6—dc22
ISBN13 978-1-58255-464-8
ISBN10 1-58255-464-1 (alk. paper)   2006012246

Contents

Contributors and consultants

Cynthia Francis Bechtel, RN, MS, CEN, EMT-1
Professor
MassBay Community College
Framingham

Laura M. Criddle, RN, MS, CCNS, CCRN, CEN
Doctoral Student, Nursing
Oregon Health & Science University
Portland

Laurie Donaghy, RN, CEN
Staff Nurse
Frankford Hospital
Philadelphia

Nancy A. Emma, RN, BSN
Officer in Charge
U.S. Army EMS Programs Office
U.S. Army DCMT
Fort Sam Houston, Tex.

Lisa Kosits, RN, BC, MSN, CCRN, CEN
Clinical Inservice Instructor
Montefiore Medical Center
Bronx, N.Y.

Charles Kunkle, PHRN, BSN, CCRN, CEN, CNA
Nurse Manager, Emergency Department
St. Mary Medical Center
Langhorne, Pa.

Sharon L. Lee, FNP, MS, CCRN, CEN
Faculty
Bryan LGH College of Health Sciences
FNP
Gastroenterologic Specialities
Lincoln, Nebr.

Ruthie Robinson, RN, PhD(C), CEN, CCRN, FAEN
Director of the Magnet Program and Clinical
    Research
Christus Hospital
Beaumont, Tex.

Donna M. Roe, RN, MS, CEN
Clinical Education Manager
St. Joseph Hospital
Nashua, N.H.

Melissa S. Wafer, RN, MSN, CEN
Instructor
Southeastern Louisiana University
Baton Rouge, La.

Robin Walsh, RN, BSN
Clinical Nurse Supervisor
University of Massachusetts
Amherst

Foreword

If there was ever a time that emergency nursing needed to be incredibly easy, it's now. With 46 million Americans living without health insurance, the baby boomer generation approaching its 60s, and the struggles associated with the continued national nursing shortage, it's no wonder that there are more people turning to emergency departments for their health care than ever before.

The 2006 National Report Card on the State of Emergency Medicine from the American College of Emergency Physicians (*www.acep.org/webportal*), which evaluates each state's emergency care systems, emphasizes the integral role that knowledgeable emergency nurses will play in "raising the grade," both nationally and locally. As such, it's crucial that emergency nurses ensure they're providing the best possible care.

One key step in emergency nursing is to quickly assess the patient's chief complaint, and act if necessary. *Emergency Nursing Made Incredibly Easy* will help the nurse hone these vital skills. This book covers the basics of triage, such as the evidence-based triage process, and holistic care issues, such as cultural and pain considerations. Subsequent chapters focus on physiological systems, covering neurologic, cardiac, respiratory, gastrointestinal, and musculoskeletal emergencies. It also discusses wound care management, genitourinary and gynecologic emergencies, maxillofacial and ocular emergencies, shock and multisystem trauma, and environmental emergencies. *Emergency Nursing Made Incredibly Easy* addresses the challenge of switching into "disaster mode," providing concise guidelines on mobilization and management for nurses facing natural and manmade events that cause mass-casualty incidents.

The clear language and illustrations will help readers anticipate and assess certain diagnoses, and prevent predictable complications. Recurring topics for each section include how to assess the patient, diagnostic tests that should be done, treatment options, and common disorders for each body system. A *Quick quiz* at the end of each chapter tests the reader's knowledge on the information presented.

In addition, icons draw your attention to important issues:

Ages and stages—highlights age-related changes and how they affect your patient's health.

Stay on the ball—focuses on critical areas involving possible dangers, risks, complications, or contraindications.

Education edge—offers patient-teaching tips.

This book can help practicing emergency department nurses learn more about their current position. It can also help nurses from other departments (or student nurses) build enough confidence to consider joining this extremely worthwhile specialty. I'm proud to introduce to you *Emergency Nursing Made Incredibly Easy*—a wonderful new tool in the challenging but rewarding world of emergency nursing.

Enjoy!

Ann White, RN, MSN, CCNS, CEN
Clinical Nurse Specialist
Emergency Services
Department of Advanced Practice Nursing
Duke University Health System
Clinical Associate Faculty
Duke University School of Nursing
Durham, N.C.

Emergency department basics

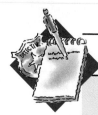

Just the facts

In this chapter, you'll learn:

♦ roles and responsibilities of an emergency nurse

♦ credentials for emergency nurses

♦ ways to work with a multidisciplinary team

♦ ways to incorporate clinical tools and best practices into your care.

What is emergency nursing?

Emergency nursing is the delivery of specialized care to a variety of ill or injured patients. Such patients may be unstable, have complex needs, and require intensive and vigilant nursing care. Others may have minor problems. No matter the reason for coming to the emergency department (ED), all patients feel that their problems are emergencies.

Common illnesses and injuries seen in patients in EDs include:
• orthopedic injuries, including fractures, strains, and sprains
• traumatic injuries from such events as car collisions and falls
• cardiovascular disorders, such as heart failure and acute coronary syndromes (unstable angina and myocardial infarction [MI])
• respiratory disorders, such as acute respiratory failure, pulmonary embolism, and asthma
• GI and hepatic disorders, such as acute pancreatitis, GI bleeding, acute liver failure, acute cholecystitis, and bowel obstructions
• renal disorders, such as acute and chronic renal failure, kidney stones, and urinary tract infections
• shock due to hypovolemia, sepsis, cardiac dysfunction, acute spinal cord injury, and anaphylaxis
• pediatric ailments, such as gastroenteritis, bronchiolitis, febrile seizures, and appendicitis
• drug overdoses

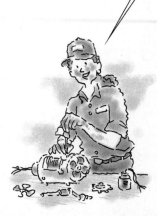

Emergency complaints come in all makes and models. This chapter will tune up your ED expertise!

- minor injuries, including lacerations and abrasions
- gynecologic and obstetric problems
- psychiatric emergencies
- injuries resulting from violence and abuse, including knife and gun injuries.

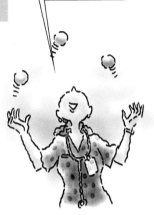

Juggling the variety of patient ailments in the ED can be tough, but we'll make sure you're prepared!

Meet the emergency nurse

An emergency nurse is responsible for making sure that all patients and members of their families receive close attention and the best care possible.

What do you do?

As an emergency nurse, you may fill many roles in the emergency setting, such as staff nurse, nurse-educator, nurse-manager, clinical nurse specialist, nurse practitioner, flight nurse, sexual assault nurse examiner, trauma care specialist, or nurse researcher. (See *Role call.*)

Where do you work?

As an emergency nurse, you may work in various settings, including:
- EDs
- flight programs
- minor care departments
- prehospital care environments
- rural clinics.

What makes you special?

A nurse who specializes in emergencies accepts a wide range of responsibilities, including:
- being an advocate
- using sound clinical judgment
- demonstrating caring practices
- collaborating with a multidisciplinary team
- demonstrating an understanding of cultural diversity
- providing patient and family teaching.

Patient advocacy is one of the most important aspects of emergency nursing.

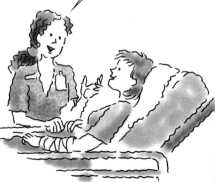

Advocacy

An advocate is a person who works on another person's behalf. As a patient advocate, you should also address the concerns of family members and the community whenever possible.

As an advocate, you're also responsible for:

Role call

By filling various nursing and management roles, an emergency nurse helps promote optimum health, prevent illness, and aid coping with illness or death. Here are various capacities in which an emergency nurse may function.

Staff nurse
- Makes independent assessments
- Plans and implements patient care
- Provides direct nursing care
- Makes clinical observations and executes interventions
- Administers medications and treatments
- Promotes activities of daily living

Nurse-educator
- Assesses patients' and families' learning needs; plans and implements teaching strategies to meet those needs
- Evaluates effectiveness of teaching
- Educates peers and colleagues
- Possesses excellent interpersonal skills

Nurse-manager
- Acts as an administrative representative of the unit
- Ensures that effective and quality nursing care is provided in a timely and fiscally sound environment

Clinical nurse specialist
- Participates in education and direct patient care
- Consults with patients and family members
- Collaborates with other nurses and health care team members to deliver high-quality care

Nurse practitioner
- Provides primary health care to patients and families; can function independently
- May obtain histories and conduct physical examinations
- Orders laboratory and diagnostic tests and interprets results
- Diagnoses disorders
- Treats patients
- Counsels and educates patients and families

Nurse researcher
- Reads current nursing literature
- Applies information in practice
- Collects data
- Conducts research studies
- Serves as a consultant during research study implementation

Flight nurse
- Performs advanced procedures in the field, such as intubation, central line placement, and chest tube placement

Sexual assault nurse examiner
- Examines patients and collects evidence in cases of known or suspected sexual assault
- May testify at trials regarding their findings

Trauma care specialist
- May function in trauma centers as staff nurse or trauma coordinator
- Maintains records related to an ED's trauma level designation

- protecting the patient's rights
- assisting the patient and his family in the decision-making process by providing education and support
- negotiating with other members of the health care team on behalf of the patient and his family
- keeping the patient and his family informed about the care plan
- advocating for flexible visitation in the ED
- respecting and supporting the decisions of the patient and his family
- serving as a liaison between the patient and family and other members of the health care team

- respecting the patient's values and cultures
- acting in the patient's best interest
- preventing injuries in the community by educating families about poison safety, use of car restraints, and safe sleeping tips for infants to prevent sudden infant death syndrome.

Stuck in the middle

Being a patient advocate can sometimes cause conflict between you and family members. For example, a patient may have an advance directive requesting no resuscitation but his family may not approve.

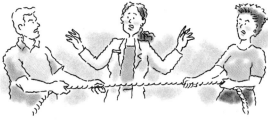

Whoa! I realize we have different ideas about emergency care, but let's do what's best for the patient, shall we?

It may also cause conflict between your professional duty and the patient's personal values. For example, the patient may be a Jehovah's Witness and refuse a blood transfusion. In this case, you should consult your facility's ethics committee as well as its policies and procedures.

Clinical judgment

An emergency nurse needs to exercise clinical judgment in a fast-paced and stressful environment. To develop sound clinical judgment, you need critical thinking skills. Critical thinking is a complex mixture of knowledge, intuition, logic, common sense, and experience.

Why be critical?

Critical thinking fosters understanding of issues and enables you to quickly find answers to difficult questions. It isn't a trial-and-error method, yet it isn't strictly a scientific problem-solving method either.

Critical thinking enhances your ability to identify a patient's needs. It also enables you to use sound clinical decision making and to determine which nursing actions best meet a patient's needs.

Developing critical thinking skills

Critical thinking skills improve with increasing clinical and scientific experience. The best way for you to develop critical thinking skills is by asking questions and learning.

Always asking questions

The first question you should find the answer to is "What are the patient's symptoms or diagnosis?" If it's a diagnosis with which

you aren't familiar, look it up and read about it. Find the answers to questions like these:
• What are the signs and symptoms?
• What's the usual cause?
• What complications can occur?
    In addition to the answers to diagnosis-related questions, also be sure to find out:
• What are the patient's physical examination findings?
• Which laboratory and diagnostic tests are necessary?
• Does the patient have risk factors? If so, are they significant? What interventions would minimize those risk factors?
• What are the patient's cultural beliefs? How can you best address the patient's cultural concerns?
• What are the possible complications? What type of monitoring is needed to watch for complications?
• What are the usual medications and treatments for the patient's condition? (If you aren't familiar with the medications or treatments, look them up in a reliable source or consult a colleague.)

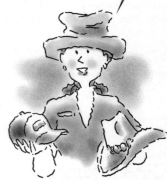

No matter what it looks like, be sure to put on your critical thinking cap for the next steps.

Critical thinking and the nursing process

Critical thinking skills are necessary when applying the nursing process—assessment, planning, implementation, and evaluation—and making patient-care decisions.

Caring practice

Caring practice is the use of a therapeutic and compassionate environment to focus on the patient's needs. Although care is based on standards and protocols, it must also be individualized to each patient.
    Caring practice also involves:
• maintaining a safe environment
• interacting with the patient and his family members in a compassionate and respectful manner throughout the ED stay
• supporting the family when a patient dies unexpectedly.

Collaboration

Collaboration allows a health care team to use all available resources for the patient. An emergency nurse is part of a multidisciplinary team in which each person contributes expertise. The collaborative goal is to optimize patient outcomes. As a nurse, you may often serve as the coordinator of such collaborative teams.

Cultural diversity

Culture is defined as the way people live and how they behave in a social group. This behavior is learned and passed on from generation to generation. Acknowledging and respecting patients' diverse cultural beliefs is a necessary part of high-quality care.

Keep an open mind

An emergency nurse is expected to demonstrate awareness and sensitivity toward a patient's religion, lifestyle, family makeup, socioeconomic status, age, gender, and values. Be sure to assess cultural factors and concerns and integrate them into the care plan.

Education

As an educator, an emergency nurse is the facilitator of patient, family, and staff education. Patient education involves teaching patients and their families about:
- the patient's illness
- the importance of managing comorbid disorders (such as diabetes, arthritis, and hypertension)
- diagnostic and laboratory testing
- planned surgical procedures, including preoperative and postoperative expectations
- instructions on specific patient care, such as wound care and range-of-motion exercises
- medications that are prescribed
- illness and injury prevention
- home care instructions and follow-up appointments.

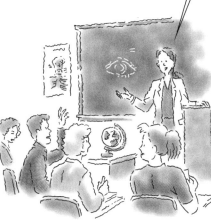

Patients, families, and staff members—everyone needs some education from an emergency nurse.

Staff as students

Emergency nurses also commonly serve as staff educators. Examples of staff teaching topics you may need to address include:
- how to use new equipment
- how to interpret diagnostic test results
- how to administer a new medication.

Becoming an emergency nurse

Most nursing students are only briefly exposed to emergency nursing. Much of the training required to become an emergency nurse is learned on the job.

Learning by doing

On-the-job training is central to gaining the extensive skills required of an emergency nurse. Your facility may provide a competency-based orientation program for new emergency nurses. In such a program, you gain knowledge and experience while working in the ED and a preceptor (a staff nurse or clinical nurse specialist with specialized training in emergency nursing) provides guidance.

An orientation period allows a nurse time to acquire the knowledge and technical skills needed to work in the emergency environment. Such technical skills include working with cardiac monitoring systems, mechanical ventilators, hemodynamic monitoring devices, autotransfusers, and intracranial pressure (ICP) monitoring devices.

Gaining credentials

The Emergency Nurses Association (ENA) is one of the world's largest specialty nursing organizations, with more than 28,000 members. The primary goal of ENA is to promote excellence in emergency nursing through leadership, education, research, and advocacy.

Through ENA, you can become certified as an emergency nurse or emergency flight nurse. Certification, demonstrated through earning your certified emergency nurse (CEN) or certified emergency flight nurse credentials, states you're a professional, with proficiency and skill in a highly specialized area of nursing. Emergency nurses can obtain certification through the Board of Certification for Emergency Nursing.

CEN certification requires renewal after 4 years. Nurses can recertify by taking the examination again or by demonstrating continuing education in emergency nursing.

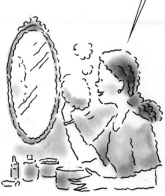

There's lots of incentive to freshen up your CEN certification over time.

Help wanted

Certification isn't mandatory to work as an emergency nurse, but it's certainly encouraged. Many units prefer to hire nurses with certification because it means that they have demonstrated expertise and commitment to emergency nursing.

Safety first

The goal of any nursing certification program is to promote safe nursing care. CEN certification is evidence that a nurse has demonstrated clinical excellence and recognizes the importance of patient safety. Certification validates the nurse's qualifications and specialized clinical knowledge.

What's in it for me?

For most nurses, the main reason for seeking CEN certification is personal fulfillment, but there are other rewards as well. Many institutions reimburse nurses for taking the examination and others offer monetary incentives to nurses with CEN certification.

Nursing responsibilities

As an emergency nurse, you're responsible for all parts of the nursing process: assessing, planning, implementing, and evaluating care of all patients in your care. Remember that each of these steps gives you an opportunity to exercise your critical thinking skills.

Assessment

Emergency nursing requires that you constantly assess the patient for subtle changes in condition and monitor all equipment being used. Caring for emergency patients may involve the use of such highly specialized equipment as cardiac monitors, hemodynamic monitoring devices, and ICP monitoring devices. As part of the patient assessment, you should also assess the patient's physical and psychological statuses and interpret laboratory data.

Planning

Planning requires you to consider the patient's psychological and physiologic needs and set realistic patient goals. The result is an individualized care plan for your patient. To ensure safe passage through the emergency environment, you must also anticipate changes in the patient's condition. For example, for a patient admitted with a diagnosis of MI, you should monitor cardiac rhythm and anticipate rhythm changes. If an arrhythmia such as complete heart block develops, you may need to change the treatment plan and establish new goals.

What's the problem?

In planning, be sure to address present and potential problems, such as:
- pain
- cardiac arrhythmias
- altered hemodynamic states
- impaired physical mobility
- impaired skin integrity
- fluid volume deficit.

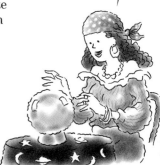

You don't need to be clairvoyant to prepare a patient care plan; just anticipate common problems.

Implementation

As a nurse, you must implement specific interventions to address existing and potential patient problems.

A call to intervene

Examples of interventions include:
- monitoring and treating cardiac arrhythmias
- managing pain
- monitoring responses to therapy.

Evaluation

It's necessary for you to continually evaluate a patient's response to interventions. Use such evaluations to change the care plan as needed to make sure that your patient continues to work toward achieving his outcome goals.

Emergency essentials

What comes to mind when you hear the word *emergency*? Do you think of a motor vehicle collision, a drowning, or a patient with cardiac arrest coming through the doors of the ED? Or, do you visualize a postoperative patient experiencing respiratory distress or a patient falling while trying to walk to the bathroom? Emergencies occur everywhere. No matter what your area of expertise, you'll encounter emergencies in your nursing career. This section will give an overview of emergency situations and your role in responding to patients who need your help.

Information station

When a patient arrives in the ED by ambulance, it's important to get as much information as you can from the prehospital care providers. For instance, if the patient was involved in an accident, you'll want to know certain information.

Danger details

- How did the accident occur?
- What type of accident was it?
- If it was a motor vehicle collision, did the vehicle sustain exterior or interior damage?

Patient particulars

- Was the patient restrained?
- Did the patient have to be extricated from the vehicle?
- Was the patient ambulatory at the scene?
- If the patient sustained a burn injury, was he found in an enclosed space?
- If the burn resulted from a fire, was the fire accompanied by an explosion?

It's quite a laundry list, but the answers to these questions provide valuable patient information.

Injuries sustained

- What injuries have the prehospital care providers identified or suspected?
- What are the patient's chief complaints?

Vital vitals

- What vital signs have care providers obtained before arriving in the ED?
- What treatment has the patient received and how did he respond?

Systematic systems

All patients with traumatic injuries should be assessed rapidly with a systematic method used consistently for all patients. The ENA has developed the Trauma Nursing Core Course to teach nurses such a method for assessing trauma patients. The ENA method uses primary and secondary surveys to rapidly identify life-threatening emergencies and prioritize care.

Primary survey

The primary survey begins with an assessment of airway, breathing, and circulation—the ABCs learned in nursing school. The ENA recommends additional assessment parameters: neurologic status—designated as *disability (D)*—and exposure and environment—designated as *E*. (See *Primary assessment of the trauma patient*.) The ABCDE primary survey consists of—you guessed it—five steps.

A is for Airway

Before you assess a trauma patient's airway, immobilize the cervical spine through initial stabilization and by applying a cervical collar. Until proven otherwise, assume that the patient who has sustained a major trauma has a cervical spine injury.

When continuing your assessment, note whether the patient can speak; if he can, he has a patent airway. Open the airway of an unresponsive patient with the head-tilt-chin-lift method or with

Primary assessment of the trauma patient

The chart below outlines the parameters for assessing the trauma patient along with their associated assessment steps and appropriate interventions.

Parameter	Assessment	Interventions
A = Airway	• Airway patency	• Institute cervical spine immobilization until X-rays determine whether the patient has a cervical spine injury. • Position the patient. • To open the airway, make sure that the neck is midline and stabilized; next, perform the jaw-thrust maneuver.
B = Breathing	• Respirations (rate, depth, effort) • Breath sounds • Chest wall movement and chest injury • Position of trachea (midline or deviation)	• Administer 100% oxygen with a bag-valve mask. • Use airway adjuncts, such as an oropharyngeal or a nasopharyngeal airway, an endotracheal tube, an esophageal-tracheal combitube, or cricothyrotomy, as indicated. • Suction the patient as needed. • Remove foreign bodies that may obstruct breathing. • Treat life-threatening conditions, such as pneumothorax or tension pneumothorax.
C = Circulation	• Pulse and blood pressure • Bleeding or hemorrhage • Capillary refill and color of skin and mucous membranes • Cardiac rhythm	• Start cardiopulmonary resuscitation, medications, and defibrillation or synchronized cardioversion. • Control hemorrhaging with direct pressure or pneumatic devices. • Establish I.V. access and fluid therapy (isotonic fluids and blood). • Treat life-threatening conditions such as cardiac tamponade.
D = Disability	• Neurologic assessment, including level of consciousness, pupils, and motor and sensory function	• Institute cervical spine immobilization until X-rays confirm the absence of cervical spine injury.
E = Exposure and environment	• Environmental exposure (extreme cold or heat) and injuries	• Examine the patient to determine the extent of injuries. • Institute appropriate therapy determined by environmental exposure (warming therapy for hypothermia or cooling therapy for hyperthermia).

modified jaw thrust in the trauma patient. Check for obstructions to the airway, such as the tongue (the most common obstruction), blood, loose teeth, or vomitus. Clear airway obstructions immediately, using the jaw thrust or chin lift technique to maintain cervical spine immobilization. You may need to use suction if blood or vomitus is present.

Insert a nasopharyngeal or oropharyngeal airway if necessary; however, remember that an oropharyngeal airway can only be used on an unconscious patient. An oropharyngeal airway stimulates the gag reflex in a conscious or semiconscious patient. If a nasopharyngeal or oropharyngeal airway fails to provide a patent airway, the patient may require intubation.

B is for Breathing

Assess the patient for spontaneous respirations, noting their rate, depth, and symmetry. Obtain oxygen saturation with pulse oximetry. Is he using accessory muscles to breathe? Do you hear breath sounds bilaterally? Do you detect tracheal deviation or jugular vein distention? Does the patient have an open chest wound? All major trauma patients require high-flow oxygen. If the patient doesn't have spontaneous respirations or if his breathing is ineffective, ventilate him by using a bag-valve-mask device until intubation can be achieved.

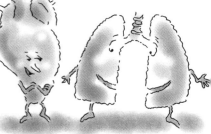

All right; just because the primary survey puts airway and breathing before circulation doesn't mean you can gloat.

C is for Circulation

Check for the presence of peripheral pulses. Determine the patient's blood pressure. What's his skin color? Does he exhibit pallor, flushing, or some other discoloration? What's his skin temperature? Is it warm, cool, or clammy to the touch? Is the patient diaphoretic? Is there obvious bleeding? All major trauma patients need at least two large-bore I.V. lines because they may require large amounts of fluids and blood. A fluid warmer should be used if possible. If the patient exhibits external bleeding, apply direct pressure over the site. If he has no pulse, initiate cardiopulmonary resuscitation immediately.

D is for Disability

Perform a neurologic assessment. Use the Glasgow Coma Scale to assess the patient's baseline status. Maintain cervical spine immobilization until X-rays confirm that there's no cervical injury. If the patient isn't alert and oriented, conduct further assessments during the secondary survey.

E is for Exposure and Environment

Expose the patient to perform a thorough assessment. Remove all clothing to assess his injuries. Remember: if the patient has bullet holes or knife tears through his clothing, don't cut through these areas. Law enforcement will count on you to preserve evidence as necessary. Environmental control means keeping the patient warm. If you've removed the patient's clothes, cover him with warm blankets. You may need to use an overhead warmer, especially with an infant or a small child. Use fluid warmers when administering large amounts of I.V. fluids. A cold patient has numerous problems with healing.

Remember that the primary ABCDE survey is a rapid assessment intended to identify life-threatening emergencies that must be treated before assessment continues.

Secondary survey

After the primary survey is completed, perform a more detailed secondary survey, which includes a head-to-toe assessment. This part of the examination identifies all injuries sustained by the patient. At this time, a care plan is developed and diagnostic tests are ordered.

Obtain a full set of vital signs initially, including respirations, pulse, blood pressure, and temperature. If you suspect chest trauma, get blood pressures in both arms.

Next, perform these five interventions:

Initiate cardiac monitoring.

Obtain continuous pulse oximetry readings. Be aware, however, that readings may be inaccurate if the patient is cold or in shock.

Insert a urinary catheter to monitor accurate intake and output measurements. Many urinary catheters also record core body temperatures. Don't insert a urinary catheter if there's blood at the urinary meatus.

Insert a nasogastric (NG) tube for stomach decompression. Injuries such as a facial fracture contraindicate the use of an NG tube; if a facial fracture is suspected, insert the tube orally instead. Depending on your facility's policy and procedures, the doctor may insert the NG tube when facial fracture is suspected.

Obtain laboratory studies as ordered, such as type and cross-matching for blood; a complete blood count or hematocrit and hemoglobin level; toxicology and alcohol screens, if indicated; a pregnancy test, if necessary; and serum electrolyte levels.

Family matters

Facilitate the presence of the patient's family. Several organizations, including the ENA and the American Heart Association, endorse the practice of allowing the patient's family to be present during resuscitation. It's important, however, to assess the family's needs before offering permission to be present. Family members may need emotional and spiritual support from you or from a member of the clergy. If a family member wishes to be present during resuscitation, assign a health care professional to explain procedures as they're performed.

Memory jogger

You may also assess a patient using this mnemonic: A Very Practical Use (AVPU).

A = Alert, oriented patient

V = responds to Voice

P = responds to Pain

U = Unresponsive patient

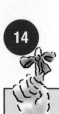

Memory jogger

The acronym SAMPLE is a mnemonic that will help you remember the types of information you'll need to obtain for the patient's history.

Subjective: What does the patient say? How did the accident occur? Does he remember? What symptoms does he report?

Allergies: Does the patient have allergies and, if so, what's he allergic to? Is he wearing a medical identification bracelet?

Medications: Does the patient take medications on a regular basis and, if so, what medications? What medications has he taken in the past 24 hours?

Past medical history: Has the patient been treated for medical conditions and, if so, which ones? Has he had surgery and if so, what type of surgery?

Last meal eaten, **L**ast tetanus shot, **L**ast menses: When was the last time the patient had anything to eat or drink? When did he have his most recent tetanus shot? (If unknown, administer one in the emergency department.) If the patient is a female of child-bearing age, when was her last menses? Could she be pregnant?

Events leading to injury: How did the accident occur? Inquire about precipitating factors, if any. For instance, the patient being seen for injuries sustained in a motor vehicle accident may have had the accident because he experienced a myocardial infarction while driving. Likewise, the patient who sustained a fall might have fallen because he tripped or became dizzy.

A little TLC

During a tense trauma situation, the urgency of the assessment and treatment processes may cause you to overlook the patient's fears. Remember to talk to the patient and explain the examination and interventions being administered. An encouraging word and tone can go a long way to comfort and calm a frightened patient. Comfort measures also include the administration of pain medication and sedation as needed.

History counts

Obtain the patient's history, remembering to obtain as much information as possible to determine the presence of coexisting conditions, or alcohol or drug use, that could affect his care or factors that might have precipitated the trauma.

Next, perform a head-to-toe assessment, starting at the patient's head and working your way down to his feet. Don't forget to check all posterior surfaces. Logroll the patient (with assistance, if necessary) to assess for injuries to the back. Address life-threatening injuries immediately.

Triage

Triage is a method of prioritizing patient care according to the type of illness or injury and the urgency of the patient's condition. It's used to ensure that each patient receives care appropriate to his need and in a timely manner.

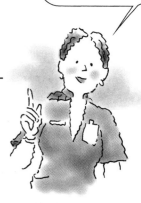

The triage method prioritizes ailments so that all patients receive appropriate care.

Many people with nonurgent conditions come to the ED because it's their only source of medical care; this increase in nonurgent cases has necessitated a means of quickly identifying and treating those patients with more serious conditions. The triage nurse must be able to rapidly assess the nature and urgency of problems for many patients and prioritize their care based on that assessment.

The ENA has established guidelines for triage based on a five-tier system:

Level I: Resuscitation—This level includes patients who need immediate nursing and medical attention, such as those with cardiopulmonary arrest, major trauma, severe respiratory distress, and seizures.

Level II: Emergent—These patients need immediate nursing assessment and rapid treatment. Patients who may be assessed as level II include those with head injuries, chest pain, stroke, asthma, and sexual assault injuries.

Level III: Urgent—These patients need quick attention, but can wait as long as 30 minutes for assessment and treatment. Such patients might report to the ED with signs of infection, mild respiratory distress, or moderate pain.

Level IV: Less urgent—Patients in this triage category can wait up to 1 hour for assessment and treatment; they may include those with an earache, chronic back pain, upper respiratory symptoms, and a mild headache.

Level V: Nonurgent—These patients can wait up to 2 hours (possibly longer) for assessment and treatment; those with sore throat, menstrual cramps, and other minor symptoms are typically assigned to level V.

If you can't decide which triage level is best for a patient, assign him the higher level.

Once divided

Carefully document the patient's chief complaint and vital signs, your triage assessment, and the triage category to which you've assigned him. It's also important to document pertinent negatives. For example, if the patient is experiencing chest pain without cardiac symptoms, be sure to note "Patient complains of nonradiating left chest pain. Denies shortness of breath, diaphoresis, or nausea. Pain increases with movement and deep inspiration." Quote the patient when appropriate.

As you perform triage, tell the patients you interview that you're the triage nurse and that you'll be performing a screening assessment. Be attentive to what's occurring beyond your current assessment because it may be necessary to leave the patient if a patient with a more critical situation arrives in the ED.

Stay in touch

Maintain communication with patients waiting to be summoned to a treatment room because a patient's status may change—improving or worsening—during an extended period in the waiting room. Patients appreciate information on the reasons for waiting-room delays.

Multidisciplinary teamwork

Nurses working with emergency patients commonly collaborate with a multidisciplinary team of health care professionals. The team approach helps caregivers to meet the diverse needs of individual patients.

The whole goal

The goal of collaboration is to provide effective and comprehensive (holistic) care. Holistic care addresses the biological, psychological, social, and spiritual dimensions of a person.

Team huddle

A multidisciplinary team providing direct patient care may consist of many professionals, including:
• registered nurses (RNs)
• doctors
• advanced practice nurses (such as clinical nurse specialists and nurse practitioners)
• licensed practical nurses (LPNs)
• respiratory therapists, paramedics, emergency department practitioners, and others. (See *Meet the team.*)

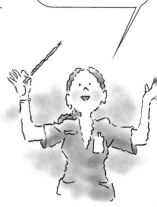

When we coordinate efforts, ED professionals make beautiful music together.

Working with registered nurses

Teamwork is essential in the stressful environment of the ED. The emergency nurse must work well with the other professional RNs in the department.

The buddy system

It's important to have a colleague to look to for moral support, physical assistance with a patient, and problem solving. No one person has all the answers, but together nurses have a better chance of solving problems.

Meet the team

Various members of the multidisciplinary team have collaborative relationships with emergency nurses. Here are some examples.

Patient-care technician
• Responsible for providing direct patient care to critically ill patients
• Bathes patients
• Obtains vital signs
• Assists with transportation of patients for testing

Pastoral caregiver
• Also known as a *chaplain*
• Meets patient's and family's spiritual and religious needs
• Provides support and empathy to the patient and his family
• Delivers patient's last rites if appropriate

Stroke team
• Assesses persons coming to the emergency department with symptoms of an acute stroke
• Assesses patients for appropriateness of thrombolytic therapy and other needed treatments
• Commonly includes a nurse, a neurologist, and a radiologist
• Can participate in hospital and community education related to stroke prevention, early signs and symptoms, and treatments

Social Services
• Assist patients and families with such problems as difficulty paying for medications, follow-up physician visits, and other health-related issues
• Assist patients with travel and housing if needed

Child Protective Services
• Designed to protect children from abusive situations
• Preserves the family unit, if possible, while ensuring the safety of children

Working with doctors

Patients in the ED are usually seen by an ED doctor who will probably have no prior knowledge of the patient. Consults made to the patient's primary care doctor can help fill in the blanks, as can assessments from specialists within your facility. Specialists commonly called to the ED to assess and treat patients include:

• cardiologists
• neurologists
• orthopedists
• gynecologists
• pediatricians.

In addition, if you work in a teaching institution, you may also interact on a regular basis with medical students, interns, and residents who are under the direction of the attending doctor.

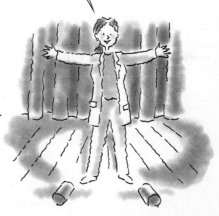

The comedy of educating, the drama of managing—a CNS plays it all!

Working with advanced practice nurses

Advanced practice nurses—clinical nurse specialists (CNSs) and acute care nurse practitioners (ACNPs)—are increasingly employed in EDs. An advanced practice nurse may be employed by a hospital and assigned to a specific unit or may be employed by a doctor to assist in caring for and monitoring patients. The advanced practice nurse assists staff nurses in clinical decision making and enhances the quality of patient care, which improves patient care outcomes.

The roles of a lifetime

The traditional roles of a CNS are:
- clinician
- educator
- researcher
- consultant
- manager.

The CNS offers support and guidance to staff nurses as they care for patients. The CNS assists with problem solving when complex care is necessary for patients and their families. In addition, the CNS may develop research projects dealing with problems identified on the unit.

On a role

An ACNP has the responsibilities traditionally held by a nurse practitioner. These responsibilities may include:
- conducting comprehensive health assessments
- diagnosing
- prescribing pharmacologic and nonpharmacologic treatments.

An ACNP may also conduct research and manage care.

Working with licensed practical nurses

In some EDs, LPNs are members of the health care team. Generally, an LPN collaborates with an RN to deliver patient care. The RN is responsible for and delegates specific tasks to the LPN, whose duties may include caring directly for patients and collecting data. The LPN may also administer approved medications, assist with procedures, and record vital signs.

Working with respiratory therapists

An emergency nurse also commonly collaborates with respiratory therapists in caring for emergency patients.

Respiration-related roles

The role of a respiratory therapist is to monitor and manage the respiratory status of patients. To do this, the respiratory therapist may:
- administer breathing treatments
- suction patients

- collect specimens
- obtain arterial blood gas values
- manage ventilator changes.

Clinical tools

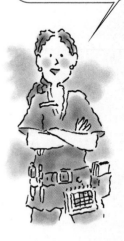

The tools of your trade? Clinical pathways, practice guidelines, and protocols.

The multidisciplinary team uses various tools to promote safe and comprehensive holistic care. These tools include clinical pathways, practice guidelines, and protocols.

Clinical pathways

Clinical pathways (also known as *critical pathways*) are care management plans for patients with a given diagnosis or condition.

Follow the path

Clinical pathways are typically generated and used by departments that deliver care for similar conditions to many patients. A multidisciplinary committee of clinicians at the facility usually develops clinical pathways. The overall goals are to:
- establish a standard approach to care for all providers in the department
- establish roles for various members of the health care team
- provide a framework for collecting data on patient outcomes.

Tried and true

Pathways are based on evidence from research and clinical practice. The committee gathers and uses information from peer-reviewed literature and experts outside the facility.

Outlines and timelines

Clinical pathways usually outline the duties of all professionals involved with patient care. They follow specific timelines for indicated actions. They also specify expected patient outcomes, which serve as checkpoints for the patient's progress and caregiver's performance.

Practice guidelines

Practice guidelines specify courses of action to be taken in response to a diagnosis or condition. Practice guidelines aid decision making by practitioners and patients. They're multidisciplinary in nature and can be used to coordinate care by multiple providers.

Let an expert be your guide

Expert health care providers usually write practice guidelines. They condense large amounts of information into easily usable formats, combining clinical expertise with the best available clinical evidence. Practice guidelines are used to:
• streamline care
• control variations in practice patterns
• distribute health care resources more effectively.

The evidence is in

Practice guidelines are valuable sources of information. They indicate which tests and treatments are appropriate and provide a framework for building a standard of care (a statement describing an expected level of care or performance).

Consider the source

Like research-based information, clinical guidelines should be evaluated for the quality of their sources. It's a good idea to read the developers' policy statement about how evidence was selected and what values were applied in making recommendations for care.

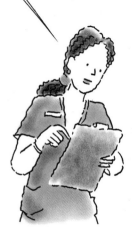

Always check where practice guidelines come from before you apply them to your patient.

Protocols

Protocols are facility-established sets of procedures for a given circumstance. Their purpose is to outline actions that are most likely to produce optimal patient outcomes.

First things first

Protocols describe a sequence of actions a practitioner should take to establish a diagnosis or begin a treatment regimen. For example, a chest pain protocol outlines a bedside strategy for managing chest pain.

Protocols facilitate delivery of consistent, cost-effective care. They're also educational resources for clinicians who strive to keep abreast of current best practices. Protocols may be either highly directive or flexible, allowing practitioners to use clinical judgment.

Input from experts

Nursing or medical experts write protocols, commonly with input from other health care providers. Protocols may be approved by legislative bodies, such as boards of nursing or medicine in some states. Hospital committees may approve other types of protocols for various facilities.

Transport

Patients who are hospitalized rarely stay in their room for their entire visit; they're transported for diagnostic tests, procedures, and surgery. The ED patient is no different. Trauma patients can experience either an interfacility or intrafacility transport journey.

Not so simple

Moving a patient from one place to another sounds simple. However, it itsn't quite so easy when a patient is hemodynamically unstable, has airway or respiratory compromise, requires continuous cardiac monitoring, continuous infusion of I.V. fluids or medications, or has an artificial airway or mechanical ventilation. In these instances, patients must be accompanied by an RN who's trained and prepared to handle any emergency situation that can happen.

Before any transport, the patient's condition must be evaluated to ensure his safety.

Interfacility transport

An *interfacility transport* is one that moves the patient from the ED to another health care facility. Interfacility transport happens on the ground with a paramedic ambulance or critical care transport, or by air (usually by helicopter, but fixed- and rotary-wing planes may also be used).

ED on wheels (or wings)

Interfacility transport vehicles are like EDs on wheels. They can safely handle the transport of critically ill patients and are staffed with critical care transport teams that include specially trained paramedics, specially trained RNs, and emergency flight nurses. The staff is trained to handle intra-aortic balloon pumps and invasive pressure and end-tidal carbon dioxide monitoring.

Sure it's costly, but you can't beat air transport for a dramatic entrance!

Movin' out

Trauma patients are moved from their original facility to another for several reasons. The patient may be moved because he requires a higher level of medical care or special services not offered at the receiving facility. Alternately, he may be moved because his physician is at another hospital, or because of family or patient convenience.

Cha-ching

Interfacility transport doesn't come without a price. Air transport can be very costly in more ways than one; it's expensive, and airplanes can only land at approved airports. This mode of travel also requires that the patient be transported via ambulance to the airplane and then from the airplane to the facility. This loading and unloading can cause the patient unneeded stress.

Helicopter transport is expensive and can cost up to four times the cost of an ambulance. Its advantage is the ability to land at the scene of an accident and at hospitals equipped with heliport pads.

Intrafacility transport

An *intrafacility transport* involves transporting the patient from the ED to another area of the receiving hospital such as an inpatient unit, the X-ray or imaging department, or the operating room.

Movin' in

Stable ED patients may be transported to another area of the hospital by ancillary support staff provided that they don't require continuous monitoring. Examples of stable patients may include pregnant patients without abdominal trauma, persistent uterine contractions, or signs of imminent birth, and patients with:
• closed head injuries
• abdominal pain, but who have stable vital signs
• closed head injuries without an alerted level of consciousness, neurologic impairment, or severe agitation
• mild injuries or illnesses that carry minimal risk of becoming unstable.

Communication

Regardless of which type of transport the patient requires, communication is vital to the patient's survival in coming to your facility, going to another facility, or just moving within your facility. Complete documentation of the patient's condition, procedures, laboratory test results, monitoring parameters, and medications is paramount.

All in the know

In fact, the Joint Commission on Accreditation of Healthcare Organizations has issued a new Sentinel Event Alert that urges paying stronger attention to the accuracy of medications given to patients as they transition from one care setting or

> Communication is key during patient transport! Of course, it's a lot easier when someone is actually listening to you!

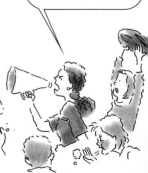

practitioner to another. Medication understanding should occur whenever a patient moves from one location to another location in a health care facility, or from one health care facility to another, or when there is a change in the caregivers responsible for the patient.

When giving report about a patient, be sure to include:
• the patient's name, age, allergies, weight, medical history, and daily medications
• when the current symptoms first occurred
• when the patient first arrived in the ED
• critical laboratory values
• diagnostic and interventional procedures that the patient received
• I.V. sites and size of catheters as well as fluids infusing, rate of infusion, and dose of any added medications
• medications given to the patient and his response
• endotracheal tube size (if the patient is intubated); depth of insertion and ventilator settings
• the patient's vital signs.

Family matters

Make sure that the patient's family is kept informed of plans to transport him. A traumatic event is stressful enough for the family, and being kept abreast of the patient's condition as well as plans for transporting him may help allay the patient's and his family's fears.

Best practices

As new procedures and medicines become available, nurses committed to excellence regularly update and adapt their practices. An approach known as *best practices* is an important tool for providing high-quality care.

Best for all concerned

The term *best practices* refers to clinical practices, treatments, and interventions that result in the best possible outcomes for the patient and your facility.

The best practice approach is generally a team effort that draws on various types of information. Common sources of information used to identify best practices are research data, personal experience, and expert opinion.

Emergency research

The goal of emergency nursing research is to improve the delivery of care and thereby improve patient outcomes. Nursing care is commonly based on evidence that's derived from research. Evidence can be used to support current practices or to change practices. (See *Research and nursing.*)

The best way to get involved in research is to be a good consumer of nursing research. You can do so by reading nursing journals and being aware of the quality of research and reported results. The Emergency Nurses Association publishes the *Journal of Emergency Nursing*, which has many pertinent research articles.

Share and share alike

Don't be afraid to share research findings with colleagues. Sharing promotes sound clinical care, and all involved may learn about easier and more efficient ways to care for patients.

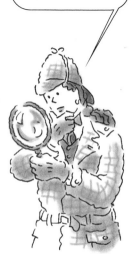

Hmmm...the evidence points to an alternate treatment.

Evidence-based care

Evidence-based care isn't based on tradition, custom, or intuition. It's derived from various concrete sources, such as:
• formal nursing research
• clinical knowledge
• scientific knowledge.

Research and nursing

All scientific research is based on the same basic process, which consists of these steps:

1. Identify a problem. Identifying problems in the emergency environment isn't difficult. An example of such a problem is maintaining body temperature in a trauma patient.

2. Conduct a literature review. The goal of this step is to see what has been published about the identified problem.

3. Formulate a research question or hypothesis. In the case of body temperature, one question is, "Which method of warming is most effective in a trauma patient?"

4. Design a study. The study may be experimental or nonexperimental. The nurse must decide what data should be collected and how to collect that data.

5. Obtain consent. The nurse must obtain consent to conduct research from the study participants. Most facilities have an internal review board that must approve such permission for studies.

6. Collect data. After the study is approved, the nurse can begin conducting the study and collecting the data.

7. Analyze the data. The nurse analyzes the data and states the conclusions derived from the analysis.

8. Share the information. Lastly, the researcher shares the collected information with other nurses through publications and presentations.

An evidence-based example

Research results may provide insight into the treatment of a patient who, for example, doesn't respond to a medication or treatment that seemed effective for other patients.

In this example, you may believe that a certain drug should be effective for pain relief, based on previous experience with that drug. The trouble with such an approach is that other factors can contribute to pain relief, such as the route of administration, the dosage, and concurrent treatments.

First, last, and always

Regardless of the value of evidence-based care, you should always use professional clinical judgment when dealing with emergency patients and their families. Remember that each patient's condition ultimately dictates treatment.

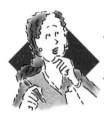

Quick quiz

1. To work in an ED, you must:
   A. have a baccalaureate degree.
   B. have certification in emergency nursing.
   C. use the nursing process in delivering nursing care.
   D. possess an advanced nursing degree.

Answer: C. The professional nurse uses the nursing process (assessment, planning, implementation, and evaluation) to care for emergency patients.

2. Professional certification in emergency nursing allows you to:
   A. function as an advanced practice nurse.
   B. validate knowledge and skills in emergency nursing.
   C. obtain an administrative position.
   D. obtain a pay raise.

Answer: B. The purpose of professional certification is to validate knowledge and skill in a particular area. Certification is a demonstration of excellence and commitment to your chosen specialty area.

3. The purpose of the multidisciplinary team is to:
   A. assist the nurse in performing patient care.
   B. replace the concept of primary care in the emergency setting.
   C. minimize lawsuits in the ED.
   D. provide holistic, comprehensive care to the patient.

Answer: D. The purpose of the multidisciplinary team is to provide comprehensive care to the emergency patient.

4. The easiest way to participate in research is to:
   A. be a good consumer of research.
   B. analyze related studies.
   C. conduct a research study.
   D. participate on your facility's internal review board.

Answer: A. Begin by reading research articles and judging whether they're applicable to your practice. Research findings aren't useful if they aren't incorporated into practice.

5. The purpose of evidence-based practice is to:
   A. validate traditional nursing practices.
   B. improve patient outcomes.
   C. refute traditional nursing practices.
   D. establish a body of knowledge unique to nursing.

Answer: B. Although evidence-based practices may validate or refute traditional practice, their purpose is to improve patient outcomes.

Scoring

☆☆☆ If you answered all five questions correctly, take a bow! You're basically a whiz when it comes to emergency nursing basics.

☆☆ If you answered three or four questions correctly, there's no room for criticism! Your critical thinking skills are basically intact.

☆ If you answered fewer than three questions correctly, the situation is emergent! Review the chapter and you'll be on the right pathway.

Holistic care

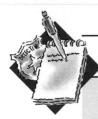

Just the facts

In this chapter, you'll learn:

♦ family dynamics to consider when you provide care

♦ issues that affect emergency patients and their families

♦ ways to assess and manage pain in emergency patients

♦ principles of ethical decision making

♦ concepts related to end-of-life decisions and how they're important to your care.

What is holistic health care?

Holistic health care revolves around a notion of totality. The goal of holistic care is to meet not only the patient's physical needs, but also his social, spiritual, and emotional needs.

A new dimension

Holistic care addresses all dimensions of a person, including:
- physical
- emotional
- social
- spiritual.

   Only by considering these dimensions can the health care team provide high-quality holistic care. You should strive to provide holistic care to all emergency patients, even if their physical needs seem more pressing than other needs.

Holistic care issues

The road to delivering the best holistic care is strewn with various issues, including:

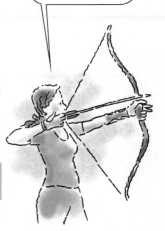

Holistic care aims to treat the entire patient from the inside out.

- patient and family issues
- cognitive issues
- ethics issues.

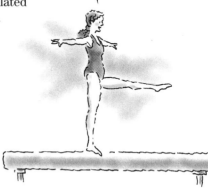

Keep in mind that the stress from a medical emergency can really throw a family off-balance.

Patient and family issues

A *family* is a group of two or more persons who possibly live together in the same household, perform certain interrelated social tasks, and share an emotional bond. Families can profoundly influence the individuals within them.

Family ties

A family is a dynamic system. During stress-free times, this system tends to maintain homeostasis, meaning that it exists in a stable state of harmony and balance. However, when a crisis sends one family member into the emergency department (ED), the rest may feel a tremendous strain and family homeostasis is thrown off. The major effects of such imbalances are:
- increased stress levels
- reorganization of family roles.

Slipping on emotional turmoil

The emergency patient's condition may change rapidly (within minutes or hours); the result of such physiological instability is emotional turmoil for the family. Family members may use whatever coping mechanisms they have, such as seeking support from friends or clergy. The longer the patient remains in the ED, however, the more stress increases for the patient and his family.

Circle out of round

When sudden critical illness or injury disrupts the family circle, a patient can no longer fulfill certain role responsibilities. Such roles are typically:
- financial (if the patient is a major contributor to the family's monetary stability)
- social (if the patient fills such roles as spouse, parent, mediator, or disciplinarian).

Unprepared for the worst

Family members may also worry about the possible death of the patient. The suddenness of the illness or injury may overwhelm the family and put it into a crisis state. The ramifications of the patient's illness or injury may cause other family members to feel hopeless and helpless.

Nursing responsibilities

The patient's family needs guidance and support during his stay in the ED and beyond. An emergency nurse's responsibility to family is to provide information about:

- nursing care
- the patient's prognosis and expected treatments.

Lend a hand

Because you're regularly exposed to members of the patient's family, you can help them during their time of crisis. For example, you can observe the family's anxiety level and, if necessary, refer them to another member of the multidisciplinary team, such as a social service agent or clergy member.

You can also help the family solve problems by helping them:

- verbalize the immediate problem
- identify support systems
- recall how they handled stress in the past.

Such assistance helps the family focus on the present issue. It also allows them to solve problems and regain a sense of control over their lives.

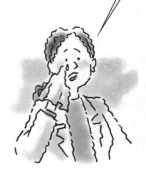

Encouraging families to express their feelings helps them relieve stress. *sniff*

Lend an ear, too

You can also help the family cope with their feelings during this stressful time. Two ways to do this are by encouraging expression of feelings (such as by crying or discussing the issue) and providing empathy.

Because you asked

During a patient's stay in the ED, families come to rely on the opinions of professionals and commonly ask for their input. They need honest information given to them in terms they can understand. In many cases, you're the health care team member who provides this information.

Living with the decision

A nurse can use phrases such as, "I know that you would like me to decide what's best for your loved one, but I can't make that decision because you're the ones who will have to live with the outcome." The emergency nurse then needs to reinforce and acknowledge the family's decision and accept their feelings about it.

Cultural considerations

Cultural influences can affect how a family copes with the hospitalization of a loved one. A patient's cultural background can also affect many aspects of care, such as:

- patient and family roles during illness

- communication between health care providers and the patient and his family
- feelings of the patient and his family regarding end-of-life issues
- family views regarding health care practices
- pain management
- nutrition
- spiritual support.

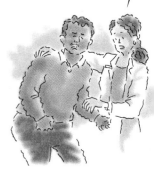

Culture affects many aspects of patient care, including pain management.

Consider culture

To provide effective holistic care, you must honor the patient's cultural beliefs and values. Because culture can impact care, you should perform a cultural assessment. (See *Assessing cultural considerations.*)

Conducting a cultural assessment enables you to:
- recognize a patient's cultural responses to illness and hospitalization
- determine how the patient and his family define health and illness
- determine the family's beliefs about the cause of the illness.

Cognitive issues

A patient in an ED may feel overwhelmed by the technology around him. Although this equipment is essential for patient care, it can create an environment that's foreign to the patient, which can result in disturbed cognition (thought-related function). In addition, the disease process can affect cognitive function in an emergency patient. For example, a patient with metabolic disturbances or hypoxia can experience confusion and changes in sensorium (mental clarity).

Fair to compare

When assessing cognitive function, the first question you should ask is, "What was your previous level of functioning?" If the patient can't answer this question, ask a family member.

It's a factor

Many factors impact a patient's cognitive function while in the ED, including:
- invasion of personal space
- medications
- pain
- sensory input.

Assessing cultural considerations

A cultural assessment yields the information you need to administer high-quality nursing care to members of various cultural populations. The goal of the cultural assessment quest is to gain awareness and understanding of cultural variations and their effects on the care you provide. For each patient, you and other members of the multidisciplinary team use the findings of a cultural assessment to develop an individualized care plan.

When performing a cultural assessment, be sure to ask questions that yield certain information about the patient and his family, including questions about:
• cultural health beliefs
• communication methods
• cultural restrictions
• social networks
• nutritional status
• religion
• values and beliefs.

Here are examples of the types of questions you should consider for each patient.

Cultural health beliefs
• What does the patient believe caused his illness? A patient may believe that his illness is the result of an imbalance in yin and yang, punishment for a past transgression, or the result of divine wrath.
• How does the patient express pain?
• What does the patient believe promotes health? Beliefs can range from eating certain foods to wearing amulets for good luck.
• In what types of healing practices (such as herbal remedies and healing rituals) does the patient engage?

Communication differences
• What language does the patient speak?
• Does the patient require an interpreter?
• How does the patient want to be addressed?
• What are the styles of nonverbal communication (for example, eye contact or touching)?

Cultural restrictions
• How does the patient's cultural group express emotion?
• How are feelings about death, dying, and grief expressed?
• How is modesty expressed?
• Does the patient have restrictions related to exposure of parts of the body?

Social networks
• What are the roles of each family member during health and illness?
• Who makes the decisions?

Nutrition
• What's the meaning of food and eating to the patient?
• What types of food does he eat?
• Does the patient's food need to be prepared a certain way?

Religion
• What's the role of religious beliefs and practices during illness?
• Does the patient believe that special rites or blessings need to be performed?
• Are there healing rituals or practices that must be followed?

Invasion of personal space

Personal space is the unmarked boundary or territory around a person. Several factors—such as cultural background and social situation—influence a patient's interpretation of personal space. A patient's personal space is limited in many ways by the emergency environment—for example, due to the confines of bed rest, lack of privacy, and use of invasive equipment.

You can try to increase your patient's sense of personal space—even within the emergency environment—by simply remembering to show common courtesy, such as:

- asking permission to perform a procedure or look at a wound or dressing
- pulling the curtain or closing the door
- knocking before you enter the patient's room.

Medications

Medications that can cause adverse central nervous system reactions and affect cognitive function include:
- inotropics—such as digoxin (Digitek), which can cause agitation, hallucinations, malaise, dizziness, vertigo, and paresthesia
- barbiturates—such as phenobarbital (Luminal), which can cause drowsiness, lethargy, hangover symptoms, physical and psychological dependence, and paradoxical excitement (in elderly patients)
- corticosteroids—such as prednisone (Hydrocortone), which can cause euphoria, psychotic behavior, insomnia, vertigo, headache, paresthesia, and seizures
- benzodiazepines—such as lorazepam (Ativan), which can cause drowsiness, sedation, disorientation, amnesia, unsteadiness, and agitation
- opioid analgesics—such as oxycodone (OxyContin), which can cause sedation, clouded sensorium, euphoria, dizziness, lightheadedness, and somnolence.

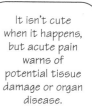

If you think finding personal space in the ED is hard, imagine what it's like for a patient!

Pain control issues

Because fear of pain is a major concern for many emergency patients, pain management is an important part of your care. Emergency patients are exposed to many types of procedures—such as I.V. procedures, cardiac monitoring, and intubation—that cause discomfort and pain. Pain is classified as acute or chronic.

Acute pain

Acute pain is caused by tissue damage due to injury or disease. It varies in intensity from mild to severe and lasts briefly. Acute pain is considered a protective mechanism because it warns of present or potential tissue damage or organ disease. It may result from a traumatic injury, surgical or diagnostic procedure, or medical disorder.

Examples include:
- pain experienced after a traumatic injury
- pain experienced during invasive procedures
- pain of acute myocardial infarction.

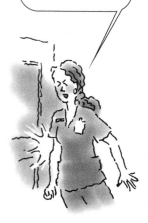

It isn't cute when it happens, but acute pain warns of potential tissue damage or organ disease.

Help is at hand

Acute pain can be managed effectively with analgesics, such as opioids and nonsteroidal anti-inflammatory drugs (NSAIDs). It generally subsides when the underlying problem is resolved.

Chronic pain

Chronic pain is ongoing pain that lasts 6 months or longer. It may be as intense as acute pain but isn't a warning of tissue damage. Some patients in the ED experience chronic as well as acute pain.

Examples of chronic pain include:
- arthritis pain
- chronic back pain
- chronic pain from cancer.

Don't be fooled

The nervous system adapts to chronic pain. This adaptation means that many typical manifestations of pain—such as abnormal vital signs and facial grimacing—cease to exist. Therefore, chronic pain should be assessed as often as acute pain (generally, at least every 2 hours or more often, depending on the patient's condition). Assess chronic pain by questioning the patient.

Pain assessment

When it comes to pain assessment for emergency patients, it's especially important for the nurse to have good assessment skills. The most valid pain assessment comes from the patient's own reports.

A pain assessment includes questions about:
- *location.* Ask the patient to tell you where the pain is; there may be more than one area of pain.
- *intensity.* Ask the patient to rate the pain using a pain scale.
- *quality.* Ask how the pain feels: sharp, dull, aching, or burning.
- *onset, duration, and frequency.* Ask when the pain started, how long it lasts, and how often it occurs.
- *alleviating and aggravating factors.* Ask what makes the pain feel better and what makes it worse.
- *associated factors.* Ask whether other problems are associated with the pain, such as nausea and vomiting.
- *effects on lifestyle.* Ask whether appetite, sleep, relationships, emotions, and work are affected.

Choose a tool

Many pain assessment tools are available. Whichever you choose, make sure it's used consistently so that everyone on the health care team is speaking the same language when addressing the patient's pain.

The three most common pain assessment tools used by clinicians are the visual analog scale, numeric rating scale, and faces scale. (See *Common pain-rating scales.*)

Silent suffering

Many patients can't verbally express feelings of pain. For example, a patient may be unable to speak due to intubation or have an altered level of consciousness ranging from confusion to unresponsiveness. In such cases, it's up to the nurse to ascertain the patient's pain level.

Body and mind

There are many physiologic and psychological responses to pain that a nurse should watch for during a pain assessment.

Some examples of the physiologic responses to pain are:
- tachycardia
- tachypnea
- dilated pupils
- increased or decreased blood pressure
- pallor
- nausea and vomiting
- loss of appetite.

Psychological responses to pain may manifest as:
- fear
- anxiety
- confusion
- depression
- sleep deprivation.

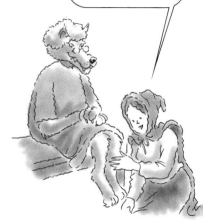

My, what a strange pallor you have, Grandma! Are you sure you aren't in any pain?

Pain particulars

When communicating aspects of a patient's pain to his doctor or other health care providers, make sure you:
- describe the pain by location, intensity, and duration
- indicate possible causes of the pain if known
- describe how the patient is responding to the pain or any treatment interventions.

Pain management

Achieving adequate pain control in the ED depends on effective pain assessment and the use of pharmacologic and nonpharmacologic treatments.

To provide the best holistic care possible, work with the doctor and other members of the health care team to develop an individualized pain management program for each patient.

Common pain-rating scales

These common pain-rating scales are examples of the rating systems you can use to help a patient quantify pain levels.

Visual analog scale

To use the visual analog scale, ask the patient to place a line across the scale to indicate the current level of pain. The scale is a 10-cm line with "No pain" at one end and "Pain as bad as it can be" at the other end. The pain rating is determined by using a ruler to measure the distance, in millimeters, from "No pain" to the patient's mark.

No pain _____ Pain as bad as it can be

Numeric rating scale

To use the numeric rating scale, ask the patient to choose a number from 0 (indicating no pain) to 10 (indicating the worst pain imaginable) to indicate his current pain level. The patient may circle the number on the scale or verbally state the number that best describes the pain.

No pain | 0   1   2   3   4   5   6   7   8   9   10 | Pain as bad as it can be

Faces scale

A pediatric or adult patient with language difficulty may not be able to describe the current pain level using the visual analog scale or the numeric rating scale. In that case, use a faces scale like the one below. Ask your patient to choose the face on a scale from 1 to 6 that best represents the severity of current pain.

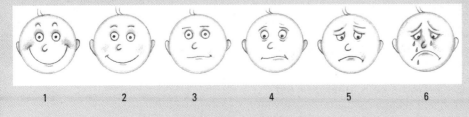

```
   1              2              3              4              5              6
```

Pharmacologic pain management

Pharmacologic pain management is common in EDs. Three classes of medications commonly used by the emergency nurse are:
- nonopioids
- opioids
- adjuvant medications.

Nonopioids are number 1

Nonopioids are the first choice for managing mild pain. They decrease pain by inhibiting inflammation at the injury site. Examples of nonopioids are:
- acetaminophen (Tylenol)

- NSAIDs, such as ibuprofen (Advil) and naproxen (Naprosyn)
- salicylates such as aspirin.

Opioid option

Opioids are narcotics that contain a derivative of the opium (poppy) plant and other synthetic drugs that imitate natural opioids. Opioids work by blocking the release of neurotransmitters involved in transmitting pain signals to the brain. There are three categories of opioids. (See *A trio of opioids*.)

Adjuvants are alright

Adjuvant analgesics are drugs that have other primary indications but are used as analgesics in some circumstances. Adjuvants may be given in combination with opioids or alone to treat patients with chronic pain. Drugs used as adjuvant analgesics include:
- anticonvulsants, such as carbamazepine (Tegretol), clonazepam (Klonopin), and gabapentin (Neurontin)
- tricyclic antidepressants, such as nortriptyline (Pamelor)
- benzodiazepines, such as alprazolam (Xanax), diazepam (Valium), and lorazepam (Ativan)
- corticosteroids, such as dexamethasone (Dexasone) and methylprednisolone (Solu-Medrol).

Adjuvant analgesics work alone or with a partner to help alleviate chronic pain.

Drug administration

A common route of pain medication administration in the ED is I.V. bolus on an as-needed basis. It's the preferred route for opioid therapy, especially when short-term pain relief is needed—for example, during procedures such as wound care. The benefit of this method is rapid pain control. On the downside, with I.V. bolus administration the patient experiences alternating periods of pain control and pain.

Nonpharmacologic pain management

Pain control isn't achieved solely with medications. Nonpharmacologic means are useful adjuncts in managing pain. Some common nonpharmacologic pain control methods are:
- distraction—such as television viewing and reading
- music therapy—a form of sound therapy using rhythmic sound to communicate, relax, and encourage healing (effective for brief periods of time)
- hypnosis—used to achieve *symptom suppression,* to block awareness of pain, or *symptom substitution,* which allows a positive interpretation of pain
- imagery—in which the patient visualizes a soothing image while the nurse describes pleasant sensations (For example, the patient may picture himself at the beach while you describe the sounds of

A trio of opioids

Opioids block the release of neurotransmitters that send pain signals to the brain. The three categories of opioids are opioid agonists (opioid analgesics), opioid antagonists (opioid reversal agents), and mixed agonist-antagonists.

Opioid agonists

Opioid agonists relieve pain by binding to pain receptors which, in effect, produces pain relief. Examples of opioid agonists are:
• morphine (Duramorph)
• fentanyl (Duragesic)
• hydromorphone (Dilaudid)
• codeine
• oxycodone (OxyContin).

Opioid antagonists

Opioid antagonists attach to opiate receptors without producing agonistic effects. They work by displacing the opioid at the receptor site and reversing the analgesic and respiratory depressant effects of the opioid. Examples of opioid antagonists are:
• naloxone (Narcan)
• naltrexone (ReVia).

Mixed opioid agonist-antagonists

Mixed opioid agonist-antagonists relieve pain by binding to opiate receptors to effect varying degrees of agonistic and antagonistic activity. They carry a lower risk of toxic effects and drug dependency than opioid agonists and opioid antagonists. Examples of mixed opioid agonist-antagonists are:
• buprenorphine (Buprenex)
• butorphanol (Stadol)
• pentazocine (Talwin).

the waves and birds and the feel of the warm sun and a breeze on the patient's skin.)
• relaxation therapy—a form of meditation used to focus attention on a single sound or image or on the rhythm of breathing
• heat application (thermotherapy)—application of dry or moist heat to decrease pain (Heat enhances blood flow, increases tissue metabolism, and decreases vasomotor tone; it also may relieve pain due to muscle aches or spasms, itching, or joint pain.)
• cold application (cryotherapy)—constricts blood vessels at the injury site, reducing blood flow to the site (Cold slows edema development, prevents further tissue damage, and minimizes bruising; it may be more effective than heat in relieving such pain as muscle aches or spasms, itching, incision pain, headaches, and joint pain.)
• transcutaneous electrical nerve stimulation—in which electrodes transmit mild electrical impulses to the brain to block pain impulses
• massage therapy—used as an aid to relaxation.

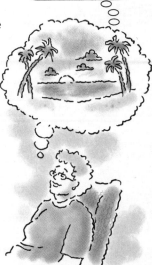

Imagery gives me a vacation away from pain.

Sensory input

Sensory stimulation in any environment may be perceived as pleasant or unpleasant and comfortable or painful. The emergency environment tends to stimulate all five senses:

- auditory
- visual
- gustatory
- olfactory
- tactile.

Too much or too little

Patients in the ED don't have control over the environmental stimulation around them. They may experience sensory deprivation, sensory overload, or both. *Sensory deprivation* can result from a reduction in the quantity and quality of normal and familiar sensory input, such as the normal sights and sounds encountered at home. *Sensory overload* results from an increase in the amount of unfamiliar sounds and sights in the emergency environment, such as beeping cardiac monitors, ringing telephones, overhead paging systems, and voices.

When environmental stimuli exceed the patient's ability to cope with the stimulation, he may experience anxiety, confusion, and panic as well as delusions.

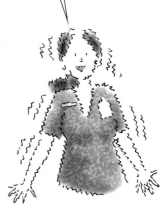

Overrrrstimulation of alllll the senses can llllead to sssssensory overload!

Ethics issues

Nurses who work in EDs routinely deal with ethical dilemmas. You'll recognize a situation as an ethical dilemma in these circumstances:
- More than one solution exists; that is, there's no clear "right" or "wrong" way to handle a situation.
- Each solution carries equal weight.
- Each solution is ethically defensible.

The value of values

Ethical dilemmas in EDs commonly revolve around quality-of-life issues for the patient, especially as they relate to end-of-life decisions—such as do-not-resuscitate orders, life support, and patients' requests for no heroic measures. When considering quality of life, make sure others don't impose their own value system on the patient. Each person has a set of personal values that are influenced by environment and culture. Nurses also have a set of professional values.

Code of ethics

The American Nurses Association (ANA) and Emergency Nurses Association have established a code of ethics. The ANA Code of Ethics for Nurses provides information that's necessary for a practicing nurse to use her professional skills in providing the most effective holistic care possible, such as serving as a patient advocate and striving to protect the health, safety, and rights of each patient.

End-of-life decisions

The threat of death is common in EDs. Perhaps at no other time is the holistic care of patients and their families as important as it is during this time. End-of-life decisions are almost always difficult for patients, families, and health care professionals to make. Nurses are in a unique position as advocates to assist patients and their families through this process.

Unsolvable mysteries

Your primary role as a patient advocate is to promote the patient's wishes. In many instances, however, a patient's wishes aren't known. That's when ethical decision making takes priority. Decisions aren't always easy to make and the answers aren't usually clear-cut. At times, such ethical dilemmas may seem unsolvable.

A question of quality

It's sometimes difficult to determine what can be done to achieve good quality of life and what can simply be achieved, technologically speaking. Technological advances sometimes seem to exceed our ability to analyze the ethical dilemmas associated with them.

Years ago, death was considered a natural part of life and most people died at home, surrounded by their families. Today, most people die in hospitals and death is commonly regarded as a medical failure rather than a natural event. Sometimes it's hard for you to know whether you're assisting in extending the patient's life or delaying the patient's death.

Consulting the committee

Most hospitals have ethics committees that review ethical dilemmas. The nurse may consider consulting the ethics committee if:
• the doctor disagrees with the patient or his family regarding treatment of the patient

- health care providers disagree among themselves about treatment options
- family members disagree about what should be done.

Determining medical futility

Medical futility refers to treatment that's hopeless or interventions that aren't likely to benefit the patient even though they may appear to be effective. For example, a patient with a terminal illness who's expected to die experiences cardiac arrest. Cardiopulmonary resuscitation may be effective in restoring a heartbeat but may still be deemed futile because it doesn't change the patient's outcome.

Dealing with cardiac arrest

In case of cardiac arrest (sudden stoppage of the heart), an emergency patient may be described by a code status. This code status describes the orders written by the doctor describing what resuscitation measures should be carried out by the nurse, and should be based on the patient's wishes regarding resuscitation measures. When cardiac arrest occurs, you must ensure that resuscitative efforts are initiated or that unwanted resuscitation doesn't take place.

Who decides?

The wishes of a competent, informed patient should always be honored. However, when a patient can't make decisions, the health care team—consisting of the patient's family, nursing staff, and doctors—may have to make end-of-life decisions for the patient.

Advance directives

Most people prefer to make their own decisions regarding end-of-life care. It's important that patients discuss their wishes with their loved ones; however, many don't. Instead, total strangers may be asked to make important health care decisions when patients can't do so. That's why it's important for people to make choices ahead of time and to make these choices known by developing advance directives.

The Patient Self-Determination Act of 1990 requires hospitals and other institutions to make information available to patients on advance directives. However, it isn't mandatory for patients to have advance directives.

Where there's a will, there's a law

There are two types of advance directives:
- treatment directive—sometimes known as a *living will*

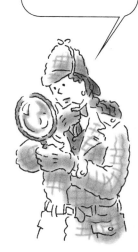

Although they aren't mandatory, advance directives can take a lot of the mystery out of end-of-life care decisions.

• appointment directive—sometimes called a *durable power of attorney for health care.*

A treatment directive, or living will, states what treatments a patient will accept and what treatments the patient will refuse in case terminal illness renders the patient unable to make those decisions at the time. For example, a patient may be willing to accept artificial nutrition but not hemodialysis.

Durable power of attorney is the appointment of a person—chosen by the patient—to make decisions on the patient's behalf if the patient can no longer do so. Durable power of attorney for health care doesn't give the chosen individual authority to access business accounts; the power is strictly related to health care decisions.

It takes two

After an advance directive is written, two witnesses must sign it. This document can be altered or canceled at any time. For more information, check the laws regarding advance directives for the state in which you practice.

Organ donation

When asked, most people say that they support organ donation. However, only a small percentage of qualified organs are ever donated. Tens of thousands of names are on waiting lists for organs in the United States alone. Organ transplantation is successful for many patients, giving them additional, high-quality years of life.

The Uniform Anatomical Gift Act governs the donation of organs and tissues. In addition, most states have legislation governing the procurement of organs and tissues. Some require medical staff to ask about organ donation on every death. Other states require staff to notify a regional organ procurement agency that then approaches the family. Become familiar with the laws of your state and the policies of the facility in which you practice.

Standards deviation

Medical criteria for organ donation vary from state to state. Many organ procurement agencies want to be notified of all deaths and imminent deaths so that they, not the medical staff, can determine if the patient is a potential candidate for organ donation.

Donations accepted

Any patient who donates organs must first be declared brain dead. Death used to be defined as the cessation of respiratory and cardiac function. However, developments in technology have made this definition obsolete. We now rely on brain death criteria to determine an individual's death.

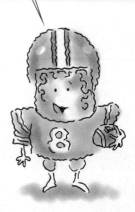

Brain death must be confirmed before a patient can donate any organs. Good thing I'm used to taking one for the team!

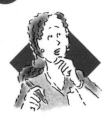

Quick quiz

1. Which statement regarding a patient's culture and his hospitalization experience is true?

A.   Culture affects a patient's experience during hospitalization because the patient has to adapt to the hospital culture.

B.   Culture doesn't affect the patient's hospitalization.

C.   Cultural factors can affect patient and family roles during illness.

D.   Culture rarely impacts decisions about health.

Answer: C. Cultural factors can have a major impact on patient and family roles during illness. Culture affects the patient's and family members' feelings about illness, pain, and end-of-life issues, among other things.

2. Factors that can impact an emergency patient's cognitive function include:

A.   medications.

B.   health condition.

C.   sleep disturbances.

D.   all of the above.

Answer: D. All of these factors can impact the patient's cognitive function while in the ED.

3. Pain assessment in an unconscious patient:

A.   isn't necessary because unconscious patients don't experience pain.

B.   requires astute assessment skills by the nurse.

C.   can be achieved through the use of visual analog scales.

D.   is treated differently from pain in a conscious patient.

Answer: B. Nurses should be especially vigilant in assessing for nonverbal signs of pain in an unconscious patient.

Scoring

✩✩✩   If you answered all three questions correctly, jump for joy! You get the whole picture of holistic care issues.

✩✩   If you answered two questions correctly, we won't issue a complaint! You're ready to join the team.

✩   If you answered fewer than two questions correctly, don't worry; it isn't an ethical dilemma! Just review the chapter and try again.

Neurologic emergencies

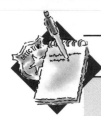

Just the facts

In this chapter, you'll learn:

♦ key areas to assess when dealing with neurologic emergencies

♦ important diagnostic tests and procedures used for neurologic emergencies

♦ common neurologic emergencies and their treatments.

Understanding neurologic emergencies

The neurologic system is a highly complex system that plays a major role in regulating many body functions. When faced with an emergency involving the neurologic system, you must assess the patient thoroughly, always being alert for subtle changes that might indicate a potential deterioration in the patient's condition. A focused assessment forms the basis for your interventions. These interventions must be instituted quickly to minimize the risks to the patient, which can be life-threatening.

Assessment

Assessment of subtle and elusive changes in the complex nervous system can be difficult. When you assess a patient for possible neurologic impairment, be sure to collect a thorough health history and investigate physical signs of impairment.

I know this is difficult, but a detailed history is the basis of neurologic emergency assessment. Now, tell me more about that childhood trauma...

Check the records

If you can't interview the patient because of his condition or impairment, you may gather history information from the patient's medical record. Family members and the emergency medical response team that transported the patient to the ED are important sources of information.

History

To collect a focused health history, gather details about the patient's current state of health, previous health status, lifestyle, and family health.

Friends and family fill in

A patient with a neurologic emergency may have trouble remembering or relating information. If the patient's family or close friends are available, include them in the assessment process. They may be able to corroborate or correct the details of the patient's health history.

Current health

Discover the patient's chief complaint by asking such questions as, "Why did you come to the hospital?" or "What has been bothering you lately?" Use the patient's words when you document these complaints.

Common complaints

If your patient is suffering from a neurologic emergency, you may hear reports of headaches, motor disturbances (such as weakness, paresis, and paralysis), seizures, sensory deviations, and altered level of consciousness (LOC).

Details, please

Encourage the patient to describe details of the current condition by asking such questions as:
• Can you describe your headache?
• When did you start feeling dizzy?
• What were you doing when the numbness started?
• Have you ever had seizures or tremors? Have you ever had weakness or paralysis in your arms or legs?
• Do you have trouble urinating, walking, speaking, understanding others, reading, or writing?
• How is your memory and ability to concentrate?

Previous health

Many chronic diseases affect the neurologic system, so ask questions about the patient's past health and what medications he's taking. Specifically, ask whether the patient has had any:
- major illnesses
- recurrent minor illnesses
- injuries
- surgical procedures
- allergies.

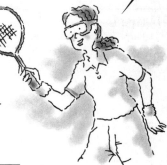

A patient's hobbies can really "play" into his neurologic assessment, so ask about them!

Lifestyle

Ask questions about the patient's cultural and social background because these affect care decisions. Note the patient's education level, occupation, and hobbies. As you gather this information, also assess the patient's self-image. Also ask about smoking, alcohol consumption, and recreational drug use.

Physical examination

A complete neurologic examination is long, detailed, and unnecessary. Because of the nature of the patient's condition, limit your examination to specific problem areas or stop your examination entirely to intervene should the patient exhibit signs and symptoms of deterioration. If your initial screening indicates a neurologic problem, you may need to conduct a more detailed assessment.

Top-to-bottom examination

Examine the patient's neurologic system in an orderly way. Beginning with the highest levels of neurologic function and working down to the lowest, assess these five areas:

 mental status

cranial nerve function

sensory function

motor function

reflexes.

Mental status

Mental status assessment begins when you talk to the patient. Responses to your questions reveal clues about the patient's orienta-

Quick check of mental status

To quickly screen your patient for disordered thought processes, ask the questions below. An incorrect answer to any question may indicate the need for a complete mental status examination. Make sure that you know the correct answers before asking the questions.

Question	Function screened
What's your name?	Orientation to person
What's your mother's name?	Orientation to other people
What year is it?	Orientation to time
What is the place that we're in?	Orientation to place
How old are you?	Memory
Where were you born?	Remote memory
What did you have for breakfast?	Recent memory
Who's President of the United States?	General knowledge
Can you count backward from 20 to 1?	Attention span and calculation skills

tion and memory. Use such clues as a guide during the physical assessment.

No easy answers

Be sure to ask questions that require more than yes-or-no answers. Otherwise, confusion or disorientation might not reveal themselves. If you have doubts about a patient's mental status, perform a screening examination. (See *Quick check of mental status*.)

Three-part exam

Use the mental status examination to check these three parameters:

 LOC

 speech

 cognitive function.

Level of consciousness

Watch for any change in the patient's LOC. It's the earliest and most sensitive indicator that his neurologic status has changed.

Descriptions and definitions

Many terms are used to describe LOC, and definitions differ widely among practitioners. To avoid confusion, clearly describe the patient's response to various stimuli and avoid using words such as:

- lethargic
- stuporous
- comatose.

Always start with a minimal stimulus, increasing intensity as necessary. The Glasgow Coma Scale offers an objective way to assess the patient's LOC. (See *Using the Glasgow Coma Scale*, page 48.)

Looking at LOC

Start by quietly observing the patient's behavior. If the patient appears to be sleeping or unconscious, try to rouse him by providing an appropriate stimulus, in this order:

 auditory

 tactile

 painful.

Speech

Listen to how well the patient expresses thoughts. Does he choose the correct words, or does he seem to have problems finding or articulating words?

It's hard to say

To assess for dysarthria (difficulty forming words), ask the patient to repeat the phrase, "No ifs, ands, or buts." Assess speech comprehension by determining the patient's ability to follow instructions and cooperate with your examination.

Language changes

Keep in mind that language performance tends to fluctuate with the time of day and changes in physical condition. A healthy person may have language difficulty when ill or fatigued. However, increasing speech difficulties may indicate deteriorating neurologic status, which warrants further evaluation.

When then who

To quickly test your patient's orientation, memory, and attention span, use the mental status screening questions. Orientation to time is usually disrupted first; orientation to person, last.

Always consider the patient's environment and physical condition when assessing orientation. For example, a patient admitted to the emergency department (ED) may not be oriented to date because of the rapid activity, events, and noise surrounding his transport to the department and the flurry of activity, bright lights,

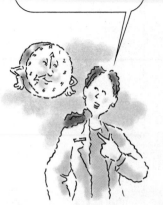

A patient's orientation to time is usually disrupted before his orientation to person.

Using the Glasgow Coma Scale

You can use the Glasgow Coma Scale to describe the patient's baseline mental status and detect and interpret changes in his level of consciousness.

To use the scale, test the patient's ability to respond to verbal, motor, and sensory stimulation and score your findings based on the scale. A patient who's alert, can follow simple commands, and is oriented to time, place, and person receives a score of 15 points. A lower score in one or more categories may signal an impending neurologic crisis. A total score of 7 or less indicates severe neurologic damage.

Test	Score	Patient's response
Eye-opening response		
Spontaneously	4	Opens eyes spontaneously
To speech	3	Opens eyes in response to verbal stimulus
To pain	2	Opens eyes only on painful stimulus
None	1	Doesn't open eyes in response to stimulus
Verbal response		
Oriented	5	Is oriented to person, place, and time
Confused	4	Tells incorrect year
Inappropriate words	3	Replies randomly with incorrect word
Incomprehensible	2	Moans or screams
None	1	Doesn't respond
Motor response		
Obeys commands	6	Responds to simple commands
Localizes pain	5	Reaches toward painful stimulus and tries to remove it
Withdraws from pain	4	Moves away from painful stimulus
Abnormal flexion	3	Assumes a decorticate posture (shown below)

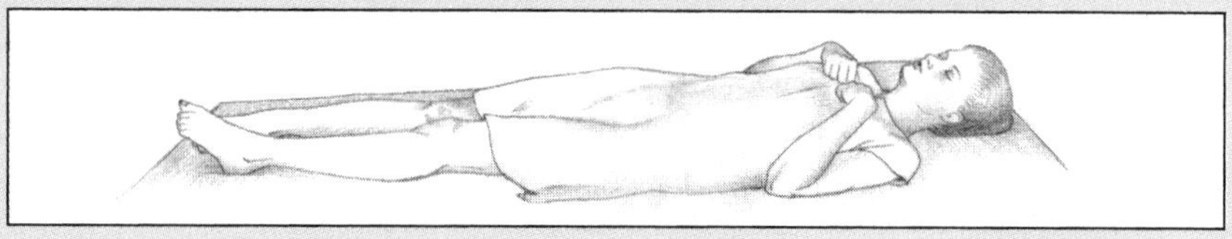

Abnormal extension	2	Assumes a decerebrate posture (shown below)

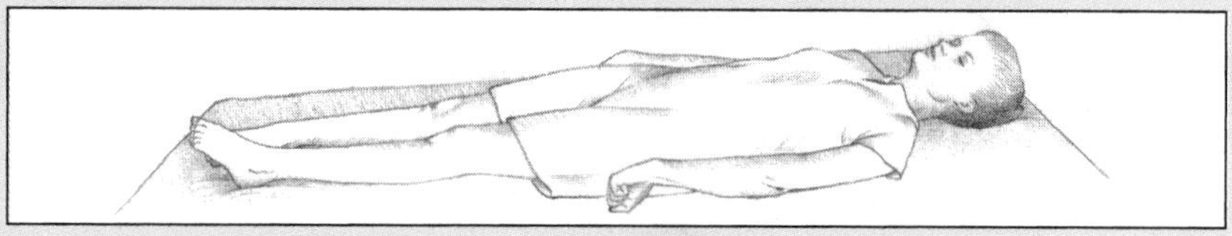

None	1	Doesn't respond; just lies flaccid

Total score

and noise in the department itself, but he can still usually remember the year.

Thought content

Disordered thought patterns may indicate delirium or psychosis. Assess thought pattern by evaluating the clarity and cohesiveness of the patient's ideas. Is his conversation smooth with logical transitions between ideas? Does he have hallucinations (sensory perceptions that lack appropriate stimuli) or delusions (beliefs not supported by reality)?

Insight on insight

Test your patient's insight by finding out whether the patient:
• has a realistic view of himself
• is aware of his illness and circumstances.
    Ask, for example, "What do you think caused your back pain?" Expect different patients to have different degrees of insight. For instance, a patient may attribute chest discomfort to indigestion rather than acknowledge that he has had a heart attack.

Lost in emotion

Throughout the interview, assess your patient's emotional status. Note his mood, emotional lability or stability, and the appropriateness of his emotional responses. Also, assess the patient's mood by asking how he feels about himself and his future. Keep in mind that signs and symptoms of depression in an elderly patient may be atypical. (See *Depression and elderly patients.*)

Cranial nerve function

Cranial nerve assessment reveals valuable information about the condition of the central nervous system (CNS), especially the brain stem. The 12 cranial nerves are the primary motor and sensory pathways between the brain and the head and neck. (See *Identifying cranial nerves*, page 50.)

Under pressure

Because of their location, some cranial nerves are more vulnerable to the effects of increasing intracranial pressure (ICP). Therefore, a neurologic screening assessment of the CNS focuses on these key nerves:
• oculomotor (III)
• abducens (VI).

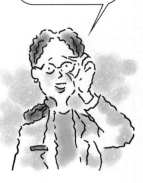

Remember that even healthy patients have different levels of inSIGHT.

Ages and stages

Depression and elderly patients

Symptoms of depression in elderly patients may be different from those found in other patients. For example, rather than the usual sad affect seen in patients with depression, elderly patients may exhibit such atypical signs as decreased function and increased agitation.

Identifying cranial nerves

The cranial nerves have sensory function, motor function, or both. They're assigned Roman numerals and written this way: *CN I, CN II, CN III,* and so on. The locations of the cranial nerves as well as their functions are shown below.

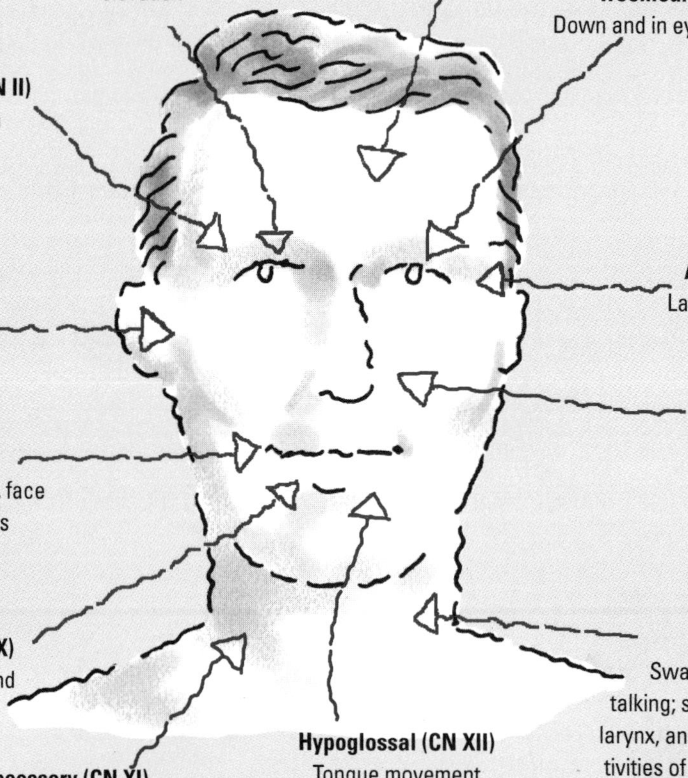

Oculomotor (CN III)
Most eye movement, pupillary constriction, upper eyelid elevation

Facial (CN VII)
Expressions in forehead, eye, and mouth; taste

Trochlear (CN IV)
Down and in eye movement

Optic (CN II)
Vision

Abducens (CN VI)
Lateral eye movement

Acoustic (CN VIII)
Hearing and balance

Olfactory (CN I)
Smell

Trigeminal (CN V)
Chewing, corneal reflex, face and scalp sensations

Glossopharyngeal (CN IX)
Swallowing, salivating, and taste

Vagus (CN X)
Swallowing, gag reflex, talking; sensations of the throat, larynx, and abdominal viscera; activities of thoracic and abdominal viscera, such as heart rate and peristalsis

Accessory (CN XI)
Shoulder movement and head rotation

Hypoglossal (CN XII)
Tongue movement

Get on some other nerves

Also evaluate other nerves if the patient's history or symptoms indicate a potential CNS emergency or when performing a complete nervous system assessment.

See about sight

Next, assess the optic (CN II) and oculomotor (CN III) nerves:

> **Memory jogger**
>
> To help you remember the names of the 12 cranial nerves, use the following mnemonic: *On old Olympus's towering tops, a Finn and German viewed some hops.*
>
> On = Olfactory   Finn = Facial
>
> Old = Optic   And = Acoustic
>
> Olympus's = Oculomotor German = Glossopharyngeal
>
> Towering = Trochlear   Viewed = Vagus
>
> Tops = Trigeminal   Some = Spinal accessory
>
> A = Abducens   Hops = Hypoglossal

• To assess the optic nerve, check visual acuity and visual fields. Do this by using a Snellen eye chart, starting with large print and moving to small print.
• To assess the oculomotor nerve, check pupil size, pupil shape, and direct and consensual response to light. When assessing pupil size, look for trends such as a gradual increase in the size of one pupil or appearance of unequal pupils. (See *Recognizing pupillary changes*, page 52.)

Funny face

To test the motor portion of the facial nerve (CN VII) to assess for possible stroke or Bell's palsy, ask the patient to:
• wrinkle his forehead
• raise and lower his eyebrows
• smile to show his teeth
• puff out his cheeks.
   Also, with the patient's eyes tightly closed, attempt to open his eyelids. As you conduct each part of this test, look for symmetry.

Now hear this

To test the vestibular portion of the acoustic nerve, observe the patient for nystagmus and disturbed balance, such as in a cerebellar stroke or Ménière's disease. Note reports of the room spinning or dizziness.

Check the pipes

Test the glossopharyngeal nerve (CN IX) and vagus nerve (CN X) together because their innervation overlaps in the pharynx:
• The glossopharyngeal nerve is responsible for swallowing, salivating, and taste perception on the posterior one-third of the tongue.

Recognizing pupillary changes

Use this table as a guide to recognize pupillary changes and identify possible causes.

Pupillary change	Possible causes
Unilateral, dilated (4 mm) fixed, and nonreactive 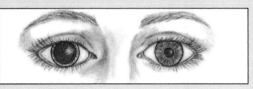	• Uncal herniation with oculomotor nerve damage • Brain stem compression • Increased intracranial pressure • Head trauma with subdural or epidural hematoma • May be normal in some people if eye has been severely damaged
Bilateral, dilated (4 mm), fixed, and nonreactive 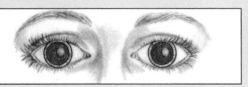	• Severe brain damage • Sympathomimetic intoxication • Anticholinergic poisoning • Cerebral ischemia or hypoxia
Bilateral, midsize (2 mm), fixed, and nonreactive 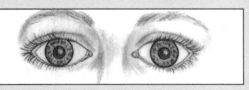	• Midbrain involvement caused by edema, hemorrhage, infarctions, lacerations, or contusions
Bilateral, pinpoint (< 1 mm), and usually nonreactive 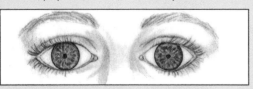	• Lesions of pons, usually after hemorrhage
Unilateral, small (1.5 mm), and nonreactive 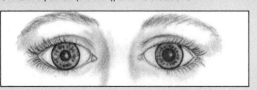	• Disruption of sympathetic nerve supply to the head caused by spinal cord lesion above the first thoracic vertebra

• The vagus nerve controls swallowing and is responsible for voice quality.

First assess these nerves by listening to the patient's voice. Then check the gag reflex by touching the tip of a tongue blade against the posterior pharynx and asking the patient to open wide and say "ah." Watch for the symmetrical upward movement of the soft palate and uvula and the midline position of the uvula. Abnormal findings may indicate stroke, expanding hematoma of the neck, palate infection, or airway foreign body.

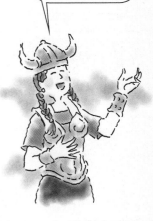

Can you see my uvula movement and position from here? I'll try again—ahhhhh!

Shrug it off

To assess for possible stroke or upper spinal cord injury, assess the spinal accessory nerve (CN XI), which controls the sternocleidomastoid muscles and the upper portion of the trapezius muscles. Press down on the patient's shoulders while he attempts to shrug against this resistance. Note shoulder strength and symmetry while inspecting and palpating the trapezius muscles.

To further test the trapezius muscles, apply resistance from one side while the patient tries to return his head to midline position.

Test tongue toughness

To assess the hypoglossal nerve (CN XII), follow these steps:
• Ask the patient to stick out his tongue. Look for any deviation from the midline, atrophy, or fasciculations.
• Test tongue strength by asking the patient to push his tongue against his cheek as you apply resistance. Observe the tongue for symmetry.
• Test the patient's speech by asking him to repeat the sentence, "Round the rugged rock that ragged rascal ran."

Sensory function

Assess the sensory system to evaluate the ability of the:
• sensory receptors to detect stimulus
• afferent nerves to carry sensory nerve impulses to the spinal cord
• sensory tracts in the spinal cord to carry sensory messages to the brain.

This is gonna hurt

To test for pain sensation, have the patient close his eyes; then touch above the area of sensory loss to find the line of demarcation, first with the sharp end of a safety pin and then with the dull end.

Motor function

Assess motor function to aid evaluation of these structures and functions:
• cerebral cortex and its initiation of motor activity by way of the pyramidal pathways
• corticospinal tracts and their capacity to carry motor messages down the spinal cord
• lower motor neurons and their ability to carry efferent impulses to the muscles
• muscles and their capacity to carry out motor commands
• cerebellum and basal ganglia and their capacity to coordinate and fine-tune movement.

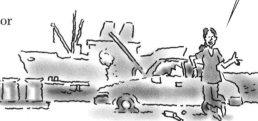

This motor functions pretty poorly, but hopefully your patient's motor functions will be in better shape!

Feats of strength

To assess arm muscle strength, ask the patient to push you away as you apply resistance. Then ask the patient to extend both arms, palms up. Have him close his eyes and maintain this position for 20 to 30 seconds. Observe the arm for downward drifting and pronation.

Assess the patient's ability to lift his leg off the bed to gauge leg strength.

Grace and gait

Assess the patient's coordination and balance. Note whether the patient can sit and stand without support. If appropriate, observe as the patient walks.

While observing the patient, note imbalances and abnormalities. When cerebellar dysfunction is present, the patient has a wide-based, unsteady gait. Deviation to one side may indicate a cerebellar lesion on the side.

Extreme coordination

Test the extremities for coordination by having the patient touch his nose and then your outstretched finger as you move it. Have him do this faster and faster. His movements should be accurate and smooth.

Test cerebellar function further by assessing rapid alternating movements. Tell the patient to use the thumb of one hand to touch each finger of the same hand in rapid sequence. Repeat with the other hand.

Abnormalities can indicate cerebellar disease, stroke, ethanol toxicity, or a cerebellar infarct.

A wide, unsteady gait might help me here, but in a patient with a neurologic emergency it signals cerebellar dysfunction.

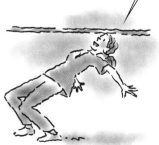

Present and absent actions

Motor responses in an unconscious patient may be appropriate, inappropriate, or absent. Appropriate responses, such as localization or withdrawal, mean that the sensory and corticospinal pathways are functioning. Inappropriate responses, such as decorticate or decerebrate posturing, indicate a dysfunction.

It can be challenging to assess motor responses in a patient who can't follow commands or is unresponsive. Make sure that you note whether any stimulus produces a response and what that response is.

Superficially speaking

You can elicit superficial reflexes using light, tactile stimulation such as stroking or scratching the skin.

Because these reflexes are cutaneous, the more you try to elicit them in succession, the less response you'll get. Therefore, observe carefully the first time you stimulate these reflexes.

Superficial reflexes include the plantar, pharyngeal, and abdominal reflexes. Here's how to test them:
• To test the *plantar reflex*, use an applicator stick, tongue blade, or key and slowly stroke the lateral side of the patient's sole from the heel to the great toe. The normal response in an adult is plantar flexion of the toes. Upward movement of the great toe and fanning of the little toes—called *Babinski's reflex*—is abnormal. (See *Babinski's reflex in infants.*)
• To test the *pharyngeal reflex* of CN IX and CN X, instruct the patient to open his mouth wide. Then, touch the back of the pharynx with a tongue blade. Normally, doing so causes the patient to gag.
• To test the *abdominal reflex* and intactness of thoracic spinal segments T8, T9, and T10, use the tip of the handle on the reflex hammer to stroke one side and then the opposite side of the patient's abdomen above the umbilicus. Repeat on the lower abdomen. Normally, the abdominal muscles contract and the umbilicus deviates toward the stimulated side.

Write it down

After you examine the patient, document your findings using a grading scale to rate each reflex. Document the rating for each reflex at the appropriate site on a stick figure.

Ages and stages

Babinski's reflex in infants

Babinski's reflex can be elicited in some normal infants—sometimes until age 2 years. However, plantar flexion of the toes is seen in more than 90% of normal infants.

Diagnostic tests

Diagnostic testing to evaluate the nervous system typically includes imaging studies. Other tests such as lumbar puncture may also be used.

Diagnostic testing may be routine for you, but it can be frightening for the patient. Try to prepare the patient and his family for each test and follow-up monitoring procedure. Some tests can be performed at the patient's bedside but many require transportation to the imaging department.

Imaging studies

The most common imaging studies used to detect neurologic disorders include angiography, computed tomography (CT) scan, magnetic resonance imaging (MRI), and spinal X-rays.

Angiography

Angiographic studies include cerebral angiography and digital subtraction angiography (DSA).

Cerebral angiography

During cerebral angiography, the technician injects a radiopaque contrast medium, usually into the brachial artery (through retrograde brachial injection) or through the femoral artery into the cerebral vessels.

Why it's done

This procedure highlights cerebral vessels, making it easier to:
• detect stenosis or occlusion associated with thrombus or spasm
• identify aneurysms and arteriovenous malformations (AVMs)
• locate vessel displacement associated with tumors, abscesses, cerebral edema, hematoma, or herniation
• assess collateral circulation.

Digital subtraction angiography

DSA highlights cerebral blood vessels. It's done this way:
• Using computerized fluoroscopy, a technician takes an image of the selected area, which is then stored in a computer's memory.
• After administering a contrast medium, the technician takes several more images.
• The computer produces high-resolution images by manipulating the two sets of images.

Sidestep stroke

Arterial DSA requires more contrast medium than cerebral angiography. However, because the dye is injected I.V., DSA doesn't increase the patient's risk of stroke.

Nursing considerations

Cerebral angiography

• Explain the procedure to the patient, and answer all questions.
• Confirm that the patient isn't allergic to iodine or shellfish because a person with such allergies may have an adverse reaction to the contrast medium. If the patient has a confirmed allergy, he may be premedicated to allow the procedure.
• Ensure that preprocedure tests have been completed and results are reviewed and available on the patient's chart, including evaluation of renal function (serum creatinine and blood urea nitrogen [BUN] levels) and coagulation studies (prothrombin time [PT], partial thromboplastin time [PTT], and platelet count). Notify the doctor of abnormal results.
• Explain that he'll probably feel a flushed sensation in his face as the dye is injected.
• Maintain bed rest, as ordered, and monitor the patient's vital signs.
• Monitor the catheter insertion site for signs of bleeding.
• As ordered, keep a pressure device such as a Femstop over the injection site; monitor the patient's peripheral pulse in the arm or leg used for catheter insertion, and mark the site.
• Unless contraindicated, encourage the patient to drink more fluids to flush the dye from the body; alternatively, increase the I.V. flow rate as ordered.
• Monitor the patient for neurologic changes and such complications as hemiparesis, hemiplegia, aphasia, and impaired LOC.
• Monitor for adverse reactions to the contrast medium, which may include restlessness, tachypnea and respiratory distress, tachycardia, facial flushing, urticaria, and nausea and vomiting.

Digital subtraction angiography

• Confirm that the patient isn't allergic to iodine or shellfish, or premedicate the patient.
• Ensure that preprocedure testing has been completed and results are reviewed and available on the patient's chart, including evaluation of renal function (serum creatinine and BUN levels) and coagulation studies (PT, PTT, and platelet count). Notify the doctor of abnormal results.

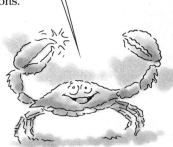

Not to sound crabby, but if your patient is allergic to me or iodine he might have an adverse reaction to the contrast medium.

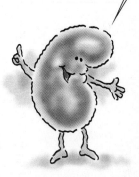

Don't forget me! Check evaluation of renal function before the procedure and report anything abnormal.

- Restrict the patient's consumption of solid food for 4 hours before the test.
- Explain that the test requires insertion of an I.V. catheter.

Steady, Freddie

- Instruct the patient to remain still during the test.
- Explain that he'll probably feel flushed or have a metallic taste in his mouth as the contrast medium is injected.
- Tell the patient to alert the doctor immediately if he feels discomfort or shortness of breath.
- Unless contraindicated, encourage the patient to drink more fluids for the rest of the day to flush the contrast medium from the body. Alternatively, increase the I.V. flow rate as ordered.

Computed tomography scan

CT scanning combines radiology and computer analysis of tissue density. CT angiogram scanning shows cerebral blood vessels.

Spine scanning

CT scanning of the spine is used to assess such disorders as herniated disk, spinal cord tumors, spinal stenosis, fractures, subluxations, and distraction injuries.

Brain scanning

CT scanning of the brain is used to detect brain contusion, brain calcifications, cerebral atrophy, hydrocephalus, inflammation, space-occupying lesions (tumors, hematomas, and abscesses), vascular anomalies, foreign bodies, and bony displacement (AVM, aneurysms, infarctions, and blood clots).

Nursing considerations

- Confirm that the patient isn't allergic to iodine or shellfish to avoid an adverse reaction to the contrast medium, if contrast is being used.
- If the test calls for a contrast medium, tell the patient that it's injected into an existing I.V. line or that a new line may be inserted. Ensure that the patient has an 18G or larger catheter as close to the heart as possible.
- Ensure that preprocedure tests, including evaluation of renal function (serum creatinine and BUN levels), are available on the patient's chart, and have been reviewed; keep in mind that the contrast medium can cause acute renal failure.
- Warn the patient and his family that he may feel flushed or notice a metallic taste in his mouth when the contrast medium is injected.

• Tell him that the CT scanner circles around him, depending on the procedure and type of equipment.
• Explain that he must lie still during the test.
• Inform the patient and his family that the contrast medium may discolor the patient's urine for 24 hours.
• Expect the doctor to write an order to increase I.V. flow rate after the test if the patient's oral intake is being restricted or oral intake is contraindicated; otherwise, suggest that the patient drink more fluids to flush the medium out of his body.

Magnetic resonance imaging

MRI generates detailed pictures of body structures. The test may involve the use of a contrast medium such as gadolinium.

Sharper images

Compared with conventional X-rays and CT scans, MRI provides superior visualization of soft tissues, sharply differentiating healthy, benign, cancerous, injured, and edematous atrophied tissue and clearly revealing blood vessels. In addition, MRI permits imaging in multiple planes, including sagittal and coronal views in regions where bones normally hamper visualization.

MRI is especially useful for studying the CNS because it can reveal structural abnormalities associated with such conditions as transient ischemic attack (TIA), tumors, multiple sclerosis, cerebral edema, and hydrocephalus.

Nursing considerations

• Confirm that the patient isn't allergic to the contrast medium (usually gadolinium).
• If the test calls for a contrast medium, tell the patient that it's injected into an existing I.V. line or that a new line may be inserted.
• Explain that the procedure can take up to $1\frac{1}{2}$ hours; tell the patient that he must remain still for intervals of 5 to 20 minutes.
• Ensure that all metallic items such as hair clips, bobby pins, jewelry (including body-piercing jewelry), watches, eyeglasses, hearing aids, and dentures are removed from the patient's body.
• Explain that the test is painless, but that the machinery may seem loud and frightening and the tunnel confining. Tell the patient that he'll receive earplugs to reduce the noise.
• Provide sedation as ordered to promote relaxation during the test.
• After the procedure, increase the I.V. flow rate as ordered, or encourage the patient to increase his fluid intake to flush the contrast medium from his system.

Spinal X-rays

The doctor may order anteroposterior and lateral spinal X-rays when spinal disease is suspected or when injury to the cervical, thoracic, lumbar, or sacral vertebral segments exists.

Depending on the patient's condition, other X-ray images may be taken from special angles, such as the open-mouth view (to identify possible odontoid fracture).

Spinal X-rays are used to detect spinal fracture; displacement and subluxation; and destructive lesions, such as primary and metastatic bone tumors.

Nursing considerations
- Reassure the patient that X-rays are painless.
- As ordered, administer an analgesic before the procedure if the patient has existing pain, so he'll be more comfortable.
- Remove the patient's cervical collar if cervical X-rays reveal no fracture and the doctor has written an order to remove it.

> Ready for a real close-up? Spinal X-rays can provide a closer look at damage to the thoracic, lumbar, or sacral vertebral segments. Hopefully you won't see a boot!

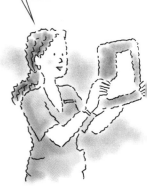

Other tests

In addition to imaging studies, lumbar puncture is another neurologic test.

Lumbar puncture

During lumbar puncture, a sterile needle is inserted into the subarachnoid space of the spinal canal, usually between the third and fourth lumbar vertebrae. A practitioner does the lumbar puncture. It requires sterile technique and careful patient positioning.

Why do it?

Lumbar puncture is used to:
- detect blood and bacteria in cerebrospinal fluid (CSF)
- obtain CSF specimens for laboratory analysis
- relieve increased ICP by removing CSF.

Contraindications and cautions

Lumbar puncture is contraindicated in patients with lumbar deformity or infection at the puncture site. It's performed cautiously in patients with increased ICP because the rapid decrease of pressure that follows withdrawal of CSF can cause tonsillar herniation and medullary compression.

Nursing considerations
- Describe lumbar puncture to the patient and his family, explaining that the procedure may cause some discomfort.

• Reassure the patient that a local anesthetic is administered before the test. Tell him to report any tingling or sharp pain he feels as the anesthetic is injected.
• Monitor the patient for neurologic deficits and complications, such as headache, fever, back spasms, or seizures, according to facility policy.

Treatments

For many of your patients with neurologic emergencies, medication or drug therapy is essential.
• Thrombolytics are used to treat patients with acute ischemic stroke.
• Anticonvulsants are used to control seizures.
• Corticosteroids are used to reduce inflammation.
    Other types of drugs commonly used to treat patients with neurologic emergencies include:
• analgesics
• anticoagulants and antiplatelets
• anticonvulsants
• benzodiazepines
• calcium channel blockers
• corticosteroids
• diuretics
• thrombolytics
• antipsychotics
• antibiotics
• antiparkinson agents.

Heads up!

When caring for a patient undergoing medication therapy, stay alert for severe adverse reactions and interactions with other drugs. (See *Selected drugs used in neurologic emergencies*, pages 62 and 63.)

Surgery

Life-threatening neurologic disorders occasionally call for emergency surgery. Surgery commonly involves craniotomy, a procedure to open the skull and expose the brain.

Be ready before and after

You'll only be responsible for the patient's care before surgery. Typically, the patient will be transferred to the intensive care unit (ICU) or neurologic ICU after surgery.

Selected drugs used in neurologic emergencies

Use this table to find out about common neurologic drugs and their indications and adverse effects.

Drug	Indications	Adverse effects
Opioid analgesics morphine (Duramorph) oxycodone (OxyContin)	• Severe pain • Mild to moderate pain	• Respiratory depression, apnea, bradycardia, seizures, sedation • Respiratory depression, bradycardia, sedation, constipation
Anticonvulsants fosphenytoin (Cerebyx) phenytoin (Dilantin)	• Status epilepticus, seizures during neurosurgery • Generalized tonic-clonic seizures, status epilepticus, nonepileptic seizures after head trauma	• Increased intracranial pressure, cerebral edema, somnolence, bradycardia, QT prolongation, heart block
Anticoagulants heparin	• Embolism prophylaxis after cerebral thrombosis in evolving stroke	• Hemorrhage, thrombocytopenia
Antiplatelets aspirin ticlopidine (Ticlid)	• Transient ischemic attacks, thromboembolic disorders • Thrombotic stroke prophylaxis	• GI bleeding, acute renal insufficiency, thrombocytopenia, hepatic dysfunction • Thrombocytopenia, agranulocytosis
Barbiturates Phenobarbital (Luminal)	• All types of seizures except absence seizures and febrile seizures in children; also used for status epilepticus, sedation, and drug withdrawal	• Respiratory depression, apnea, bradycardia, angioedema, Stevens-Johnson syndrome
Benzodiazepines diazepam (Valium) lorazepam (Ativan)	• Status epilepticus, anxiety, acute alcohol withdrawal, muscle spasm • Status epilepticus, anxiety, agitation	• Respiratory depression, bradycardia, cardiovascular collapse, drowsiness, acute withdrawal syndrome • Drowsiness, acute withdrawal syndrome
Calcium channel blockers nimodipine (Sular)	• Neurologic deficits caused by cerebral vasospasm after congenital aneurysm rupture	• Decreased blood pressure, tachycardia, edema

Selected drugs used in neurologic emergencies *(continued)*

Drug	Indications	Adverse effects
Corticosteroids dexamethasone (Dexone), methylprednisolone (Solu-Medrol)	• Cerebral edema, severe inflammation	• Heart failure, cardiac arrhythmias, edema, circulatory collapse, thromboembolism, pancreatitis, peptic ulceration
Diuretics furosemide (loop) (Lasix)	• Edema, hypertension	• Renal failure, thrombocytopenia, agranulocytosis, volume depletion, dehydration
mannitol (osmotic) (Osmitrol)	• Cerebral edema, increased intracranial pressure	• Heart failure, seizures, fluid and electrolyte imbalance
Thrombolytics alteplase (recombinant tissue plasminogen activator) (Activase)	• Acute ischemic stroke	• Cerebral hemorrhage, spontaneous bleeding, allergic reaction
Serotonin inhibitors sumatriptan (Imitrex)	• Acute migraine or cluster-type headache	• Blood pressure alterations

Craniotomy

During craniotomy, a surgical opening into the skull exposes the brain. This procedure allows various treatments, such as ventricular shunting, excision of a tumor or abscess, hematoma aspiration, and aneurysm clipping (placing one or more surgical clips on the neck of an aneurysm to destroy it).

Condition and complexity count

The degree of risk depends on your patient's condition and the complexity of the surgery. Craniotomy raises the risk of having various complications, such as:
• infection
• hemorrhage
• respiratory compromise
• increased ICP.

Nursing considerations

• Encourage the patient and his family to ask questions about the procedure. Provide clear answers to the family to reduce their confusion and anxiety and enhance effective coping.
• Explain that the patient's head will most likely be shaved before surgery.

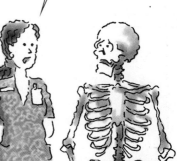

You should know that we'll probably have to shave your head before surgery. Oh, wait...

• Explain that he'll probably be transferred to the ICU initially for close monitoring, he'll awaken with a dressing on his head to protect the incision, and he might have a surgical drain.
• Provide emotional support to the patient and his family as they cope with the concept of surgery.

Cerebral aneurysm repair

Surgical intervention is the only sure way to prevent rupture or rebleeding of a cerebral aneurysm.

Expose and attack

In cerebral aneurysm repair, a craniotomy is performed to expose the aneurysm. Depending on the aneurysm's shape and location, the surgeon then uses one of several corrective techniques, such as:
• clamping the affected artery
• wrapping the aneurysm wall with a biological or synthetic material
• clipping or ligating the aneurysm.

Nursing considerations

• Tell the patient and his family that, after surgery, he'll probably be transferred to the ICU for close monitoring. Explain that several I.V. lines, intubation, and mechanical ventilation may be needed.
• Give emotional support to the patient and his family to help them cope with the upcoming surgery.

Common disorders

In the ED, you're likely to encounter patients with common neurologic emergencies, especially head trauma, increased ICP, seizures, spinal cord injury, stroke, subarachnoid hemorrhage, and subdural hematoma. Regardless of the disorder, your priority is always to ensure vital functioning—that is, airway, breathing, and circulation.

Head trauma

Head trauma is any traumatic insult to the brain that causes physical, intellectual, emotional, social, or vocational changes. Children ages 6 months to 2 years, adults ages 15 to 24, and elderly adults are most at risk for head trauma.

To put it bluntly

Head trauma is generally categorized as *blunt trauma* (closed or open) or *penetrating trauma*. Blunt trauma is more common. It typically occurs when the head strikes a hard surface or a rapidly moving object strikes the head. The dura may be intact, and no brain tissue is exposed to the external environment.

Open and exposed

In penetrating trauma, as the name suggests, an opening in the scalp, skull, meninges, or brain tissue exposes the cranial contents to the environment. The risk of infection is high. Possible complications include:
- increased ICP due to edema or hematoma formation
- infection (in open wounds)
- respiratory depression and failure
- brain herniation.

> Extra, extra! Brain exposed in penetrating trauma scandal!

On the decline

Mortality from head injury has declined as a result of:
- advances in preventive measures such as air bags, seat belts, and helmet laws
- quicker emergency response and transport times
- improved treatment measures.

What causes it

Head injury commonly results from:
- motor vehicle collisions (the most common cause)
- falls
- sports-related injuries
- interpersonal violence.

> Never fear—the cranial vault is here! It protects the brain from physical blows.

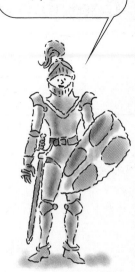

How it happens

The brain is shielded by the cranial vault (composed of skin, bone, meninges, and CSF), which intercepts the force of a physical blow. Below a certain level of force, the cranial vault prevents energy from damaging the brain.

The degree of traumatic head injury is usually proportional to the amount of force reaching the intracranial tissues. In addition, until they're ruled out, you must presume that neck injuries are present in patients with traumatic head injuries.

Case closed

Blunt trauma is typically a sudden acceleration-deceleration or coup-contrecoup injury. In a coup-contrecoup injury, the head hits a more stationary object or a moving object, injuring cranial tissues near the point of impact (coup); the remaining force then pushes the brain against the opposite side of the skull, causing a second impact and injury on the opposite surface (contrecoup).

Contusions and lacerations also occur as the brain's soft tissues slide over the rough bone of the skull base. The brain may also endure rotational shear, damaging the upper midbrain and areas of the frontal, temporal, parietal, and occipital lobes.

What to look for

Types of head trauma include:
- concussion
- contusion
- epidural hematoma
- intraparenchymal hematoma
- skull fractures
- subdural hematoma.

Each type is associated with specific signs and symptoms. (See *Hidden Hematoma* and *Types of head injury*, pages 68 to 71.)

What tests tell you

These diagnostic tests are used for head injury:
- A CT scan will show a fracture of the cranial vault and shows intracranial hemorrhage from ruptured blood vessels, ischemic or necrotic tissue, cerebral edema, a shift in brain tissue, and subdural, epidural, and intracerebral hematomas.
- Cerebral angiography shows the location of vascular disruption due to internal pressure or injuries that result from cerebral contusion or skull fracture.
- MRI can assess diffuse axonal injuries.

How it's treated

Treatment may be surgical or supportive.

It's surgical

Surgical treatment includes:
- craniotomy and decompression craniectomy
- evacuation of a hematoma.

Surgery aims to remove fragments driven into the brain and to evacuate hematomas and control bleeding. Such measures reduce the risk of infection and further brain damage due to fractures.

It's supportive

Provide supportive treatment, which includes:
- close observation to detect changes in neurologic status suggesting further damage

Ages and stages

Hidden hematoma

An older person with cerebral atrophy can tolerate a larger subdural hematoma for a longer time than a younger person before the hematoma causes neurologic changes. Thus, a hematoma in an older patient can become rather large before signs or symptoms occur, even in an acute condition.

• cleaning and debridement of any wounds associated with skull fractures
• diuretics, such as mannitol, to reduce cerebral edema
• analgesics to relieve complaints of headache
• anticonvulsants such as phenytoin to prevent seizures
• respiratory support, including mechanical ventilation and endo-tracheal (ET) tube intubation, for any patient with a Glasgow Coma Scale score of 8 or less or respiratory failure from brain stem involvement.

What to do

• Institute cardiac monitoring and be alert for cardiac changes or arrhythmias.
• Maintain a patent airway. Monitor oxygen saturation levels through pulse oximetry and arterial blood gas (ABG) analysis as ordered.
• Any patient with a Glasgow Coma Scale score of less than or equal to 8 should have an ET tube and mechanical ventilation in place.
• In a moderate injury, insert an oral gastric tube to decompress the stomach. Avoid using a nasogastric tube.
• Initially, monitor vital signs continuously and check for additional injuries; continue to check vital signs and neurologic status, including LOC and pupil size, every 15 minutes.
• Maintain spinal immobilization until the spine has been cleared.
• Assess hemodynamic parameters to help evaluate cerebral perfusion pressure (CPP). CPP should be maintained at 70 mm Hg at all times.

Metabolic medicine

• Administer medications as ordered. If necessary, use continuous infusions of such agents as midazolam (Versed), fentanyl (Sublimaze), or morphine to reduce metabolic demand and the risk of increased ICP.
• Observe the patient closely for signs of hypoxia or increased ICP, such as headache, dizziness, irritability, anxiety, and such changes in behavior as agitation.
• Carefully monitor the patient for CSF leakage. Check the bedsheets for a blood-tinged spot surrounded by a lighter ring (halo sign). Elevate the head of the bed 30 degrees.
• Position the patient so that secretions drain properly. If you detect CSF leakage from the nose, place a gauze pad under the nostrils. Don't suction through the nose, but use the mouth. If CSF leaks from the ear, position the patient so his ear drains naturally.

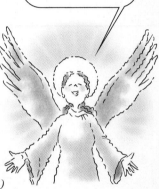

Sometimes it's divine, but after head trauma a halo signals CSF leakage.

(Text continues on page 70.)

Types of head injury

Here's a summary of the signs and symptoms and diagnostic test findings for different types of head injury.

Type	Description
Concussion (closed head injury)	• A blow to the head hard enough to move the brain within the skull, but not hard enough to cause a cerebral contusion; causes temporary neural dysfunction. • Recovery is usually complete within 24 to 48 hours, but headache can persist for months. • Repeated injuries have a cumulative effect on the brain. • Unconsciousness lasts less than six hours, frequently only a few minutes
Contusion (bruising of brain tissue; more serious than concussion)	• Acceleration-deceleration or coup-contrecoup injuries disrupt normal nerve function in bruised area. • Injury is directly beneath the site of impact when the brain rebounds against the skull from the force of a blow (a beating with a blunt instrument, for example), when the force of the blow drives the brain against the opposite side of the skull, or when the head is hurled forward and stopped abruptly (as in an automobile crash when the driver's head strikes a the windshield). • Brain continues moving and slaps against the skull (acceleration), then rebounds (deceleration). • Bone may strike bony prominences inside the skull (especially the sphenoidal ridges), causing intracranial hemorrhage that may result in tentorial herniation.
Diffuse axonal injury	• This condition involves severe brain injury with extensive damage to the brain structures, primarily the white matter of the brain. • Axon damage in the cerebral hemispheres, corpus callosum, and brain stem result as well as axonal swelling and disconnection. • This condition is commonly accompanied by damage to blood vessels and tissues. • This condition may be categorized as mild, moderate, or severe.
Subdural hematoma	• Accumulation of blood in the subdural space (between dura mater and arachnoid). • This condition may be acute, subacute, or chronic and unilateral or bilateral. • It's usually associated with torn connecting veins in the cerebral cortex or venous sinus bleeds, but rarely from arteries. • Acute hematomas are a surgical emergency.

Signs and symptoms

- Short-term loss of consciousness secondary to disruption of the reticular activating system, possibly due to abrupt pressure changes in the areas responsible for consciousness, changes in polarity of the neurons, ischemia, or structural distortion of neurons
- Vomiting from localized injury and brainstem compression
- Anterograde and retrograde amnesia (in which the patient can't recall events immediately after the injury or events that led up to the traumatic incident) correlating with severity of injury; all related to disruption of reticular activating system
- Irritability or lethargy from localized injury and compression
- Behavior out of character due to focal injury
- Complaints of dizziness, nausea, or severe headache due to focal injury and brainstem compression

- Severe scalp wounds from direct injury may or may not be present
- Labored respiration and loss of consciousness secondary to increased pressure from bruising
- Drowsiness, confusion, disorientation, agitation, or violence from increased intracranial pressure (ICP) associated with trauma
- Hemiparesis related to interrupted blood flow to the site of injury
- Decorticate or decerebrate posturing from cortical damage or hemispheric dysfunction
- Unequal pupillary response from brain stem involvement

- *Mild:* Loss of consciousness for 6 to 24 hours with possible decerebrate or decorticate posture; rapid improvement within 24 hours with return to baseline neurologic function; possible residual period of amnesia
- *Moderate:* Almost immediate and complete loss of consciousness; coma state lasting over 24 hours to days without any lucid intervals; immediate decorticate and decerebrate postures continuing until the patient awakens; residual neurologic dysfunction
- *Severe:* nonresolving brain stem impairment; coma state ranging from days to weeks; accompanying autonomic dysfunction

- Worsening headache from enlarging hematoma
- Unilateral pupil abnormality from increased ICP
- Gradual or rapidly deteriorating level of consciousness from drowsiness, slow cerebration, and confusion to coma

Diagnostic test findings

- Computed tomography (CT) scan reveals no sign of fracture, bleeding, or other nervous system lesion.

- CT scan shows changes in tissue density, possible displacement of the surrounding structures, and evidence of ischemic tissue, hematomas, and fractures.

- CT scan or magnetic resonance imaging (MRI) reveals extent of tissue damage and widespread cerebral edema.

- CT scan and arteriography reveal mass and altered blood flow in the area, confirming a hematoma.
- CT scan or MRI evidence of subdural mass and brain tissue shifting.
- The cerebrospinal fluid (CSF) is yellow and has relatively low protein (chronic subdural hematoma).

(continued)

Types of head injury (continued)

Type	Description
Intracerebral hematoma	• Subacute hematomas have a better prognosis because venous bleeding tends to be slower. • Depending on the site and amount of bleeding, traumatic or spontaneous disruption of cerebral vessels in brain parenchyma cause neurologic deficits. • Shear forces from brain movement commonly cause vessel laceration and hemorrhage into the parenchyma. • Frontal and temporal lobes are common sites. Trauma is associated with few intracerebral hematomas; most are caused by hypertension. However, patients with severe head injuries almost always have intraparenchymal bleeds.
Skull fracture	• Types of skull fractures include: linear, comminuted, and depressed. • Fractures of the anterior and middle fossae are associated with severe head trauma and are more common than posterior fossa fractures. • A blow to the head causes one or more of the types. This condition may not be problematic unless the brain is exposed or bone fragments are driven into neural tissue or the dura is torn.

Seizure watch

• Institute seizure precautions as necessary. Use safety precautions to minimize the risk of injury.
• Prepare the patient for craniotomy as indicated depending on the underlying injury.
• After the patient is stabilized, clean and dress superficial scalp wounds using strict sterile technique.
• Explain all procedures and treatments to the patient and his family.
• Provide instructions for follow-up care for the patient with a concussion who will be discharged. (See *After a concussion*, page 72.)

Signs and symptoms	Diagnostic test findings
• Unresponsive immediately or may experience a lucid period before lapsing into a coma from increasing ICP and mass effect of hemorrhage • Possible motor deficits and decorticate or decerebrate responses from compression of corticospinal tracts and brain stem	• CT scan identifies the bleeding site.
• May not produce symptoms, depending on underlying brain trauma • Discontinuity and displacement of bone structure with severe fracture • Motor sensory and cranial nerve dysfunction with associated facial fractures • Persons with anterior fossa basilar skull fractures may have periorbital ecchymosis (raccoon eyes), anosmia (loss of smell due to first cranial nerve involvement) and pupil abnormalities (second and third cranial nerve involvement) • CSF rhinorrhea (leakage through the nose), CSF otorrhea (leakage from the ear), hemotympanium (blood accumulation at the tympanic membrane), ecchymosis over the mastoid bone (Battle sign), and facial paralysis (seventh cranial nerve injury) accompany middle fossa basilar skull fractures • Signs of medullary dysfunction, such as cardiovascular and respiratory failure, accompanying posterior fossa basilar skull fracture	• CT scan and MRI reveal swelling and intracranial hemorrhage from ruptured blood vessels. • CT scan may reveal a fracture.

Increased intracranial pressure

ICP refers to the pressure exerted within the intact skull, a rigid structure, by the three components of intracranial volume, which are:

 blood

 CSF

 brain tissue.

Tip the scales

Normally the body can maintain a balance of intracranial volume. However, any condition that alters the normal balance of intracranial components can increase ICP. Significant or rapid elevations in ICP aren't well tolerated by the brain and may result in herniation.

Education edge

After a concussion

The patient with a concussion may be discharged from the emergency department (ED). In such cases, the patient and his family need instructions on how to monitor the patient at home and when the patient should seek medical care. Include the following in your discharge teaching:
• Ensure that a responsible person, such as a family member, will be with the patient at home for the next 24 hours.
• Teach the family member how to check the patient's neurologic status, such as observing for confusion, difficulty walking, changes in level of consciousness, projectile vomiting, unequal pupils, lethargy, irritability, difficulty arousing, failure to feed, or continuous crying.
• Advise the family member to notify their family doctor or bring the patient back to the ED if any of these signs and symptoms occur.

What causes it

Increased ICP can be caused by any condition that decreases any of the three components of the intracranial vault. Some causes may include:
• hemorrhage
• bleeding or edema
• hydrocephalus
• space-occupying lesions (tumors, abscesses, cysts, foreign bodies, and AVMs).

How it happens

Under normal circumstances, a change in the volume of one of the intracranial contents triggers a reciprocal change in one or more of the components to maintain a consistent pressure. When this balance becomes altered, ICP increases. Initially, the body compensates by regulating the volume of the three substances via:
• displacing CSF into the spinal canal
• increasing absorption or decreasing production of CSF
• limiting blood flow to the head
• forcing brain tissue out of the skull.
    When these compensatory mechanisms become overtaxed, small changes in volume lead to big changes in pressure.

What to look for

Signs and symptoms of increased ICP can be subtle early on. Typically, signs and symptoms are manifested in the patient's LOC, pupils, motor responses, and vital signs.

Early symptoms

- Headache
- Increased blood pressure (intermittently)
- Nausea and vomiting
- Muscle weakness or motor changes on the side opposite the lesion, and positive pronator drift
- Varied LOC (initially) (The patient may become restless, anxious, or quiet, or you may note that he needs increased stimulation to be aroused.)

Further compromise

- Hemiparesis
- Hemiplegia
- Increased systolic blood pressure, profound bradycardia, and abnormal respirations
- Can't be aroused (as ICP continues to increase)
- Pupillary changes (may reveal constriction of one pupil and not the other, a sluggish reaction by both pupils, pupillary changes only on one side, or unequal pupils)
- Seizures

Severe increased ICP

- Absent doll's eye reflex
- Bradycardia
- Systolic hypertension
- Hyperthermia
- Widened pulse pressure
- Profound weakness
- Pupils fixed and dilated

What tests tell you

The patient with increased ICP typically undergoes diagnostic testing to determine the underlying cause of the problem. Such tests may include:

- cerebral angiography to evaluate cerebral blood flow and evidence of vascular disruptions
- CT or MRI imaging to evaluate for hematomas, lesions, ischemic tissue, or fractures.

How it's treated

Treatment focuses on correcting the underlying problem and controlling ICP and may include:
- I.V. normal saline (only in severe head trauma)
- osmotic diuretics.

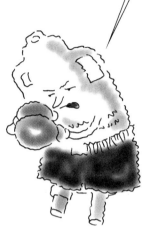

I.V. saline solution can help knock out increased ICP.

What to do

- Institute cardiac monitoring and be alert for cardiac changes or arrhythmias.
- Initially, monitor vital signs continuously and continue to check vital signs and neurologic status, including LOC and pupil size, every 15 minutes.
- Maintain a patent airway. Monitor oxygen saturation levels through pulse oximetry and ABG analysis as ordered.
- Assist with insertion of a CSF drainage system or an ICP monitoring device as appropriate.
- Assess hemodynamic parameters to aid in evaluating CPP.
- Administer medications as ordered. If necessary, use continuous infusions of such agents as Versed, fentanyl, morphine, or Diprivan to reduce metabolic demand.
- If an ICP monitoring system is inserted, continuously monitor ICP waveforms and pressure.
- Elevate the head of the bed 30 degrees.
- Institute seizure precautions as necessary. Use safety precautions to minimize the risk of injury.
- Explain all procedures and treatments to the patient and his family.
- Prepare to transfer the patient to the ICU when indicated.

What to avoid

- Avoid extreme hip and knee flexion because these actions can increase intra-abdominal and intrathoracic pressures.
- Minimize procedures that might increase ICP, such as suctioning.

Seizures

Seizures are paroxysmal events associated with abnormal electrical discharges of neurons in the brain. They aren't an actual disorder but, rather, an indication of an underlying problem. Seizure disorder, or *epilepsy*, is a condition of the brain characterized by recurrent seizures. However, many seizures aren't a part of a seizure disorder but may result from isolated events such as fever, toxin exposure, alcohol withdrawal, or a concussion.

Primary and secondary

Primary seizure disorder or epilepsy is idiopathic without apparent structural changes in the brain. Secondary epilepsy, characterized by structural changes or metabolic alterations of the neuronal membranes, causes increased automaticity.

Who's affected...

Epilepsy affects 1% to 2% of the population; approximately 2 million people live with epilepsy. The incidence is highest in children and older adults. The prognosis is good if the patient adheres strictly to the prescribed treatment.

...and how

Complications of epilepsy may include hypoxia or anoxia due to airway occlusion, traumatic injury, brain damage, and depression and anxiety.

What causes it

In about one-half of seizure disorder cases, the cause is unknown. Some possible causes are:
• anoxia
• birth trauma (such as inadequate oxygen supply to the brain, blood incompatibility, or hemorrhage)
• infectious diseases (meningitis, encephalitis, or brain abscess)
• head injury or trauma
• perinatal infection.

How it happens

Some neurons in the brain may depolarize easily or be hyperexcitable, firing more readily when stimulated than normally happens. On stimulation, the electric current spreads to surrounding cells, which fire in turn. The impulse thus cascades to:
• one area of the brain (a partial seizure)
• both sides of the brain (a generalized seizure)
• cortical, subcortical, and brain stem areas.

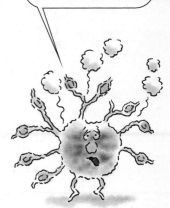

Boy, am I burned out. When neurons get hyperexcited, we fire more readily than usual, causing cells to retaliate and leading to seizures.

Increase O$_2$ or else

The brain's metabolic demand for oxygen increases dramatically during a generalized seizure. If this demand isn't met, hypoxia and brain damage result.

Firing of inhibitory neurons causes the excited neurons to slow their firing and eventually stop. Without this inhibitory action, the result is status epilepticus (continuous seizures or seizures occurring one right after another). Without treatment, the resulting anoxia is fatal.

What to look for

The hallmark of a seizure disorder is recurring seizures, which can be classified as partial or generalized. Some patients are affected by more than one type. (See *Identifying types of seizures.*)

What tests tell you

Here are possible primary diagnostic results of tests for seizure disorders:
• CT scan to show density readings of the brain and may indicate abnormalities in internal brain structures such as a tumor or cyst.
• MRI may indicate abnormalities in internal brain structures.
• EEG is used to confirm the diagnosis of epilepsy by providing evidence of the continuing tendency to have seizures.

How it's treated

Generally, treatment consists of drug therapy specific to the type of seizures. The goal is to reduce seizures using a combination of the fewest drugs.

For tonic-clonic seizures

The most commonly prescribed drugs for generalized tonic-clonic seizures (alternating episodes of muscle spasm and relaxation) include phenytoin, carbamazepine (Tegretol), Phenobarbital (Luminal), and primidone (Mysoline).

Surgery and emergencies

If drug therapy fails, treatment may include surgical removal of a focal lesion or neural pathway in an attempt to stop seizures.

Continuous

In some cases, a patient may experience continuous seizures or recurrent seizures lasting at least 20 to 30 minutes. If these seizures occur, immediate intervention is necessary. (See *Status epilepticus*, page 78.)

What to do

• Ensure patient safety.
• Protect the patient's airway but never place anything in the patient's mouth.
• Administer oxygen as needed.
• Obtain a blood glucose level as indicated.
• Initiate I.V. or intraosseous (I.O.) access.
• Administer naloxone (Narcan) if opioid toxicity is suspected.

Identifying types of seizures

Use these guidelines to understand different seizure types. Keep in mind that some patients may be affected by more than one type.

Partial seizures
Arising from a localized area in the brain, they may spread to the entire brain, causing a generalized seizure. Types include *Jacksonian, sensory, complex partial,* and *secondarily generalized.*

Jacksonian seizures
These begin as localized motor seizures with stiffening or jerking in one extremity, and a tingling sensation in the same area. The patient seldom loses consciousness unless the seizure progresses to a generalized tonic-clonic seizure.

Sensory seizure
Symptoms include hallucinations, flashing lights, tingling sensations, vertigo, déjà vu, and smelling a foul odor.

Complex partial seizure
Signs and symptoms vary but usually include purposeless behavior, such as a glassy stare, picking at clothes, aimless wandering, lip-smacking or chewing motions, and unintelligible speech.

An aura may occur first, and seizures may last a few seconds to 20 minutes. Afterward, mental confusion may last for several minutes. The patient has no memory of his actions during the seizure.

Secondarily generalized partial seizure
This can be simple or complex and can progress to a generalized seizure. An aura may occur first, with loss of concentration immediately or 1 to 2 minutes later.

Generalized seizures
Types include *absence, myoclonic, clonic, tonic, generalized tonic-clonic,* and *atonic.*

Absence seizure
Absence seizure (*petit mal seizure*) is most common in children. It usually begins with a brief change in the level of consciousness, signaled by blinking or rolling of the eyes, a blank stare, and slight mouth movements. The patient retains his posture and continues preseizure activity without difficulty.

Such seizures last 1 to 10 seconds. If not properly treated, seizures can recur up to 100 times per day and progress to a generalized tonic-clonic seizure.

Myoclonic seizure
This is marked by brief, involuntary muscle jerks of the body or extremities and typically occurs in early morning.

Clonic seizure
This is characterized by bilateral rhythmic movements.

Tonic seizure
This is characterized by a sudden stiffening of muscle tone, usually of the arms, but may also include the legs.

Generalized tonic-clonic seizure
Typically begins with a loud cry caused by air rushing from the lungs and through the vocal cords. The patient falls to the ground, losing consciousness. The body stiffens (tonic phase) and then alternates between episodes of muscle spasm and relaxation (clonic phase). Tongue biting, incontinence, labored breathing, apnea, and cyanosis may also occur.

The seizure stops in 2 to 5 minutes. Afterward, the patient regains consciousness but is somewhat confused. He may have difficulty talking and may have drowsiness, fatigue, headache, muscle soreness, and arm or leg weakness. He may fall into a deep sleep afterward.

Atonic seizure
This is characterized by a general loss of postural tone and temporary loss of consciousness. It occurs in children and is sometimes called a *drop attack* because the child falls.

Stay on the ball

Status epilepticus

Status epilepticus is a continuous seizure state that must be interrupted by emergency measures. It can occur during all types of seizures.

Always an emergency

Status epilepticus is accompanied by a continuous generalized tonic-clonic seizure. It can result from withdrawal of antiepileptic medications, hypoxic or metabolic encephalopathy, acute head trauma, or septicemia secondary to encephalitis, meningitis, toxins, or hypothermia.

Act fast

Emergency treatment usually consists of lorazepam (Ativan) or diazepam (Valium); I.V. dextrose 50% is given when seizures are secondary to hypoglycemia; and I.V. thiamine in patients with chronic alcoholism or those who are undergoing withdrawal. After the seizure has stopped, administer fosphenytoin (Cerebyx) or phenytoin (Dilantin).

• Administer diazepam (Valium) or lorazepam (Ativan) I.V., I.O., or rectally as ordered, to control seizures.
• Institute cardiac monitoring and be alert for cardiac changes or arrhythmias.
• Monitor a patient receiving anticonvulsants for signs of toxicity, such as nystagmus, ataxia, lethargy, dizziness, drowsiness, slurred speech, irritability, nausea, and vomiting.
• When administering fosphenytoin (Cerebyx) I.V., use a large vein, administer it according to the guidelines (not more than 150 mg/phenytoin equivalent/minute). Monitor vital signs continuously during the infusion and for 10 to 20 minutes after the infusion is complete. Be alert for signs of hypotension.
• If the patient has a history of anticonvulsant medication use, draw a therapeutic level and send it to the laboratory.

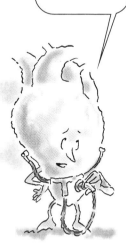

Be alert for cardiac changes after seizures.

Tonic-clonic interventions

If the patient has a generalized tonic-clonic seizure, follow these steps:
• Avoid restraining the patient during a seizure.
• Help the patient to a lying position if not already in that position, loosen any tight clothing, and place something flat and soft, such as a pillow, under his head.
• Clear the area of hard objects.
• Don't force anything into the patient's mouth.
• Turn the patient's head or turn him on his side to allow secretions to drain.
• After the seizure, reassure the patient that he's okay, orient him to time and place, and tell him that he had a seizure.

Spinal cord injury

Spinal injuries include fractures, contusions, and compressions of the vertebral column. They usually result from trauma to the head or neck. Fractures of the 5th, 6th, or 7th cervical; 12th thoracic; and 1st lumbar vertebrae are most common.

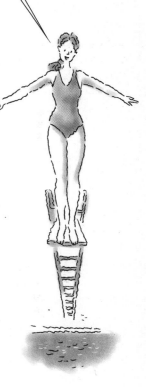

Look out below! Diving into shallow water is a top cause of serious spinal cord trauma.

Dangerous damage

The real danger with spinal injury is spinal cord damage due to cutting, pulling, swelling, twisting, and compression. Spinal cord injury can occur at any level, and the damage it causes may be partial or involve the entire cord. Complications of spinal cord injury include neurogenic shock and spinal shock.

What causes it

The most serious spinal cord trauma typically results from motor vehicle collisions, falls, sports injuries, dives into shallow water, and gunshot or stab wounds. Less serious injuries commonly occur from lifting heavy objects and minor falls. Spinal cord dysfunction may also result from hyperparathyroidism and neoplastic lesions.

How it happens

Spinal cord trauma results from deforming forces. Types of trauma include:
- hyperextension
- hyperflexion
- rotational twisting, which adds shearing forces
- vertebral compression from downward force from the top of the cranium or from the sacrum upward, along the vertical axis, and through the vertebra.

During spinal cord trauma

- An injury causes microscopic hemorrhages in the gray matter and pia-arachnoid, or macroscopic damage, tearing, compression, and disruption.
- The hemorrhages gradually increase in size until all of the gray matter is filled with blood, which causes necrosis.
- From the gray matter, the blood enters the white matter, where it impedes circulation within the spinal cord.
- Resulting edema causes compression and decreases the blood supply.
- The spinal cord loses perfusion and becomes ischemic. The edema and hemorrhage are usually greatest in the two segments above and below the injury.

• The edema temporarily adds to the patient's dysfunction by increasing pressure and compressing the nerves. For example, edema near the 3rd to 5th cervical vertebrae may interfere with respiration.

After acute trauma

• In the white matter, circulation usually returns to normal within 24 hours after injury if the cord wasn't transected.
• In the gray matter, an inflammatory reaction prevents restoration of circulation.
• Phagocytes appear at the site within 35 to 48 hours after injury.
• Macrophages engulf degenerating axons and collagen replaces the normal tissue.
• Scarring and meningeal thickening leaves the nerves in the area blocked or tangled.

What to look for

In your assessment, look for:
• history of trauma, a neoplastic lesion, or an infection that could produce a spinal abscess
• muscle spasm and back or neck pain that worsens with movement; in cervical fractures, pain that causes point tenderness; in dorsal and lumbar fractures, pain that may radiate to other areas, such as the legs
• sensory loss ranging from mild paresthesia to quadriplegia and shock, if the injury damages the spinal cord; in milder injury, symptoms that may be delayed several days or weeks
• ecchymosis, pain, edema, guarding, tenderness, and crepitus over the spine and paraspinal area
• loss of the bulbocavernous reflex with complete cord transection as evidenced by a lack of anal sphincter response when a finger placed in the rectum and then the clitoris or glans is tugged (or when an indwelling urinary catheter is pulled)
• loss of rectal tone
• cough tenderness (coughing can induce neck pain)
• feeling of hot water or an electric shock running down the patient's back
• mouth breathing because of a loss of diaphragmatic control
• arms folded across the chest in a guarded position or outstretched above the head, which may indicate a C5 to C6 injury.

Specifically speaking

Specific signs and symptoms depend on the type and degree of injury. (See *Types of spinal cord injury.*)

Types of spinal cord injury

Spinal cord injury may be classified as complete or incomplete. Incomplete injury may be an anterior cord syndrome, central cord syndrome, or Brown-Séquard syndrome, depending on which area of the cord is affected. To help you assess your patient, here are the characteristic signs and symptoms of each.

Type	Description	Signs and symptoms
Complete injury	• All tracts of the spinal cord completely disrupted • All functions involving the spinal cord below the level of injury lost • Complete and permanent loss	• Loss of motor function (quadriplegia or tetraplegia) with cervical cord transection; paraplegia with thoracic cord transection • Muscle flaccidity • Loss of all reflexes and sensory function below the level of injury • Bladder and bowel atony • Paralytic ileus • Loss of vasomotor tone in lower body parts with low and unstable blood pressure • Loss of perspiration below level of injury • Dry, pale skin • Respiratory impairment
Incomplete injury: Central cord syndrome	• Center position of cord affected • Typically from cervical hyperextension injury	• Motor deficits greater in upper than in lower extremities • Variable degree of bladder dysfunction
Incomplete injury: Anterior cord syndrome	• Occlusion of anterior spinal artery • Occlusion from pressure of bone fragments	• Loss of motor function below the level of injury • Loss of pain and temperature sensations below the level of injury • Intact touch, pressure, position, and vibration senses
Incomplete injury: Brown-Séquard syndrome	• Hemisection of cord affected (damage to cord on only one side) • Most common in stabbing and gunshot wounds	• Ipsilateral paralysis or paresis below the level of injury • Ipsilateral loss of touch, pressure, vibration, and position sense below the level of injury • Contralateral loss of pain and temperature sensations below the level of injury

What tests tell you

Diagnosis of acute spinal cord injuries are based on the results of these diagnostic tests:
• Spinal X-rays (the most important diagnostic measure) reveal fracture.
• CT scan and MRI show the location of the fracture, site of compression, spinal cord edema, and a possible spinal cord mass.
• Neurologic evaluation is used to locate the level of injury and detect cord damage.

How it's treated

The primary treatment after spinal injury is immediate immobilization to stabilize the spine and prevent further cord damage. Other treatment is supportive.

Cervical injuries require immobilization, using head support on both sides of the patient's head, a hard cervical collar, or skeletal traction with skull tongs, a halo device, or surgical fixations.

What to do

• Immediately stabilize the patient's spine. As with all spinal injuries, suspect cord damage until proven otherwise. Use a rigid cervical collar, lateral head immobilizer, and backboard.
• If the patient has a helmet in place, remove it if possible, according to facility policy. Ensure that at least two persons are present during the removal.
• Check the patient's airway and his respiratory rate and rhythm.
• Evaluate the patient's LOC.
• Perform a neurologic assessment to establish baseline motor and sensory status and continually reassess neurologic status for changes.
• Assess respiratory status closely at least every hour initially. Obtain baseline tidal volume, pulse oximetry, and capnography, and reassess frequently. Auscultate breath sounds and check secretions as necessary.
• Monitor oxygen saturation levels and administer supplemental oxygen as indicated.
• Begin cardiac monitoring and assess cardiac status frequently, at least every hour initially. Monitor blood pressure and hemodynamic status frequently.
• If your patient becomes hypotensive, prepare to administer fluids and vasopressors.
• Administer methylprednisolone as ordered if the patient's injury has occurred within the past 8 hours.
• Anticipate gastric tube insertion and low intermittent suctioning. Assess the abdomen for distention.

Distention prevention

• Insert an indwelling urinary catheter as ordered. To prevent bladder distention, monitor intake and output.
• Institute measures to keep the patient warm, such as applying warmed blankets, keeping the patient covered when possible, and administering warmed I.V. fluids.
• Begin measures to prevent skin breakdown due to immobilization.

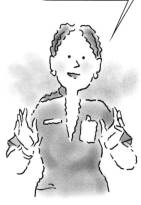

Immediate immobilization after the injury helps prevent further spinal cord damage.

• Obtain and monitor laboratory and diagnostic test results, including electrolytes, BUN and creatinine levels, complete blood count (CBC), and urinalysis.
• Assess for signs of neurogenic shock, such as bradycardia, pink and warm skin below the injury and cold and pale skin above it, and for signs of spinal shock, such as flaccid paralysis and loss of deep tendon and perianal reflexes.
• Prepare the patient for surgical stabilization if necessary.
• Provide emotional support to the patient and his family.

Stroke

Stroke, also known as a *cerebrovascular accident* or *brain attack*, is a sudden impairment of cerebral circulation in one or more blood vessels. Stroke interrupts or diminishes oxygen supply and commonly causes serious damage or necrosis in the brain tissues.

The sooner the better

The sooner circulation returns to normal after a stroke, the better your patient's chances are for a complete recovery. However, about one-half of patients who survive a stroke remain permanently disabled and experience a recurrence within weeks, months, or years.

Number three

Stroke is the third most common cause of death in the United States and the most common cause of neurologic disability. It affects more than 500,000 people each year and is fatal in about one-half of these cases.

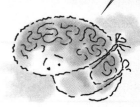

It's sad, but true; one-half of all stroke survivors remain permanently disabled.

What causes it

Stroke typically results from one of three causes:

thrombosis of the intracranial vessels, occluding blood flow, or the cerebral arteries supplying the brain

embolism from thrombus outside the brain, such as in the heart, aorta, or common carotid artery

hemorrhage from an intracranial artery or vein, such as from hypertension, ruptured aneurysm, AVM, trauma, or hemorrhagic disorder.

Risk factor facts

Risk factors that predispose a patient to stroke include:
• cardiac disease, including arrhythmias, coronary artery disease, myocardial infarction, dilated cardiomyopathy, and valvular disease
• cigarette smoking
• diabetes
• familial hyperlipidemia
• family history of stroke
• history of TIA (see *TIA and elderly patients*)
• hypertension
• increased alcohol intake
• obesity and a sedentary lifestyle
• use of hormonal contraceptives.

How it happens

Regardless of the cause, the underlying event leading to stroke is oxygen and nutrient deprivation in the brain cells. Here's what happens:
• Normally, arterial flow is interrupted and autoregulatory mechanisms maintain cerebral circulation until collateral circulation develops to deliver blood to the affected area.
• If the compensatory mechanisms become overworked or cerebral blood flow remains impaired for more than a few minutes, oxygen deprivation leads to infarction of brain tissue.
• The brain cells cease to function because they can't engage in anaerobic metabolism or store glucose or glycogen for later use.

Ischemic stroke

Here's what happens when a thrombotic or embolic stroke causes ischemia:
• Some of the neurons served by the occluded vessel die from lack of oxygen and nutrients.
• Cerebral infarction then occurs, in which tissue injury triggers an inflammatory response that in turn increases ICP.
• Injury to the surrounding cells disrupts metabolism and leads to changes in ionic transport, localized acidosis, and free radical formation.
• Calcium, sodium, and water accumulate in the injured cells, and excitatory neurotransmitters are released.
• Consequent continued cellular injury and swelling set up a cycle of further damage.

Hemorrhagic stroke

Here's what happens when a hemorrhage causes a stroke:

Ages and stages

TIA and elderly patients

To help assess for a history of transient ischemic attack (TIA), ask an elderly patient about recent falls—especially frequent falls. Doing so is important because an older patient is less likely to forget about or minimize frequent falls than he is to report other signs of a TIA.

Cellular swelling is one consequence of ischemic stroke.

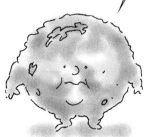

• Impaired cerebral perfusion causes infarction, and the blood acts as a space-occupying mass, exerting pressure on the brain tissues.
• The brain's regulatory mechanisms attempt to maintain equilibrium by increasing blood pressure to maintain CPP. The increased ICP forces CSF out, thus restoring equilibrium.
• If the hemorrhage is small, the patient may have minimal neurologic deficits. If the bleeding is heavy, ICP increases rapidly and perfusion stops. Even if the pressure returns to normal, many brain cells die.
• Initially, the ruptured cerebral blood vessels may constrict to limit the blood loss. This vasospasm further compromises blood flow, leading to more ischemia and cellular damage.
• If a clot forms in the vessel, decreased blood flow also promotes ischemia. If the blood enters the subarachnoid space, meningeal irritation occurs.
• Blood cells that pass through the vessel wall into the surrounding tissue may break down and block the arachnoid villi, causing hydrocephalus.

What to look for

Clinical features of stroke vary, depending on the artery affected (and, consequently, the portion of the brain it supplies), the severity of the damage, and the extent of collateral circulation that develops to help the brain compensate for decreased blood supply. (See *Stroke signs and symptoms*, page 86.)

Left is right and right is left

A stroke in the left hemisphere produces symptoms on the right side of the body; in the right hemisphere, symptoms on the left side. Common signs and symptoms of stroke include sudden onset of:
• hemiparesis on the side opposite the affected side of the brain (may be more severe in the face and arm than in the leg)
• unilateral sensory defect (such as numbness, or tingling) generally on the same side as the hemiparesis (left middle cerebral artery stroke)
• slurred or indistinct speech or the inability to understand speech
• blurred or indistinct vision, double vision, or vision loss in one eye (usually described as a curtain coming down or "gray-out" of vision)
• mental status changes or loss of consciousness (particularly if associated with one of the above symptoms)
• very severe headache with hemorrhagic stroke (subarachnoid hemorrhage stroke).

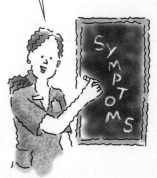

Blurred vision, slurred speech, and hemiparesis are just three stroke symptoms.

Stroke signs and symptoms

With stroke, functional loss reflects damage to the area of the brain that's normally perfused by the occluded or ruptured artery. Although one patient may experience only mild hand weakness, another may develop unilateral paralysis.

Hypoxia and ischemia may produce edema that affects distal parts of the brain, causing further neurologic deficits. Here are the signs and symptoms that accompany stroke at different sites.

Site	Signs and symptoms	Site	Signs and symptoms
Middle cerebral artery	• Aphasia • Dysphasia • Dyslexia (reading problems) • Dysgraphia (inability to write) • Visual field cuts • Hemiparesis on the affected side, which is more severe in the face and arm than in the leg	Anterior cerebral artery	• Confusion • Weakness • Numbness on the affected side (especially in the arm) • Paralysis of the contralateral foot and leg • Incontinence • Poor coordination • Impaired motor and sensory functions • Personality changes, such as flat affect and distractibility
Internal carotid artery	• Headaches • Weakness • Paralysis • Numbness • Sensory changes • Vision disturbances such as blurring on the affected side • Altered level of consciousness • Bruits over the carotid artery • Aphasia • Dysphagia • Ptosis	Vertebral or basilar artery	• Mouth and lip numbness • Dizziness • Weakness on the affected side • Vision deficits, such as color blindness, lack of depth perception, and diplopia • Poor coordination • Dysphagia • Slurred speech • Amnesia • Ataxia
		Posterior cerebral artery	• Visual field cuts • Sensory impairment • Dyslexia • Coma • Blindness from ischemia in the occipital area

What tests tell you

Here are some test findings that help diagnose a stroke:
• CT scanning discloses structural abnormalities, edema, and lesions, such as nonhemorrhagic infarction and aneurysms. Results

are used to differentiate a stroke from other disorders, such as a tumor and hematoma. Patients with TIA generally have a normal CT scan. CT scanning shows evidence of hemorrhagic stroke immediately and of ischemic (thrombotic or embolic) stroke within 72 hours after the onset of symptoms. CT scans should be obtained within 25 minutes after the patient arrives in the ED, and results should be available within 45 minutes of arrival to determine whether hemorrhage is present. (If hemorrhagic stroke is present, thrombolytic therapy is contraindicated.)
• Cerebral angiography shows details of disruption or displacement of the cerebral circulation by occlusion or hemorrhage.
• DSA is used to evaluate patency of the cerebral vessels and shows evidence of occlusion of the cerebral vessels, a lesion, or vascular abnormalities.
• Carotid duplex scan is a high-frequency ultrasound that shows blood flow through the carotid arteries and reveals stenosis due to atherosclerotic plaque and blood clots.

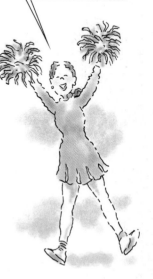

Give me a CT scan and a DSA! These two tests can help you diagnose a stroke today!

Go with the flow
• Brain scan shows ischemic areas but may not be conclusive for up to 2 weeks after stroke.
• No laboratory tests confirm the diagnosis of stroke, but some tests aid diagnosis and some are used to establish a baseline for thrombolytic treatment. A blood glucose test shows whether the patient's symptoms are related to hypoglycemia. Hemoglobin level and hematocrit may be elevated in severe occlusion. Baselines obtained before thrombolytic therapy begins include CBC, platelet count, PTT, PT, fibrinogen level, and chemistry panel.

How it's treated
The goal is to begin treatment within 60 minutes after your patient arrives in the ED. (See *Suspected stroke algorithm*, page 88.)

Drugs of choice
Thrombolytics (also called *fibrinolytics*) are the drugs of choice in treating a stroke patient. The patient must first meet certain criteria to be considered for this type of treatment. (See *Who's suited for thrombolytic therapy?* page 89.)

Drugs for management
Drug therapy for the management of stroke includes:
• thrombolytics for emergency treatment of ischemic stroke
• aspirin or ticlopidine (Ticlid) as an antiplatelet agent to prevent recurrent ischemic stroke
• benzodiazepines to treat patients with seizure activity

Suspected stroke algorithm

Identify signs of possible stroke

Critical EMS assessments and actions

- Support ABCs; give **oxygen** if needed
- Perform prehospital stroke assessment
- Establish time when patient last known normal (Note: therapies may be available beyond 3 hours from onset)

- Transport; consider triage to a center with a stroke unit if appropriate; consider bringing a witness, family member, or caregiver
- Alert hospital
- Check glucose if possible

Immediate general assessment and stabilization

- Assess ABCs, vital signs
- Provide **oxygen** if hypoxemic
- Obtain I.V. access and blood samples
- Check glucose; treat if indicated

- Perform neurologic screening assessment
- Activate stroke team
- Order emergency computed tomography (CT) scanning of brain
- Obtain 12-lead electrocardiogram

Immediate neurologic assessment by stroke team or designee

- Review patient history
- Establish symptom onset
- Perform neurologic examination (NIH Stroke Scale or Canadian Neurologic Scale)

Does CT scan show any hemorrhage?

No hemorrhage

**Probable acute ischemic stroke;
consider fibrinolytic therapy**

- Check for fibrinolytic exclusions
- Repeat neurologic exam: are deficits rapidly improving to normal?

Hemorrhage

Consult neurologist or neurosurgeon;
consider transfer if not available

Patient remains candidate for fibrinolytic therapy?	**Not a candidate** →	Administer **aspirin**

Candidate

**Review risks/benefits with patient and family:
If acceptable**

- Give **tPA**
- No anticoagulants or antiplatelet treatment for 24 hours

- Begin stroke pathway
- Admit to stroke unit if available
- Monitor blood pressure; treat if indicated

- Monitor neurologic status; emergency CT scan if deterioration
- Monitor blood glucose; treat if needed
- Initiate supportive therapy; treat comorbidities

Stay on the ball

Who's suited for thrombolytic therapy?

Not every stroke patient is a candidate for thrombolytic therapy. Each is evaluated to see whether established criteria are met.

Criteria that must be present

Criteria that must be present for a patient to be considered for thrombolytic therapy include:
• age 18 or older
• acute ischemic stroke associated with significant neurologic deficit
• onset of symptoms less than 3 hours before treatment begins.

Criteria that must *not* be present

In addition to meeting the above criteria, the patient must not:
• show evidence of intracerebral hemorrhage during pretreatment evaluation
• exhibit evidence of subarachnoid hemorrhage during pretreatment evaluation even if computed tomography (CT) scan is normal
• have a history of recent (within 3 months) intracranial or intraspinal surgery, serious head trauma, or previous stroke
• have a history of intracranial hemorrhage

• have uncontrolled hypertension at the time of treatment (blood pressure remaining at greater than 185 mm Hg systolic and greater than 110 mm Hg diastolic)
• have experienced a seizure at the onset of stroke
• have active internal bleeding or acute trauma
• have an intracranial neoplasm, arteriovenous malformation, or aneurysm
• have known bleeding diathesis involving, but not limited to:
  – current use of oral anticoagulants, such as warfarin (Coumadin), International Normalized Ratio greater than 1.7, or prothrombin time greater than 15 seconds
  – receipt of heparin within 48 hours before the onset of stroke and an elevated partial thromboplastin time
  – platelet count less than 100,000/ml
• have a CT scan showing a multilobar infarction
• have experienced arterial puncture at a noncompressible site within the last 7 days.

• anticonvulsants to treat patients with seizures or to prevent them after the patient's condition has stabilized
• antihypertensives and antiarrhythmics to treat patients with risk factors for recurrent stroke
• corticosteroids to minimize associated cerebral edema
• analgesics to relieve the headaches that may follow a hemorrhagic stroke.

Under the knife

Depending on the cause and extent of the stroke, the patient may undergo:
• craniotomy to remove a hematoma

• carotid endarterectomy to remove atherosclerotic plaques from the inner arterial wall
• extracranial bypass to circumvent an artery that's blocked by occlusion or stenosis.

What to do

Your facility may have a stroke protocol and stroke team composed of specially trained practitioners who respond to potential stroke patients. When a patient shows signs and symptoms of a stroke, first evaluate the patient and complete a stroke screening tool such as the Cincinnati Stroke Scale. Then assess the patient using a stroke assessment tool such as the NIH Stroke Scale.

After your initial assessment, call the stroke team if your facility has one. They will evaluate the patient, complete a neurologic assessment, report findings, and facilitate rapid and appropriate care of the patient. Such care includes emergency interventions, diagnostic tests, and transfer to the ICU. During this time, do the following:
• Secure and maintain the patient's airway and anticipate the need for ET intubation and mechanical ventilation.

> Once you've assessed, call for the best—the stroke team! They'll be able to provide further evaluation.

Multiple monitors

• Monitor oxygen saturation levels via pulse oximetry and ABG levels as ordered. Administer supplemental oxygen as ordered to maintain oxygen saturation greater than 90%.
• Place the patient on a cardiac monitor, and monitor for cardiac arrhythmias.
• Assess the patient's neurologic status frequently; at least every 15 to 30 minutes initially, then hourly as indicated. Observe for signs of increased ICP.
• Obtain laboratory studies as ordered, such as CBC, PT, International Normalized Ratio, and PTT.
• Prepare to administer labetalol (Normodyne) as ordered to maintain the patient's blood pressure at less than 185 mm Hg systolic and less than 110 mm Hg diastolic.
• Assess hemodynamic status frequently. Give fluids as ordered and monitor I.V. infusions to avoid overhydration, which may increase ICP.
• Assess the patient receiving thrombolytic therapy for signs and symptoms of bleeding every 15 to 30 minutes and institute bleeding precautions. Monitor results of coagulation studies.

Anticonvulsant, antiplatelet, anticoagulation

• Monitor the patient for seizures and administer anticonvulsants as ordered. Institute safety precautions to prevent injury.
• If the patient had a TIA, administer antiplatelet agents. Administer anticoagulants such as heparin if he shows signs of stroke progression, unstable signs of stroke (such as TIA), or evidence of embolic stroke. Monitor coagulation studies closely.
• If the patient isn't a candidate for thrombolytic therapy, prepare to administer heparin anticoagulation as ordered.
• Initiate steps to prevent skin breakdown.
• Provide meticulous eye and mouth care.
• Maintain communication with the patient. If he's aphasic, set up a simple method of communicating.
• Provide psychological support.
• Anticipate transfer to the ICU or interventional radiology as appropriate.

Subarachnoid hemorrhage

Subarachnoid hemorrhage refers to bleeding that occurs into the subarachnoid space. CSF normally occupies this space. This major complication is associated with cerebral aneurysms.

It's cerebral

A cerebral aneurysm is a weakness in the wall of a cerebral artery that causes that area of the artery to dilate or bulge. The most common form is a *berry aneurysm*, a saclike outpouching in a cerebral artery. Cerebral aneurysms usually arise at an arterial junction in the circle of Willis, the circular anastomosis forming the major cerebral arteries at the base of the brain.

Women more prone

The incidence of cerebral aneurysm is slightly higher in women than in men, especially those in their late 40s or early to mid-50s, but a cerebral aneurysm can occur at any age in either gender.

What causes it

The major cause of a subarachnoid hemorrhage is rupture of a cerebral aneurysm. A cerebral aneurysm may result from a congenital defect such as an AVM, from a degenerative process, or both. The most common cause is trauma.

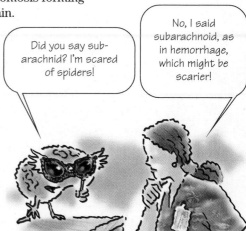

How it happens

Subarachnoid hemorrhage happens when blood flow exerts pressure against a weak arterial wall, stretching it like an overblown balloon and making it likely to rupture. Rupture is followed by hemorrhage, in which blood spills into the subarachnoid space normally occupied by CSF. Sometimes, blood also spills into brain tissue, where a clot can cause potentially fatal increased ICP and brain tissue damage.

What to look for

Occasionally, your patient may exhibit signs and symptoms due to blood oozing into the subarachnoid space. These signs and symptoms, which may have persisted for several days, include:
- headache
- intermittent nausea and vomiting
- nuchal rigidity
- photophobia
- stiff back and legs.

Without warning

Aneurysm rupture usually occurs abruptly and without warning, causing:
- sudden, severe headache from increased pressure due to bleeding into a closed space
- nausea and projectile vomiting related to increased ICP
- altered LOC (possibly including deep coma, depending on the severity and location of bleeding) due to increased pressure caused by increased cerebral blood volume
- meningeal irritation due to bleeding into the meninges and resulting in nuchal rigidity, back and leg pain, fever, restlessness, irritability, occasional seizures, photophobia, and blurred vision
- hemiparesis, hemisensory defects, dysphagia, and vision defects due to bleeding into the brain tissues
- diplopia, ptosis, dilated pupil, and inability to rotate the eye caused by compression on the oculomotor nerve if the aneurysm is near the internal carotid artery.

Making the grade

Typically, the severity of a ruptured intracranial aneurysm is graded according to the patient's signs and symptoms. (See *Grading cerebral aneurysm rupture*.)

What tests tell you

The following tests aid in the diagnosis of cerebral aneurysm:

Grading cerebral aneurysm rupture

The severity of cerebral aneurysm symptoms varies from patient to patient, depending on the site and amount of bleeding. Five grades characterize ruptured cerebral aneurysm:
- *Grade I: minimal bleeding*—The patient is alert, with no neurologic deficit; he may have a slight headache and nuchal rigidity.
- *Grade II: mild bleeding*—The patient is alert, with a mild to severe headache and nuchal rigidity; he may have third-nerve palsy.
- *Grade III: moderate bleeding*—The patient is confused or drowsy, with nuchal rigidity and, possibly, a mild focal deficit.
- *Grade IV: severe bleeding*—The patient is stuporous, with nuchal rigidity and, possibly, mild to severe hemiparesis.
- *Grade V: moribund (usually fatal)*—If the rupture is nonfatal, the patient is in a deep coma or decerebrate.

• Cerebral angiography confirms a cerebral aneurysm that isn't ruptured and reveals altered cerebral blood flow, vessel lumen dilation, and differences in arterial filling.
• CT scan reveals evidence of aneurysm and possible hemorrhage.
• Lumbar puncture and analysis of CSF will reveal blood in the CSF.
• MRI is used to detect vasospasm and locate the bleeding.

How it's treated

Emergency treatment begins with oxygenation and ventilation. Then, to reduce the risk of rebleeding, the neurosurgeon or neuroradiologist may attempt to repair the aneurysm. Surgical repair usually includes clipping, ligating, or wrapping the aneurysm neck with muscle.

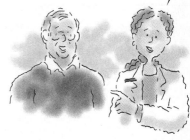

Elderly patients, or ones with serious diseases, may opt for conservative treatment instead of surgery.

Staging an intervention

Other techniques for surgery include interventional radiology in conjunction with endovascular balloon therapy. This technique occludes the aneurysm or vessel and uses cerebral angiography to treat arterial vasospasm.

It's electric!

In some cases, a type of nonsurgical repair called *electrothrombosis* is used. This method involves the insertion of electrically charged platinum coils into the aneurysm. The positively charged platinum is believed to attract negatively charged blood elements, such as white and red blood cells, platelets, and fibrinogen, resulting in intra-aneurysmal thrombosis. Additionally, the coils protect against further hemorrhage by reducing blood pulsations in the vessel and sealing the hole or weak area of the wall. Eventually clots form and the aneurysm is separated from the parent vessel by the formation of new connective tissue.

Being conservative

The patient may receive conservative treatment when surgical correction poses too much risk, such as when the patient is elderly or has heart, lung, or other serious disease, when the aneurysm is in a dangerous location, or when vasospasm necessitates a delay in surgery.

Conservative treatment methods include:
• bed rest (possibly for 4 to 6 weeks) in a quiet, darkened room with the head of the bed flat or raised less than 30 degrees
• avoidance of coffee, other stimulants, and aspirin to reduce the risk of rupture and elevation of blood pressure
• administration of an analgesic

• administration of antihypertensives, if the patient is hypertensive
• administration of corticosteroids to reduce edema
• administration of phenobarbital or other sedative
• administration of a vasoconstrictor to maintain an optimum blood pressure level (20 to 40 mm Hg above normal), if necessary.

What to do

• Establish and maintain a patent airway and anticipate the need for supplementary oxygen or mechanical ventilatory support. Monitor ABG levels.
• Initiate cardiac monitoring and be alert for cardiac changes and arrhythmias.
• Position the patient to promote pulmonary drainage and prevent upper airway obstruction. If intubated, preoxygenate with 100% oxygen before suctioning.
• Impose aneurysm precautions (such as bed rest, limited visitors, and avoidance of coffee and physical activity) to minimize the risk of rebleeding and avoid increased ICP.
• Monitor LOC and vital signs frequently. Avoid taking temperatures rectally.
• Accurately measure intake and output.

Watch out

• Be alert for danger signs and symptoms that may indicate an enlarging aneurysm, rebleeding, intracranial clot, increased ICP, or vasospasm. These signs and symptoms include decreased LOC, unilateral enlarged pupil, onset or worsening of hemiparesis or motor deficit, increased blood pressure, slowed pulse rate, worsening of headache or sudden onset of a headache, renewed or worsened nuchal rigidity, and renewed or persistent vomiting.
• If the patient develops vasospasm—evidenced by focal motor deficits, increasing confusion, and worsening headache—initiate hypervolemic-hemodilution therapy as ordered, such as the administration of normal or hypertonic saline, whole blood, packed red cells, albumin plasma protein fraction, and crystalloid solution. The calcium channel blocker nimodipine (Sular) may reduce smooth-muscle spasm and maximize perfusion during spasm. During therapy, assess the patient for fluid overload.
• Turn the patient often and institute measures to reduce the risks associated with bed rest.

Rebound effects

• Inform the patient and his family about the condition, planned treatments, and possible complications.

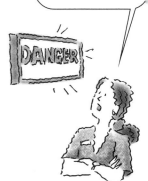

These danger signs may indicate an enlarging aneurysm or other problems.

• Prepare the patient for surgery or transfer him to the ICU as appropriate; provide preoperative teaching if the patient's condition permits.

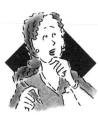

Quick quiz

1. Which finding would lead the nurse to suspect that a patient with spinal cord injury is experiencing spinal shock?

    A.   Orthostatic hypotension
    B.   Bradycardia
    C.   Flaccid paralysis
    D.   Lack of sweating below the level of injury

Answer: C. Signs of spinal shock include flaccid paralysis, loss of deep tendon and perianal reflexes, and loss of motor and sensory function.

2. A patient with significant neurologic deficits comes to the ED and is diagnosed with an acute ischemic stroke. Which indication would make the patient a candidate for thrombolytic therapy?

    A.   His symptoms started about 2 hours ago.
    B.   He has uncontrolled hypertension.
    C.   His platelet count is 88,000/uL.
    D.   He had a seizure when his symptoms began.

Answer: A. To be considered for thrombolytic therapy, the patient must have an acute ischemic stroke associated with significant neurologic deficits, and the onset of the symptoms must have occurred less than 3 hours before beginning treatment.

3. A patient with a head injury is admitted to the ED. Emergency response personnel report that the patient suffered a brief period of loss of consciousness after the injury but is now lucid and complaining of vomiting and a severe headache. Which condition would the nurse suspect?

    A.   Concussion
    B.   Skull fracture
    C.   Subdural hematoma
    D.   Diffuse axonal injury

Answer: B. A brief period of loss of consciousness followed by a lucid period and complaints of vomiting and a severe headache may indicate a concussion.

4. During a neurologic examination, the patient can't raise his eyebrows or close his eyes tightly against resistance. Which cranial nerve might be damaged?

    A.   CN II
    B.   CN V
    C.   CN VII
    D.   CN XII

Answer: C. The facial nerve, CN VII, controls facial expression and taste in the anterior two-thirds of the tongue.

Scoring

☆☆☆ If you answered all four questions correctly, pat yourself on the back! You're a neurologic emergency know-it-all.

☆☆ If you answered three questions correctly, stand tall! You're emerging as an emergency expert.

☆ If you answered fewer than three questions correctly, don't worry! Just "head" back to the beginning of the chapter and try again.

Cardiac emergencies

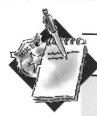

Just the facts

In this chapter, you'll learn:

♦ emergency assessment of the cardiovascular system

♦ diagnostic tests and procedures for cardiovascular emergencies

♦ cardiovascular disorders in the emergency department and their treatments.

Understanding cardiac emergencies

The cardiovascular system is a major control system in the body, playing a key role in cellular nutrition and circulation. It's responsible for carrying life-sustaining oxygen and nutrients via the blood to all cells of the body. When faced with an emergency involving the cardiovascular system, you must assess the patient thoroughly, always being alert for subtle changes that might indicate a potential deterioration in the patient's condition. A thorough nursing assessment forms the basis for your interventions, which must be instituted quickly to minimize potentially life-threatening risks to the patient.

Assessment

Assessment of a patient's cardiovascular system includes a health history and physical examination. If you can't interview the patient because of his condition, you may gather history information from the patient's family members, the patient's primary nurse or other health care providers, or the emergency medical response team.

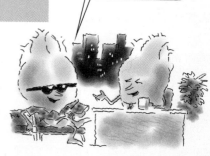

I don't wanna brag here, Bob, but my system happens to be one of the body's major players.

Health history

To obtain the health history of a patient's cardiovascular system, begin by introducing yourself and then obtain information on the patient's chief complaint, personal and family health, and chest pain, if any.

Chief complaint

Use the seven attributes of a symptom, listed below, to obtain details about the patient's chief complaint:

location (Where is it? Does it radiate?)

quality (What's it like?)

quantity or severity (How bad is it on a 1-to-10 scale?)

timing (When does it start? How long does it last? How often does it occur?)

setting or environmental factors (including personal activities and contributing factors, such as climbing stairs and exercising)

factors that make it better or worse

associated manifestations.

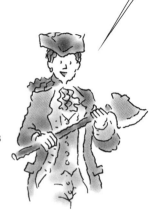

Hail to the chief! Chief complaint, that is. Make sure to get details about all of these symptoms when conducting your assessment.

Personal and family health

Ask the patient for details about his family history and past medical history. Also ask about:
• current health habits, such as smoking, alcohol intake, caffeine intake, exercise, and dietary intake of fat and sodium
• stressors in the patient's life and coping strategies he uses to deal with them
• environmental or occupational factors
• activities of daily living
• drugs the patient is taking, including prescription drugs, over-the-counter drugs, and herbal preparations
• menopause (if applicable)
• previous surgeries.

Complaints of chest pain

Many patients with cardiovascular problems complain of chest pain. Use the seven attributes of a symptom to get a complete picture of the patient's pain.

Cardiac questions

To thoroughly assess your patient's cardiac function, be sure to ask these questions:
• Are you in pain?
• Where's the pain located?
• Does the pain feel like a burning, tight, or squeezing sensation?
• Does the pain radiate to your arm, neck, back, or jaw?

• When did the pain begin?
• What relieves or aggravates it?
• Are you experiencing nausea, dizziness, or sweating?
• Do you feel short of breath? Has breathing trouble ever awakened you from sleep?
• Does your heart ever pound or skip a beat? When?

• Do you ever get dizzy or faint? When?
• Do you experience swelling in your ankles or feet? When? Does anything relieve the swelling?
• Do you urinate frequently at night?
• Have you had to limit your activities?

Where, what, and why

If the patient isn't in distress, ask questions that require more than a yes-or-no response. Use familiar expressions rather than medical terms whenever possible. (See *Cardiac questions*.)

In his own words

Let the patient describe his condition in his own words. Ask him to describe the location, radiation, intensity, and duration of pain and precipitating, exacerbating, or relieving factors to obtain an accurate description of chest pain. (See *Differentiating chest pain*, page 100.)

Physical examination

Cardiac emergencies affect people of all ages, ethnicities, and cultures and can take many forms. To best identify abnormalities, use a consistent, methodical approach to the physical examination. Because of the emergency nature of the patient's condition, remember that you may need to limit your examination to specific problem areas or stop your examination entirely to intervene if the patient exhibits signs or symptoms that his condition is deteriorating. If your initial screening indicates a cardiac problem, you may need to conduct a more detailed assessment.

The heart of it

When performing an assessment of a patient's heart health, proceed in this order:

 inspection

 palpation

Stay on the ball

Differentiating chest pain

Use this table to help you more accurately assess chest pain.

What it feels like	Where it's located	What makes it worse	What causes it	What makes it better
Aching, squeezing, pressure, heaviness, burning pain; usually subsides within 10 minutes	Substernal; may radiate to jaw, neck, arms, and back	Eating, physical effort, smoking, cold weather, stress, anger, hunger, lying down	Angina pectoris	Rest, nitroglycerin (*Note:* Unstable angina appears even at rest.)
Tightness or pressure; burning, aching pain, possibly accompanied by shortness of breath, diaphoresis, weakness, anxiety, or nausea; sudden onset; lasts ½ hour to 2 hours	Typically across chest but may radiate to jaw, neck, arms, or back	Exertion, anxiety	Acute myocardial infarction	Nitroglycerin and opioid analgesics such as morphine
Sharp and continuous; may be accompanied by friction rub; sudden onset	Substernal; may radiate to neck or left arm	Deep breathing, supine position	Pericarditis	Sitting up, leaning forward, anti-inflammatory drugs
Excruciating, tearing pain; may be accompanied by blood pressure difference between right and left arm; sudden onset	Retrosternal, upper abdominal, or epigastric; may radiate to back, neck, or shoulders	Not applicable	Dissecting aortic aneurysm	Analgesics, surgery
Sudden, stabbing pain; may be accompanied by cyanosis, dyspnea, or cough with hemoptysis	Over lung area	Inspiration	Pulmonary embolus	Analgesics
Sudden, severe pain; sometimes accompanied by dyspnea, increased pulse rate, decreased breath sounds, or deviated trachea	Lateral thorax	Normal respiration	Pneumothorax	Analgesics, chest tube insertion

percussion

 auscultation.

Inspection

First, take a moment to assess the patient's general appearance.

First impressions

Is the patient too thin or obese? Is he alert? Does he appear anxious? Note the patient's skin color. Are his fingers clubbed? (Clubbing is a sign of chronic hypoxia caused by a lengthy cardiovascular or respiratory disorder.) If the patient is dark-skinned, inspect his mucous membranes for pallor.

Check the chest

Next, inspect the chest. Note landmarks you can use to describe your findings as well as structures underlying the chest wall. Look for pulsations, symmetry of movement, retractions, or heaves (strong outward thrusts of the chest wall that display during systole).

Arms and legs, too

Also inspect the patient's arms or legs, noting color, hair distribution, and lesions, ulcers, or edema.

Light the way

Then position a light source, such as a penlight, so that it casts a shadow on the patient's chest. Note the location of the apical impulse. This location is also usually the point of maximal impulse (PMI) and should be located in the fifth intercostal space medial to the left midclavicular line.

The apical impulse indicates how well the left ventricle is working because it corresponds to the apex of the heart. To find the apical impulse in a woman with large breasts, displace the breasts during the examination.

Neck next

Continue your inspection by observing the vessels in the neck. Note the carotid artery pulsations, which should be brisk and localized and don't decrease when the patient is upright, when he inhales, or when palpated. Also inspect the jugular veins. The internal jugular vein has a softer, undulating pulsation, which changes in response to position, breathing, and palpation.

> **Memory jogger**
>
> To remember the order in which you should perform assessment of the cardiovascular system, just think, "I'll Properly Perform Assessment."
>
> I—Inspection
>
> P—Palpation
>
> P—Percussion
>
> A—Auscultation

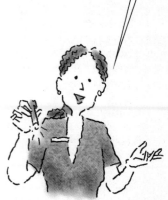

Using a light to cast a shadow on a patient's chest helps locate the apical impulse.

Then go for the jugular

Check the jugular venous pulse by having the patient lie on his back. Elevate the head of the bed 30 to 45 degrees, and turn the patient's head slightly away from you. Normally, the highest pulsation takes place no more than 1½" (3.8 cm) above the sternal notch. If pulsations appear higher, it indicates elevation in central venous pressure (CVP) and jugular vein distention.

Abnormal findings

Here are some of the abnormal findings you may note on inspection and what such findings tell you:
• Cyanosis, pallor, or cool or cold skin may indicate poor cardiac output and tissue perfusion.
• Skin may be flushed if the patient has a fever.
• Absence of body hair on the arms or legs may indicate diminished arterial blood flow to those areas.
• Swelling, or *edema*, may indicate heart failure or venous insufficiency. It may also be caused by varicosities or thrombophlebitis.
• Chronic right-sided heart failure may cause ascites and generalized edema.
• Inspection may reveal barrel chest (rounded thoracic cage caused by chronic obstructive pulmonary disease), scoliosis (lateral curvature of the spine), or kyphosis (convex curvature of the thoracic spine). If severe enough, these conditions can impair cardiac output by preventing chest expansion and inhibiting heart muscle movement.
• Retractions (visible indentations of the soft tissue covering the chest wall) or the use of accessory muscles to breathe typically result from a respiratory disorder, but a congenital heart defect or heart failure may also cause them.

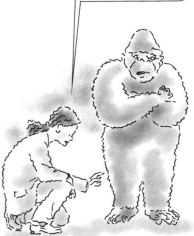

Hmmm...well, since diminished arterial blood flow is usually signaled by lack of arm or leg hair, I think you're probably safe.

Palpation

Note skin temperature, turgor, and texture. Using the ball of your hand and then your fingertips, gently palpate over the precordium to find the apical impulse. Note heaves or thrills (fine vibrations that feel like the purring of a cat). (See *Palpating the apical impulse.*)

Palpate the potentials

Also palpate the sternoclavicular, aortic, pulmonic, tricuspid, and epigastric areas for abnormal pulsations. Pulsations aren't usually felt in these areas. However, an aortic arch pulsation in the sternoclavicular area or an abdominal aorta pulsation in the epigastric area may be a normal finding in a thin patient.

Palpating the apical impulse

The apical impulse is associated with the first heart sound and carotid pulsation. To ensure that you're feeling the apical impulse and not a muscle spasm or some other pulsation, use one hand to palpate the patient's carotid artery and the other to palpate the apical impulse. Then compare the timing and regularity of the impulses. The apical impulse should roughly coincide with the carotid pulsation.

Note the amplitude, size, intensity, location, and duration of the apical impulse. You should feel a gentle pulsation in an area about ½" to ¾" (1.5 to 2 cm) in diameter.

Elusive impulse

The apical impulse may be difficult to palpate in patients who are obese or pregnant and in patients with thick chest walls. If it's difficult to palpate with the patient lying on his back, have him lie on his left side or sit upright.

Refill, please

Check capillary refill and time by assessing the nail beds on the fingers and toes. Refill time should be no more than 3 seconds, or long enough to say "capillary refill." If you are unable to obtain capillary refill and time because of patient injuries or disease, firmly press in the sternal area and assess for blanching in 3 seconds.

And compare

Palpate for the pulse on each side of the neck, comparing pulse volume and symmetry. Don't palpate both carotid arteries at the same time or press too firmly. If you do, the patient may faint or become bradycardic.

Regular and equal

All pulses should be regular in rhythm and equal in strength. Pulses are graded on a scale from 0 to 4+:
- 4+ is bounding.
- 3+ is increased.
- 2+ is normal.
- 1+ is weak.
- 0 is absent.

Abnormal findings

Abnormal findings on palpation may reveal:
- weak pulse, indicating low cardiac output or increased peripheral vascular resistance such as in arterial atherosclerotic disease (note that elderly patients commonly have weak pedal pulses)

- strong bounding pulse, commonly found in hypertension and in high cardiac output states, such as exercise, pregnancy, anemia, and thyrotoxicosis
- apical impulse that exerts unusual force and lasts longer than one-third of the cardiac cycle—a possible indication of increased cardiac output
- displaced or diffuse impulse, possibly indicating left ventricular hypertrophy
- pulsation in the aortic, pulmonic, or right ventricular area, which is a sign of chamber enlargement or valvular disease
- pulsation in the sternoclavicular or epigastric area, which is a sign of an aortic aneurysm

What a thrill!

- palpable thrill, which is an indication of blood flow turbulence and is usually related to valvular dysfunction (Determine how far the thrill radiates and make a mental note to listen for a murmur at this site during auscultation.)
- heave along the left sternal border, which is an indication of right ventricular hypertrophy
- heave over the left ventricular area, which is a sign of a ventricular aneurysm (A thin patient may experience a heave with exercise, fever, or anxiety because of increased cardiac output and more forceful contraction.)
- displaced PMI, which is a possible indication of left ventricular hypertrophy caused by volume overload from mitral or aortic stenosis, septal defect, acute myocardial infarction (MI), or another disorder.

Percussion

Percussion is less useful than other assessment methods, but it may help you locate the cardiac borders.

Border patrol

Begin percussing at the anterior axillary line and continue toward the sternum along the fifth intercostal space. The sound changes from resonance to dullness over the left border of the heart, normally at the midclavicular line. The right border of the heart is usually aligned with the sternum and can't be percussed.

Auscultation

You can learn a great deal about the heart by auscultating for heart sounds. Cardiac auscultation requires a methodical approach.

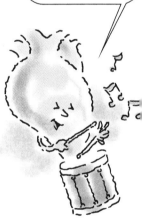

Percussion isn't the best way to assess, but it's definitely the catchiest!

Heart sound sites

When auscultating for heart sounds, place the stethoscope over the four different sites illustrated here.

Auscultation sites are identified by the names of heart valves but aren't located directly over the valves. Rather, these sites are located along the pathway blood takes as it flows through the heart's chambers and valves.

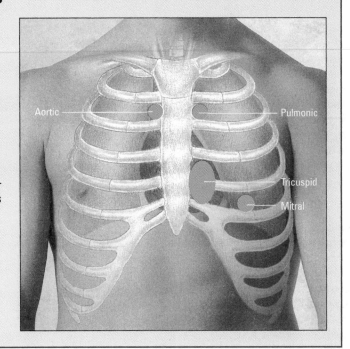

Aortic — Pulmonic — Tricuspid — Mitral

Erb and friends

First, identify the auscultation sites, including the sites over the four cardiac valves, at Erb's point, and at the third intercostal space at the left sternal border. Use the bell to hear low-pitched sounds and the diaphragm to hear high-pitched sounds. (See *Heart sound sites.*)

Auscultate for heart sounds with the patient in three positions:

 lying on his back with the head of the bed raised 30 to 45 degrees

 sitting up

lying on his left side.

Upward, downward, zigward, zagward

Use a zigzag pattern over the precordium. Start at the apex and work upward, or at the base and work downward. Whichever approach you use, be consistent. Use the diaphragm to listen as you go in one direction; use the bell as you come back in the other direction. Be sure to listen over the entire precordium, not just over the valves. Note the patient's heart rate and rhythm.

1, 2, 3, 4, and more

Systole is the period of ventricular contraction:
• As pressure in the ventricles increases, the mitral and tricuspid valves snap closed. The closure produces the first heart sound, S_1.
• At the end of ventricular contraction, the aortic and pulmonic valves snap shut. This snap produces the second heart sound, S_2.
• Always identify S_1 and S_2, and then listen for adventitious sounds, such as the third and fourth heart sounds (S_3 and S_4).
• Also listen for murmurs (vibrating, blowing, or rumbling sounds) and rubs (harsh, scratchy, scraping, or squeaking sounds).

Listen for the "dub"

Start auscultating at the aortic area where the S_2 is loudest. An S_2 is best heard at the base of the heart at the end of ventricular systole. It occurs when the pulmonic and aortic valves close and is generally described as sounding like "dub." Its sound is shorter, higher-pitched, and louder than S_1. When the pulmonic valve closes later than the aortic valve during inspiration, you hear a split S_2.

Listen for the "lub"

From the base of the heart, move to the pulmonic area and then down to the tricuspid area. Then move to the mitral area, where S_1 is the loudest.

An S_1 is best heard at the apex of the heart. It results from closure of the mitral and tricuspid valves and is generally described as sounding like "lub." It's low-pitched and dull. An S_1 occurs at the beginning of ventricular systole. It may be split if the mitral valve closes just before the tricuspid valve.

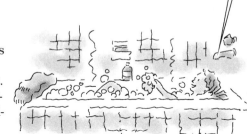

Rub-a-"dub"-"lub"! The S_2 sound is high-pitched and loud, whereas the S_1 sound is low-pitched and dull.

Major auscultation, man!

Also auscultate the major arteries, such as the carotid, femoral, and popliteal arteries, using the bell of the stethoscope to assess for bruits.

Abnormal findings

On auscultation, you may detect S_1 and S_2 heart sounds that are accentuated, diminished, or inaudible. Other abnormal heart sounds—such as S_3, S_4, and murmurs—may result from pressure changes, valvular dysfunctions, and conduction defects. (See *Interpreting abnormal heart sounds*.)

Third heart sound

The third heart sound—known as S_3, or *ventricular gallop*—is a low-pitched noise best heard by placing the bell of the stethoscope at the apex of the heart.

Kentucky galloper

Its rhythm resembles a horse galloping, and its cadence resembles the word "Ken-tuc-ky" (lub-dub-by). Listen for S_3 with the patient in a supine or left-lateral decubitus position.

An S_3 usually sounds during early diastole to middiastole, at the end of the passive-filling phase of either ventricle. Listen for this sound immediately after S_2. It may signify that the ventricle isn't compliant enough to accept the filling volume without additional force.

Fourth heart sound

The fourth heart sound, or S_4, is abnormal and occurs late in diastole, just before the pulse upstroke. It immediately precedes the S_1 of the next cycle. Known as the *atrial* or *presystolic gallop*, it occurs during atrial contraction.

Tennessee walker

An S_4 shares the same cadence as the word "Ten-nes-see" (le-lub-dub). It's heard best with the bell of the stethoscope and with the patient in the supine position.

What S₄ says

An S_4 may indicate cardiovascular disease, such as:
• acute MI
• anemia
• angina
• aortic stenosis
• cardiomyopathy
• coronary artery disease (CAD)
• elevated left ventricular pressure
• hypertension.

If the S_4 sound persists, it may indicate impaired ventricular compliance or volume overload.

Murmurs

A murmur, which is longer than a heart sound, makes a vibrating, blowing, or rumbling noise. Just as turbulent water in a stream babbles as it passes through a narrow point, turbulent blood flow produces a murmur.

Ages and stages

Interpreting abnormal heart sounds

An S_3 may occur normally in a child or young adult. In a patient older than age 30, however, it usually indicates a disorder, such as:
• right-sided heart failure
• left-sided heart failure
• pulmonary congestion
• intracardiac blood shunting
• myocardial infarction
• anemia
• thyrotoxicosis.

Common S₄
S_4 commonly appears in elderly patients with age-related systolic hypertension and aortic stenosis.

Identifying heart murmurs

To identify a heart murmur, first listen closely to determine its timing in the cardiac cycle. Then determine its other characteristics, including quality, pitch, and location, as well as possible causes.

Timing	Quality and pitch	Location	Possible causes
Midsystolic (systolic ejection)	Harsh and rough with medium to high pitch	Pulmonic	Pulmonic stenosis
	Harsh and rough with medium to high pitch	Aortic and suprasternal notch	Aortic stenosis
Holosystolic (pansystolic)	Harsh with high pitch	Tricuspid	Ventricular septal defect
	Blowing with high pitch	Mitral, lower left sternal border	Mitral insufficiency
	Blowing with high pitch	Tricuspid	Tricuspid insufficiency
Early diastolic	Blowing with high pitch	Mid-left sternal edge (not aortic area)	Aortic insufficiency
	Blowing with high pitch	Pulmonic	Pulmonic insufficiency
Middiastolic to late diastolic	Rumbling with low pitch	Apex	Mitral stenosis
	Rumbling with low pitch	Tricuspid, lower right sternal border	Tricuspid stenosis

If you detect a murmur, identify where it's loudest, pinpoint when it sounds during the cardiac cycle, and describe its pitch, pattern, quality, and intensity. (See *Identifying heart murmurs*.)

Location, location, and...timing

Murmurs can start in any cardiac auscultatory site and may radiate from one site to another. To identify the radiation area, auscultate from the site where the murmur seems loudest to the farthest site where it's still heard. Note the anatomic landmark of this farthest site.

Pinpoint its presence

Determine whether the murmur happens during systole (between S_1 and S_2) or diastole (between S_2 and the next S_1). Then pinpoint when in the cardiac cycle the murmur takes place—for example, during middiastole or late systole. A murmur heard throughout systole is called a *holosystolic* (or *pansystolic*) *murmur*, and a murmur heard throughout diastole is called a *pandiastolic mur-*

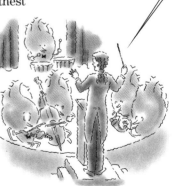

Just for fun, let's keep this piece down to a murmur and see if the audience can identify it. Ready?

mur. Occasionally, murmurs run through both portions of the cycle (continuous murmur).

Pitch

Depending on the rate and pressure of blood flow, pitch may be high, medium, or low. You can best hear a low-pitched murmur with the bell of the stethoscope, a high-pitched murmur with the diaphragm, and a medium-pitched murmur with both.

Pattern

Crescendo is produced when the velocity of blood flow increases and the murmur becomes louder. Decrescendo is produced when velocity decreases and the murmur becomes quieter. A crescendo-decrescendo pattern describes a murmur with increasing loudness followed by increasing softness.

Quality

The volume of blood flow, the force of the contraction, and the degree of valve compromise all contribute to murmur quality. Terms used to describe quality include *musical, blowing, harsh, rasping, rumbling,* or *machinelike.*

Intensity

Use a standard, six-level grading scale to describe the intensity of the murmur:

grade I—extremely faint; barely audible even to the trained ear

grade II—soft and low; easily audible to the trained ear

grade III—moderately loud; about equal to the intensity of normal heart sounds

grade IV—loud with a palpable thrill at the murmur site

grade V—very loud with a palpable thrill; audible with the stethoscope in partial contact with the chest

grade VI—extremely loud, with a palpable thrill; audible with the stethoscope over, but not in contact with, the chest.

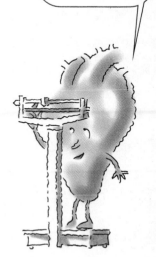

Just like using a regular scale, the heart murmur scale involves a lot of intensity.

Rubs
To detect a pericardial friction rub, use the diaphragm of the stethoscope to auscultate in the third left intercostal space along the lower left sternal border.

Rubbed the wrong way

Listen for a harsh, scratchy, scraping, or squeaking sound throughout systole, diastole, or both. To enhance the sound, have the patient sit upright and lean forward or exhale. A rub usually indicates pericarditis.

Bruits

Sounds aren't normally heard over the carotid arteries. A bruit, which sounds like buzzing or blowing, could indicate arteriosclerotic plaque formation. When you auscultate for the femoral and popliteal pulses, check for a bruit or other abnormal sounds. A bruit over the femoral or popliteal artery usually indicates narrowed vessels.

Bothersome bruits

During auscultation of the central and peripheral arteries, you may notice a continuous bruit caused by turbulent blood flow. A bruit over the abdominal aorta usually indicates an aneurysm (weakness in the arterial wall that allows a sac to form) or a dissection (a tear in the layers of the arterial wall).

Diagnostic tests

Advances in diagnostic testing allow for earlier and easier diagnosis and treatment of cardiac emergencies. For example, in some patients, echocardiography—a noninvasive, risk-free test—can provide as much diagnostic information on valvular heart disease as cardiac catheterization, an invasive, high-risk test.

Cardiac monitoring

Cardiac monitoring is a form of electrocardiography (ECG) that enables continuous observation of the heart's electrical activity. It's an essential assessment tool in the emergency department (ED) and is used to continually monitor the patient's cardiac status to enable rapid identification and treatment of abnormalities in rate, rhythm, or conduction.

A test with 12 views

The 12-lead ECG measures the heart's electrical activity and records it as waveforms. It's one of the most valuable and commonly used diagnostic tools; however, it isn't 100% diagnostic and is used in conjunction with other tests. The standard 12-lead ECG uses a series of electrodes placed on the patient's extremities and chest wall to assess the heart from

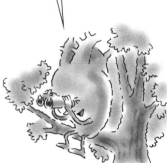

Cardiac monitoring lets you assess the heart from the vantage of 12 different views.

12 different views (leads). The 12 leads include three bipolar limb leads (I, II, and III), three unipolar augmented limb leads (aV_R, aV_L, and aV_F), and six unipolar precordial limb leads (V_1 to V_6). The limb leads and augmented leads show the heart from the frontal plane. The precordial leads show the heart from the horizontal plane. (See *Precordial lead placement*, page 112.)

Up, down, and across...

Scanning up, down, and across the heart, each lead transmits information about a different area. The waveforms obtained from each lead vary depending on the location of the lead in relation to the wave of electrical stimulus, or *depolarization*, passing through the myocardium.

...from top to bottom...

The six limb leads record electrical activity in the heart's frontal plane. This plane is a view through the middle of the heart from top to bottom. Electrical activity is recorded from the anterior to the posterior axis.

...and, finally, horizontal

The six precordial leads provide information on electrical activity in the heart's horizontal plane, a transverse view through the middle of the heart, dividing it into upper and lower portions. Electrical activity is recorded from a superior or an inferior approach.

Practice pointers

• Use a systematic approach to interpret the ECG recording. Compare the patient's previous ECG with the current one, if available, to help identify changes.
• P waves should be upright; however, they may be inverted in lead aV_R or biphasic or inverted in leads III, aV_L, and V_1.
• PR intervals should always be constant, just like QRS-complex durations.
• QRS-complex deflections vary in different leads. Observe for pathologic Q waves.
• ST segments should be isoelectric or have minimal deviation.
• ST-segment elevation greater than 1 mm above the baseline and ST-segment depression greater than 0.5 mm below the baseline are considered abnormal. Leads facing an injured area have ST-segment elevations, and leads facing away show ST-segment depressions.
• The T wave normally deflects upward in leads I, II, and V_3 through V_6. It's inverted in lead aV_R and variable in the other leads. T-wave changes have many causes and aren't always a reason for

Precordial lead placement

To record a 12-lead ECG, place electrodes on the patient's arms and left leg and place a ground lead on the patient's right leg. The three standard limb leads (I, II, and III) and the three augmented leads (aV_R, aV_L, and aV_F) are recorded using these electrodes. Then, to record the precordial chest leads, place electrodes as follows:

- V_1—fourth intercostal space (ICS), right sternal border
- V_2—fourth ICS, left sternal border
- V_3—midway between V_2 and V_4
- V_4—fifth ICS, left midclavicular line
- V_5—fifth ICS, left anterior axillary line
- V_6—fifth ICS, left midaxillary line.

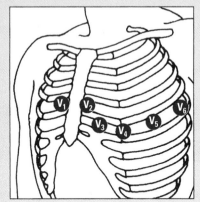

Right precordial lead placement

Right precordial leads can provide specific information about the function of the right ventricle. Place the six leads on the right side of the chest in a mirror image of the standard precordial lead placement, as follows:

V_{1R}—fourth ICS, left sternal border
V_{2R}—fourth ICS, right sternal border
V_{3R}—halfway between V_{2R} and V_{4R}
V_{4R}—fifth ICS, right midclavicular line
V_{5R}—fifth ICS, right anterior axillary line
V_{6R}—fifth ICS, right midaxillary line.

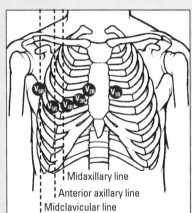

Midaxillary line
Anterior axillary line
Midclavicular line

Posterior lead placement

Posterior leads can be used to assess the posterior side of the heart. To ensure an accurate reading, make sure the posterior electrodes V_7, V_8, and V_9 are placed at the same horizontal level as the V_6 lead at the fifth intercostal space. Place lead V_7 at the posterior axillary line, lead V_9 at the paraspinal line, and lead V_8 halfway between leads V_7 and V_9.

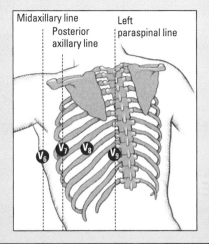

Midaxillary line
Posterior axillary line
Left paraspinal line

alarm. Excessively tall, flat, or inverted T waves accompanying such symptoms as chest pain may indicate ischemia.
• A normal Q wave generally has a duration of less than 0.04 second. An abnormal Q wave has a duration of 0.04 second or more, a depth greater than 4 mm, or a height one-fourth of the R wave. Abnormal Q waves indicate myocardial necrosis, developing when depolarization can't follow its normal path because of damaged tissue in the area.
• Remember that aV_R normally has a large Q wave, so disregard this lead when searching for abnormal Q waves.

Cardiac marker studies

Analysis of cardiac markers (proteins) aids diagnosis of acute MI.

Release those enzymes!

After infarction, damaged cardiac tissue releases significant amounts of enzymes into the blood. Serial measurement of enzyme levels reveals the extent of damage and helps monitor the progress of healing.

Heart enzymes

Cardiac enzymes include creatine kinase (CK), CK's isoenzyme MB (found specifically in heart muscle), lactate dehydrogenase (LD), and LD's isoenzymes LD_1 and LD_2 that are found in heart muscle. (See *Release of cardiac enzymes and proteins*, page 114.)

Troponin T and I and myoglobin are more specific tests of cardiac muscle and can be used to detect damage more quickly, allowing faster and more effective treatment.

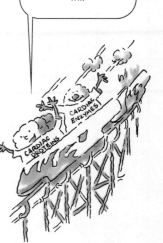

LD$_1$ and LD$_2$ are just two enzymes along for the bloodstream ride that occurs after MI!

Practice pointers

• Before CK measurement, make certain that the patient hasn't ingested alcohol, aminocaproic acid, or lithium. If the patient has recently taken these substances, note this on the laboratory request.
• Avoid administering I.M. injections because they can cause muscle damage and elevate some cardiac markers.
• After any cardiac enzyme test, handle the collection tube gently to prevent hemolysis and send the sample to the laboratory immediately. A delay can affect test results.

Echocardiography

Echocardiography is used to examine the size, shape, and motion of cardiac structures. It's done using a transducer placed at

Release of cardiac enzymes and proteins

Because they're released by damaged tissue, serum proteins and isoenzymes (catalytic proteins that vary in concentration in specific organs) can help identify the compromised organ and assess the extent of damage. After an acute myocardial infarction (MI), cardiac enzymes and proteins rise and fall in characteristic patterns, as shown in the graph.

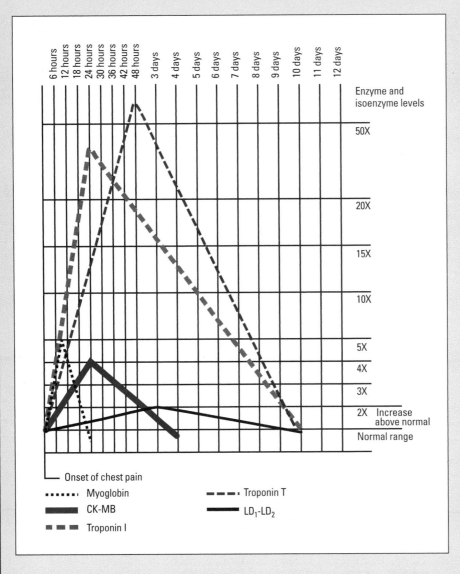

What's it all mean?

Here's what the results of cardiac marker studies indicate:

• CK-MB levels increase 4 to 8 hours after the onset of acute MI, peak after 20 hours, and may remain elevated for up to 72 hours.

• LD_1 and LD_2 levels increase 8 to 12 hours after acute MI, peak in 24 to 48 hours, and return to normal in 10 to 14 days, if tissue necrosis doesn't persist.

• Troponin levels increase within 3 to 6 hours after myocardial damage. Troponin I peaks in 14 to 20 hours, with a return to baseline in 5 to 7 days. Troponin T peaks in 12 to 24 hours, with a return to baseline in 10 to 15 days. Because troponin levels stay elevated for a long time, they can be used to detect an infarction that occurred several days earlier.

• Myoglobin levels may increase within 30 minutes to 4 hours after myocardial damage, peak within 6 to 7 hours, and return to baseline after 24 hours. However, because skeletal muscle damage may cause myoglobin levels to increase, it isn't specific to myocardial injury.

an acoustic window (an area where bone and lung tissue are absent) on the patient's chest. The transducer directs sound waves toward cardiac structures, which reflect these waves.

Echo, echo

The transducer picks up the echoes, converts them to electrical impulses, and relays them to an echocardiography machine for display on a screen and for recording on a strip chart or videotape. The most commonly used echocardiography techniques are motion mode (M-mode) and two-dimensional.

Motion mode

In *M-mode echocardiography*, a single, pencil-like ultrasound beam strikes the heart, producing an "ice pick," or vertical, view of cardiac structures. This mode is especially useful for precisely viewing cardiac structures.

Echo in 2-D

In *two-dimensional echocardiography*, the ultrasound beam rapidly sweeps through an arc, producing a cross-sectional, or fan-shaped, view of cardiac structures. This technique is useful for recording lateral motion and providing the correct spatial relationship between cardiac structures. In many cases, both techniques are performed to complement each other. Patients who come to the ED with atrial fibrillation who require an echocardiogram may have mildly distorted images because of the rapid motion of the heart.

TEE combination

In *transesophageal echocardiography (TEE)*, ultrasonography is combined with endoscopy to provide a better view of the heart's structures. (See *A closer look at TEE.*)

Echo abnormalities

The echocardiogram may detect mitral stenosis, mitral valve prolapse, aortic insufficiency, wall motion abnormalities, and pericardial effusion (excess pericardial fluid).

Practice pointers

• Explain the procedure to the patient, and advise him to remain still during the test because movement can distort results.
• Tell the patient that conductive gel is applied to the chest and that a quarter-sized transducer is placed directly over it. Because pressure is exerted to keep the transducer in contact with the skin, warn the patient that he may feel minor discomfort.
• After the procedure, remove the conductive gel from the skin.

A closer look at TEE

In transesophageal echocardiography (TEE), a small transducer is attached to the end of a gastroscope and inserted into the esophagus so that images of the heart's structure can be taken from the posterior of the heart. This test causes less tissue penetration and interference from chest wall structures and produces high-quality images of the thoracic aorta (except for the superior ascending aorta, which is shadowed by the trachea).

TEE is used to diagnose or evaluate:
• congenital heart disease
• endocarditis
• intracardiac thrombi
• thoracic and aortic disorders
• tumors
• valvular disease or repairs.

Hemodynamic monitoring

Hemodynamic monitoring is an invasive procedure used to assess cardiac function and determine the effectiveness of therapy by measuring:
- blood pressure
- cardiac output
- intracardiac pressures
- mixed oxygen saturation. (See *Putting hemodynamic monitoring to use.*)

Getting involved

Hemodynamic monitoring involves insertion of a catheter into the vascular system. The types of hemodynamic monitoring include:
- arterial blood pressure monitoring
- pulmonary artery pressure monitoring (PAP), using the internal and external jugular and subclavian veins. (Femoral and antecubital veins may be used but aren't the sites of choice.)

Controversial contraindications

As an invasive procedure, hemodynamic monitoring remains controversial in some EDs because of the risks involved, including sepsis, pneumothorax, air embolism, and pulmonary artery infarction.

Arterial blood pressure monitoring

In arterial blood pressure monitoring, the practitioner inserts a catheter into the radial or femoral artery to measure blood pressure or obtain samples of arterial blood for diagnostic tests such as arterial blood gas (ABG) studies. A transducer transforms the flow of blood during systole and diastole into a waveform, which appears on an oscilloscope.

Pulmonary artery pressure monitoring

Continuous PAP and intermittent pulmonary artery wedge pressure (PAWP) measurements provide important information about left ventricular function and preload. Use this information for monitoring, aiding diagnosis, refining assessment, guiding interventions, and projecting patient outcomes.

PAP purposes

PAP monitoring is indicated for patients who:
- are hemodynamically unstable
- need fluid management or continuous cardiopulmonary assessment

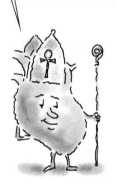

An audience with the PAP reveals important info about left ventricular function.

Putting hemodynamic monitoring to use

Hemodynamic monitoring provides information on intracardiac pressures, arterial pressure, and cardiac output. To understand intracardiac pressures, picture the heart and vascular system as a continuous loop with constantly changing pressure gradients that keep the blood moving. Hemodynamic monitoring records the gradients within the vessels and heart chambers. Cardiac output indicates the amount of blood ejected by the heart each minute.

Pressure and description	Normal values	Causes of increased pressure	Causes of decreased pressure
Central venous pressure or right atrial pressure The central venous pressure or right atrial pressure shows right ventricular function and end-diastolic pressure.	Normal mean pressure ranges from 1 to 6 mm Hg (1.34 to 8 cm H_2O).	• Right-sided heart failure • Volume overload • Tricuspid valve stenosis or insufficiency • Constrictive pericarditis • Pulmonary hypertension • Cardiac tamponade • Right ventricular infarction	• Reduced circulating blood volume
Right ventricular pressure Typically, the doctor measures right ventricular pressure only when initially inserting a pulmonary artery catheter. Right ventricular systolic pressure normally equals pulmonary artery systolic pressure; right ventricular end-diastolic pressure, which reflects right ventricular function, equals right atrial pressure.	Normal systolic pressure ranges from 20 to 30 mm Hg; normal diastolic pressure, from 0 to 5 mm Hg.	• Mitral stenosis or insufficiency • Pulmonary disease • Hypoxemia • Constrictive pericarditis • Chronic heart failure • Atrial and ventricular septal defects • Patent ductus arteriosus	• Reduced circulating blood volume
Pulmonary artery pressure Pulmonary artery systolic pressure shows right ventricular function and pulmonary circulation pressures. Pulmonary artery diastolic pressure reflects left ventricular pressures, specifically left ventricular end-diastolic pressure, in a patient without significant pulmonary disease.	Systolic pressure normally ranges from 20 to 30 mm Hg. The mean pressure usually ranges from 10 to 15 mm Hg.	• Left-sided heart failure • Increased pulmonary blood flow (left or right shunting, as in atrial or ventricular septal defects) • Any condition causing increased pulmonary arteriolar resistance (such as pulmonary hypertension, volume overload, mitral stenosis, or hypoxia)	• Reduced circulating blood volume
Pulmonary artery wedge pressure Pulmonary artery wedge pressure (PAWP) reflects left atrial and left ventricular pressures, unless the patient has mitral stenosis. Changes in PAWP reflect changes in left ventricular filling pressure.	The mean pressure normally ranges from 6 to 12 mm Hg.	• Left-sided heart failure • Mitral stenosis or insufficiency • Pericardial tamponade	• Reduced circulating blood volume

• are receiving multiple or frequently administered cardioactive drugs
• are experiencing shock, trauma, pulmonary or cardiac disease, or multiple organ dysfunction syndrome.

PAP's parts

A pulmonary artery (PA) catheter has up to six lumens that gather hemodynamic information. In addition to distal and proximal lumens used to measure pressures, a PA catheter has a balloon inflation lumen that inflates the balloon for PAWP measurement and a thermistor connector lumen that allows cardiac output measurement. Some catheters also have a pacemaker wire lumen that provides a port for pacemaker electrodes and measures continuous mixed venous oxygen saturation.

PAP and PAWP procedures

In PAP or PAWP measurement, the practitioner inserts the balloon-tipped, multilumen catheter into the patient's internal jugular or subclavian vein. When the catheter reaches the right atrium, the balloon is inflated to float the catheter through the right ventricle into the pulmonary artery. When the catheter is in the pulmonary artery, PAWP measurement is possible through an opening at the catheter's tip. The catheter is then deflated and rests in the pulmonary artery, allowing diastolic and systolic PAP readings.

The balloon should be totally deflated except when taking a PAWP reading because prolonged wedging can cause pulmonary infarction.

Practice pointers

Nursing considerations depend on the type of hemodynamic monitoring conducted.

Arterial blood pressure monitoring
• Explain the procedure to the patient and his family, if possible.
• After catheter insertion, observe the pressure waveform to assess arterial pressure.
• Assess the insertion site for signs of infection, such as redness and swelling. Notify the practitioner immediately if you note such signs.
• Document the date and time of catheter insertion, catheter insertion site, type of flush solution used, type of dressing applied, and patient's tolerance of the procedure.

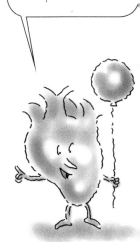

Careful…overinflating a PA catheter balloon can distend the pulmonary artery and rupture vessels.

PAP monitoring

- After catheter insertion, you may inflate the balloon with a syringe to take PAWP readings. Be careful not to inflate the balloon with more than 1.5 cc of air. Overinflation could distend the pulmonary artery, causing vessel rupture. Don't leave the balloon wedged for a prolonged period because prolonged wedging could lead to a pulmonary infarction.
- After each PAWP reading, flush the line per facility policy. If you encounter difficulty, notify the practitioner.
- Maintain 300 mm Hg pressure in the pressure bag to permit a flush flow of 3 to 6 ml/hour.
- Make sure that stopcocks are properly positioned and connections are secure. Loose connections may introduce air into the system or cause blood backup, leakage of deoxygenated blood, or inaccurate pressure readings. Also make sure the lumen hubs are properly identified to serve the appropriate catheter ports.

Irritation prevention

- Because the catheter can slip back into the right ventricle and irritate it, check the monitor for a right ventricular waveform to detect this problem promptly.
- To minimize valvular trauma, make sure the balloon is deflated whenever the catheter is withdrawn from the pulmonary artery to the right ventricle or from the right ventricle to the right atrium.
- Document the date and time of catheter insertion, the practitioner who performed the procedure, the catheter insertion site, pressure waveforms and values for the various heart chambers, the balloon inflation volume required to obtain a wedge tracing, arrhythmias that took place during or after the procedure, the type of flush solution used and its heparin concentration (if any), the type of dressing applied, and the patient's tolerance of the procedure.

Cardiac output monitoring

Cardiac output—the amount of blood ejected by the heart in 1 minute—is monitored to evaluate cardiac function. The normal range for cardiac output is 4 to 8 L/minute. The most widely used method for monitoring cardiac output is the bolus thermodilution technique. Other methods include the Fick method and the dye dilution test.

On the rocks or room temperature

To measure cardiac output, a solution is injected into the right atrium through a port on a PA catheter. Iced or room-temperature injectant may be used depending on your facility's policy and the patient's status.

This indicator solution mixes with the blood as it travels through the right ventricle into the pulmonary artery, and a thermistor on the catheter registers the change in temperature of the flowing blood. A computer then plots the temperature change over time as a curve and calculates flow based on the area under the curve.

To be continued

Some PA catheters contain a filament that permits continuous cardiac output monitoring. Using such a device, an average cardiac output value is determined over a 3-minute span; the value is updated every 30 to 60 seconds. This type of monitoring allows close scrutiny of the patient's hemodynamic status and prompt intervention in case problems arise.

Better assessor

Cardiac output is better assessed by calculating cardiac index, which takes body size into account. To calculate the patient's cardiac index, divide his cardiac output by his body surface area, a function of height and weight. The normal cardiac index ranges from 2.5 to 4.2 L/minute/m^2 for adults or 3.5 to 6.5 L/minute/m^2 for pregnant women.

Physiologic changes can affect the cardiac output and the cardiac index; they include:
- decreased preload
- increased preload
- vasoconstriction (changes in afterload)
- vasodilation (changes in afterload)
- hypothermia.

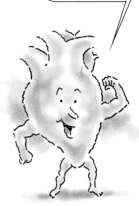

Lucky for me, cardiac index takes body size into account!

Practice pointers

- Make sure your patient doesn't move during the procedure because movement can cause an error in measurement.
- Perform cardiac output measurements and monitoring at least every 2 to 4 hours, especially if the patient is receiving vasoactive or inotropic agents or if fluids are being added or restricted.
- Discontinue cardiac output measurements when the patient is hemodynamically stable and weaned from his vasoactive and inotropic medications.
- Monitor the patient for signs and symptoms of inadequate perfusion, including restlessness, fatigue, changes in level of consciousness (LOC), decreased capillary refill time, diminished peripheral pulses, oliguria, and pale, cool skin.

• Add the fluid volume injected for cardiac output determinations to the patient's total intake.
• Record the patient's cardiac output, cardiac index, and other hemodynamic values and vital signs at the time of measurement. Note the patient's position during measurement.

Treatments

Many treatments are available for patients with cardiac emergencies. Commonly used treatment measures include drug therapy, surgery, balloon catheter treatments, and other treatments, such as defibrillation, synchronized cardioversion, and pacemaker insertion.

Drug therapy

Types of drugs used to improve cardiovascular function include adrenergics, adrenergic blockers, antianginals, antiarrhythmics, anticoagulants, antihypertensives, cardiac glycosides and phosphodiesterase (PDE) inhibitors, diuretics, and thrombolytics.

Adrenergics

Adrenergic drugs are also called *sympathomimetics* because they produce effects similar to those produced by the sympathetic nervous system.

Classified by chemical

Adrenergic drugs are classified in two groups based on their chemical structure—catecholamines (naturally occurring and synthetic) and noncatecholamines. (See *Understanding adrenergics*, page 122.)

Which receptor

Therapeutic use of adrenergic drugs depends on which receptors they stimulate and to what degree. Adrenergic drugs can affect:
• alpha-adrenergic receptors
• beta-adrenergic receptors
• dopamine receptors.

Mimicking norepinephrine and epinephrine

Most of the adrenergic drugs produce their effects by stimulating alpha- and beta-adrenergic receptors. These drugs mimic the action of norepinephrine or epinephrine.

Understanding adrenergics

Adrenergic drugs produce effects similar to those produced by the sympathetic nervous system. They can affect alpha-adrenergic receptors, beta-adrenergic receptors, or dopamine receptors. However, most of the drugs stimulate the alpha- and beta-receptors, mimicking the effects of norepinephrine and epinephrine. Dopaminergic drugs act on receptors typically stimulated by dopamine. Use this table to learn about the indications and adverse reactions associated with these drugs.

Drugs	Indications	Adverse reactions
Catecholamines		
dobutamine (Dobutrex)	• Increase cardiac output in short-term treatment of cardiac decompensation from depressed contractility	• Headache • Tachycardia • Cardiac arrhythmias (premature ventricular contractions) • Hypertension
dopamine	• Adjunct in shock to increase cardiac output, blood pressure, and urine flow	• Dyspnea • Bradycardia • Palpitations • Tachycardia • Cardiac arrhythmias (ventricular) • Hypotension • Widened QRS • Angina
epinephrine	• Anaphylaxis • Bronchospasm • Hypersensitivity reactions • Restoration of cardiac rhythm in cardiac arrest	• Restlessness • Anxiety • Headache • Tachycardia • Palpitations • Cardiac arrhythmias (ventricular fibrillation) • Precordial pain (in patients with ischemic heart disease)
norepinephrine (Levophed)	• GI bleeding • Maintain blood pressure in acute hypotensive states	• Headache • Bradycardia • Hypertension
Noncatecholamines		
ephedrine	• Maintain blood pressure in acute hypotensive states, especially with spinal anesthesia • Treatment of orthostatic hypotension and bronchospasm	• Restlessness • Anxiety • Dizziness • Headache • Cardiac arrhythmias (ventricular fibrillation) • Nausea

Understanding adrenergics (continued)

Drugs	Indications	Adverse reactions
Noncatecholamines (continued)		
phenylephrine (Neo-Synephrine)	• Maintain blood pressure in hypotensive states, especially hypotensive emergencies with spinal anesthesia	• Restlessness • Anxiety • Dizziness • Headache • Palpitations • Cardiac arrhythmias

Doing it like dopamine

Dopaminergic drugs act primarily on receptors in the sympathetic nervous system that are stimulated by dopamine.

Catecholamines

Because of their common basic chemical structure, catecholamines share certain properties. They stimulate the nervous system, constrict peripheral blood vessels, increase heart rate, and dilate the bronchi. They can be manufactured in the body or in a laboratory.

Excitatory or inhibitory

Catecholamines primarily act directly. When catecholamines combine with alpha- or beta-receptors, they cause an excitatory or inhibitory effect. Typically, activation of alpha-receptors generates an excitatory response except for intestinal relaxation. Activation of the beta-receptors mostly produces an inhibitory response except in the cells of the heart, where norepinephrine produces excitatory effects.

How heartening

The clinical effects of catecholamines depend on the dosage and the route of administration. Catecholamines are potent inotropes, meaning they make the heart contract more forcefully. As a result, the ventricles empty more completely with each heartbeat, increasing the workload of the heart and the amount of oxygen it needs to do this harder work.

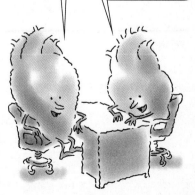

You know, I'm working my arteries off taking on this extra workload, but does the boss even notice? Nope!

Hey, you're the one who took the catecholamines.

Rapid rates

Catecholamines also produce a positive chronotropic effect, which means they cause the heart to beat faster. The heart beats faster because catecholamines increase the depolarization rate of pacemaker cells in the sinoatrial (SA) node of the heart. As catecholamines cause blood vessels to constrict and blood pressure to increase, the heart rate decreases as the body tries to prevent an excessive increase in blood pressure.

Fascinating rhythm

Catecholamines can cause the Purkinje fibers (an intricate web of fibers that carry electrical impulses into the ventricles of the heart) to fire spontaneously, possibly producing abnormal heart rhythms, such as premature ventricular contractions and fibrillation. Epinephrine is likelier than norepinephrine to produce this spontaneous firing.

Noncatecholamines

Noncatecholamine adrenergic drugs have a variety of therapeutic uses because of the many effects these drugs can have on the body, such as the local or systemic constriction of blood vessels by phenylephrine.

Alpha active

Direct-acting noncatecholamines that stimulate alpha activity include methoxamine (Vasoxyl) and phenylephrine. Those that selectively exert $beta_2$ activity include:
- albuterol (Proventil)
- isoetharine
- metaproterenol (Alupent).
    Ephedrine is a dual-acting noncatecholamine that combines both actions.

Adrenergic blockers

Adrenergic blocking drugs, also called *sympatholytic drugs,* are used to disrupt sympathetic nervous system function. (See *Understanding adrenergic blockers.*)

Impending impulses

Adrenergic blockers work by blocking impulse transmission (and thus sympathetic nervous system stimulation) at adrenergic neurons or adrenergic receptor sites. The action of the drugs at these sites can be exerted by:
- interrupting the action of sympathomimetic (adrenergic) drugs
- reducing available norepinephrine

Understanding adrenergic blockers

Adrenergic blockers block impulse transmission at adrenergic receptor sites by interrupting the action of adrenergic drugs, reducing the amount of norepinephrine available, and blocking the action of cholinergics. Use this table to learn the indications and adverse reactions associated with these drugs.

Drugs	Indications	Adverse reactions
Alpha-adrenergic blockers		
phentolamine and prazosin (Minipress)	• Hypertension • Peripheral vascular disorders • Pheochromocytoma	• Orthostatic hypotension • Severe hypertension • Bradycardia • Tachycardia • Edema • Difficulty breathing • Light-headedness • Flushing • Arrhythmias • Angina • Heart attack • Shock
Beta-adrenergic blockers		
Nonselective carvedilol (Coreg), labetalol (Normodyne), nadolol (Corgard), penbutolol (Levatol), pindolol (Visken), propranolol (Inderal), sotalol (Betapace), and timolol (Blocadren) **Selective** acebutolol (Sectral), atenolol (Tenormin), betaxolol (Kerlone), bisoprolol (Zebeta), esmolol (Brevibloc), and metoprolol (Lopressor)	• Prevention of complications after myocardial infarction, angina, hypertension, supraventricular arrhythmias, anxiety, essential tremor, cardiovascular symptoms associated with thyrotoxicosis, migraine headaches, pheochromocytoma	• Hypotension • Bradycardia • Peripheral vascular insufficiency • Heart failure • Bronchospasm • Sore throat • Atrioventricular block

• preventing the action of cholinergic drugs.

Classified information

Adrenergic blockers are classified according to their site of action as alpha-adrenergic blockers or beta-adrenergic blockers.

Alpha-adrenergic blockers

Alpha-adrenergic blockers work by interrupting the actions of sympathomimetic drugs at alpha-adrenergic receptors. This interruption results in:
• relaxation of the smooth muscle in the blood vessels
• increased dilation of blood vessels
• decreased blood pressure.
    Drugs in this class include:
• phentolamine
• prazosin.

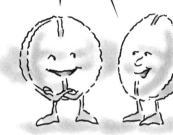

A mixed bag

Ergotamine is a mixed alpha agonist and antagonist. At high doses, it acts as an alpha-adrenergic blocker. Alpha-adrenergic blockers work in one of two ways:

They interfere with or block the synthesis, storage, release, and reuptake of norepinephrine by neurons.

They antagonize epinephrine, norepinephrine, or adrenergic (sympathomimetic) drugs at alpha receptor sites.

Not very discriminating

Alpha receptor sites are either alpha$_1$ or alpha$_2$ receptors. Alpha-adrenergic blockers include drugs that block stimulation of alpha$_1$ receptors and that may block alpha$_2$ stimulation.

Reducing resistance

Alpha-adrenergic blockers occupy alpha receptor sites on the smooth muscle of blood vessels, which prevents catecholamines from occupying and stimulating the receptor sites. As a result, blood vessels dilate, increasing local blood flow to the skin and other organs. The decreased peripheral vascular resistance (resistance to blood flow) helps to decrease blood pressure.

Beta-adrenergic blockers

Beta-adrenergic blockers, the most widely used adrenergic blockers, prevent stimulation of the sympathetic nervous system by inhibiting the action of catecholamines and other sympathomimetic drugs at beta-adrenergic receptors.

Selective (or not)

Beta-adrenergic drugs are selective or nonselective. Nonselective beta-adrenergic drugs affect:
• beta$_1$-receptor sites (located mainly in the heart)

• beta$_2$-receptor sites (located in the bronchi, blood vessels, and uterus).

Nonselective beta-adrenergic drugs include carvedilol, timolol, nadolol, penbutolol, labetalol, pindolol, sotalol, and propranolol.

Highly discriminating

Selective beta-adrenergic drugs primarily affect the beta$_1$-adrenergic sites. They include atenolol, esmolol, acebutolol, and metoprolol.

Intrinsically sympathetic

Some beta-adrenergic blockers, such as pindolol and acebutolol, have intrinsic sympathetic activity. This sympathetic activity means that, instead of attaching to beta-receptors and blocking them, these beta-adrenergic blockers attach to beta-receptors and stimulate them. These drugs are sometimes classified as *partial agonists*.

Widely effective

Beta-adrenergic blockers have widespread effects in the body because they produce their blocking action not only at the adrenergic nerve endings but also in the adrenal medulla. Effects on the heart include:
• increased peripheral vascular resistance
• decreased blood pressure
• decreased force of contractions of the heart
• decreased oxygen consumption by the heart
• slowed conduction of impulses between the atria and ventricles
• decreased cardiac output.

Selective or nonselective

Some of the effects of beta-adrenergic blocking drugs depend on whether the drug is classified as selective or nonselective. Selective beta-adrenergic blockers, which preferentially block beta$_1$ receptor sites, reduce stimulation of the heart. They're commonly called *cardioselective beta-adrenergic blockers*.

Nonselective beta-adrenergic blockers, which block beta$_1$ and beta$_2$ receptor sites, reduce stimulation of the heart and cause the bronchioles of the lungs to constrict. This constriction causes bronchospasm in patients with chronic obstructive lung disorders.

Antianginals

When the oxygen demands of the heart exceed the amount of oxygen being supplied, areas of heart muscle become ischemic (not receiving enough oxygen). When the heart muscle is ischemic, a person experiences chest pain. This condition is known as *angina* or *angina pectoris*.

Reduce demand, increase supply

Although angina's cardinal symptom is chest pain, the drugs used to treat angina aren't typically analgesics. Instead, antianginal drugs correct angina by reducing myocardial oxygen demand (the amount of oxygen the heart needs to do its work), increasing the supply of oxygen to the heart, or both.

The top three

The three classes of commonly used antianginal drugs include:

 nitrates (for acute angina)

 beta-adrenergic blockers (for long-term prevention of angina)

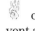 calcium channel blockers (used when other drugs fail to prevent angina). (See *Understanding antianginal drugs*.)

Nitrates

Nitrates are the drug of choice for relieving acute angina.

Anti-angina effect

Nitrates cause the smooth muscle of the veins and, to a lesser extent, the arteries to relax and dilate. Here's what happens:
• When the veins dilate, less blood returns to the heart.
• Decreased blood return reduces the amount of blood in the ventricles at the end of diastole, when the ventricles are full. (This blood volume in the ventricles just before contraction is called *preload.*)
• By reducing preload, nitrates reduce ventricular size and ventricular wall tension so the left ventricle doesn't have to stretch as much to pump blood. This reduction in size and tension in turn reduces the oxygen requirements of the heart.
• As the coronary arteries dilate, more blood is delivered to the myocardium, improving oxygenation of the ischemic tissue.

Reducing resistance

The arterioles provide the most resistance to the blood pumped by the left ventricle (called *peripheral vascular resistance*). Nitrates decrease afterload by dilating the arterioles, reducing resistance, easing the heart's workload, and easing oxygen demand.

Beta-adrenergic blockers

Beta-adrenergic blockers are used for long-term prevention of angina and are one of the main types of drugs used to treat hypertension.

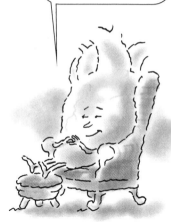

Nitrates help the smooth muscles of my veins relax, kick back, and forget all about angina.

Understanding antianginal drugs

Antianginal drugs are effective in treating patients with angina because they reduce myocardial oxygen demand, increase the supply of oxygen to the heart, or both. Use this table to learn about the indications and adverse reactions associated with these drugs.

Drugs	Indications	Adverse reactions
Nitrates		
isosorbide dinitrate (Isordil), isosorbide mononitrate (Imdur), and nitroglycerin (Nitro-Bid)	• Relief and prevention of angina	• Dizziness • Headache • Hypotension • Increased heart rate
Beta-adrenergic blockers		
atenolol (Tenormin), metoprolol (Lopressor), nadolol (Corgard), and propranolol (Inderal)	• First-line therapy for hypertension • Long-term prevention of angina	• Angina • Arrhythmias • Bradycardia • Bronchial constriction • Diarrhea • Fainting • Fluid retention • Heart failure • Nausea • Shock • Vomiting
Calcium channel blockers		
amlodipine (Norvasc), diltiazem (Cardizem), nicardipine (Cardene), nifedipine (Procardia), and verapamil (Calan)	• Long-term prevention of angina (especially Prinzmetal's angina)	• Arrhythmias • Dizziness • Flushing • Headache • Heart failure • Hypotension • Orthostatic hypotension • Persistent peripheral edema • Weakness

Down with everything

Beta-adrenergic blockers decrease blood pressure and block beta-adrenergic receptor sites in the heart muscle and conduction system. These actions decrease the heart rate and reduce the force of the heart's contractions, resulting in lower demand for oxygen.

Calcium channel blockers

Calcium channel blockers are commonly used to prevent angina that doesn't respond to nitrates or beta-adrenergic blockers. Some calcium channel blockers are also used as antiarrhythmics.

Preventing passage

Calcium channel blockers prevent the passage of calcium ions across the myocardial cell membrane and vascular smooth-muscle cells, causing dilation of the coronary and peripheral arteries. This dilation in turn decreases the force of the heart's contractions and reduces the workload of the heart.

Rate reduction

By preventing arterioles from constricting, calcium channel blockers also reduce afterload. In addition, decreasing afterload decreases oxygen demands of the heart.

Conduction reduction

Calcium channel blockers also reduce the heart rate by slowing conduction through the SA and atrioventricular (AV) nodes. A slower heart rate reduces the heart's need for oxygen.

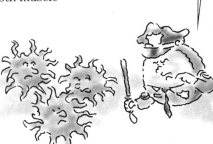

Sorry, folks...this cell membrane has been blocked until further notice. Move along—nothing to see here.

Antiarrhythmics

Antiarrhythmics are used to treat arrhythmias, which are disturbances of the normal heart rhythm. (See *Understanding antiarrhythmics.*)

Benefits vs. risks

Unfortunately, many antiarrhythmic drugs can worsen or cause arrhythmias, too. In any case, the benefits of antiarrhythmic therapy must be weighed against its risks.

Four classes plus...

Antiarrhythmics are categorized into four major classes: I (which includes IA, IB, and IC), II, III, and IV. The mechanisms of action of antiarrhythmic drugs vary widely, and a few drugs exhibit properties common to more than one class. One drug, adenosine, doesn't fall into any of these classes.

Class I antiarrhythmics

Class I antiarrhythmics are sodium channel blockers. This group is the largest group of antiarrhythmic drugs. Class I agents are commonly subdivided into classes IA, IB, and IC.

Understanding antiarrhythmics

Antiarrhythmics are used to restore normal heart rhythm in patients with arrhythmias. Use this table to learn about the indications and adverse reactions associated with these drugs.

Drugs	Indications	Adverse reactions
Class IA antiarrhythmics		
disopyramide (Norpace), procainamide (Procanbid), quinidine sulfate, and quinidine gluconate	• Atrial fibrillation • Atrial flutter • Paroxysmal atrial tachycardia • Ventricular tachycardia	• Abdominal cramping • Anorexia • Bitter taste • Diarrhea • Nausea • Vomiting
Class IB antiarrhythmics		
lidocaine (Xylocaine) and mexiletine (Mexitil)	• Ventricular tachycardia, ventricular fibrillation	• Bradycardia • Drowsiness • Hypotension • Light-headedness • Paresthesia • Sensory disturbances
Class IC antiarrhythmics		
flecainide (Tambocor), moricizine (Ethmozine), and propafenone (Rythmol)	• Ventricular tachycardia, ventricular fibrillation, supraventricular arrhythmias	• Bronchospasm (propafenone) • New arrhythmias
Class II antiarrhythmics		
acebutolol (Sectral), esmolol (Brevibloc), and propranolol (Inderal)	• Atrial flutter, atrial fibrillation, paroxysmal atrial tachycardia	• Arrhythmias • Bradycardia • Bronchoconstriction • Diarrhea • Heart failure • Hypotension • Nausea and vomiting
Class III antiarrhythmics		
amiodarone (Cordarone)	• Life-threatening arrhythmias resistant to other antiarrhythmics	• Aggravation of arrhythmias • Anorexia • Hypotension • Severe pulmonary toxicity

(continued)

Understanding antiarrhythmics *(continued)*

Drugs	Indications	Adverse reactions
Class IV antiarrhythmics		
diltiazem (Cardizem) and verapamil (Calan)	• Supraventricular arrhythmias	• Atrioventricular block • Bradycardia • Dizziness • Flushing (with diltiazem) • Hypotension • Peripheral edema
Miscellaneous antiarrhythmics		
adenosine (Adenocard)	• Paroxysmal supraventricular tachycardia	• Chest discomfort • Dyspnea • Facial flushing • Shortness of breath

Class IA antiarrhythmics

Class IA antiarrhythmics control arrhythmias by altering the myocardial cell membrane and interfering with autonomic nervous system control of pacemaker cells.

No (para)sympathy

Class IA antiarrhythmics also block parasympathetic stimulation of the SA and AV nodes. Because stimulation of the parasympathetic nervous system causes the heart rate to slow down, drugs that block the parasympathetic nervous system increase the conduction rate of the AV node.

Rhythmic risks

This increase in the conduction rate can produce dangerous increases in the ventricular heart rate if rapid atrial activity is present, as in a patient with atrial fibrillation. In turn, the increased ventricular heart rate can offset the ability of the antiarrhythmics to convert atrial arrhythmias to a regular rhythm.

Class IB antiarrhythmics

Lidocaine, a class IB antiarrhythmic, is one of the antiarrhythmics commonly used in treating patients with acute ventricular arrhythmias. Another IB antiarrhythmic is mexiletine.

Talk about overbearing! Class IA antiarrhythmics interfere with myocardial cell membrane, parasympathetic stimulation of SA nodes, and more!

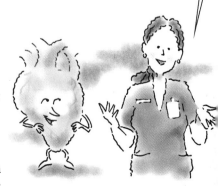

Class IB drugs work by blocking the rapid influx of sodium ions during the depolarization phase of the heart's depolarization-repolarization cycle. This blocking action results in a decreased refractory period, which reduces the risk of arrhythmia.

Make a IB-line for the ventricle

Because class IB antiarrhythmics especially affect the Purkinje fibers and myocardial cells in the ventricles, they're used only in treating patients with ventricular arrhythmias.

Class IC antiarrhythmics

Class IC antiarrhythmics are used to treat patients with certain severe, refractory (resistant) ventricular arrhythmias. Class IC antiarrhythmics include flecainide, moricizine, and propafenone.

Slowing the seeds of conduction

Class IC antiarrhythmics primarily slow conduction along the heart's conduction system. Moricizine decreases the fast inward current of sodium ions of the action potential. This decrease depresses the depolarization rate and effective refractory period.

Class II antiarrhythmics

Class II antiarrhythmics include the beta-adrenergic antagonists, also known as *beta-adrenergic blockers*.

Receptor blockers

Class II antiarrhythmics block beta-adrenergic receptor sites in the conduction system of the heart. As a result, the ability of the SA node to fire spontaneously (automaticity) is slowed. The ability of the AV node and other cells to receive and conduct an electrical impulse to nearby cells (conductivity) is also reduced.

Strength reducers

Class II antiarrhythmics also reduce the strength of the heart's contractions. When the heart beats less forcefully, it doesn't require as much oxygen to do its work.

Class III antiarrhythmics

Class III antiarrhythmics are used to treat patients with ventricular arrhythmias. Amiodarone is the most widely used class III antiarrhythmic.

One-way to two-way

Although the exact mechanism of action isn't known, class III antiarrhythmics are thought to suppress arrhythmias by converting a unidirectional block to a bidirectional block. They have little or no effect on depolarization.

Miscellaneous antiarrhythmics

The class IV antiarrhythmics include calcium channel blockers. These drugs block the movement of calcium during phase 2 of the action potential and slow conduction and the refractory period of calcium-dependent tissues, including the AV node. The calcium channel blockers used to treat patients with arrhythmias are verapamil and diltiazem. Miscellaneous antiarrhythmics also include adenosine.

Adenosine

Adenosine is an injectable antiarrhythmic drug indicated for acute treatment of paroxysmal supraventricular tachycardia.

Depressing the pacemaker

Adenosine depresses the pacemaker activity of the SA node, reducing the heart rate and the ability of the AV node to conduct impulses from the atria to the ventricles.

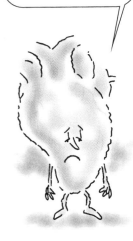

Adenosine depresses me. Well, it depresses my pacemaker activity, to be exact.

Anticoagulants

Anticoagulants are used to reduce the ability of the blood to clot. (See *Understanding anticoagulants*.) Major categories of anticoagulants include antiplatelet drugs, heparin, and oral anticoagulants.

Antiplatelet drugs are used to prevent arterial thromboembolism, especially in patients at risk for MI, stroke, and arteriosclerosis (hardening of the arteries). They interfere with platelet activity in different drug-specific and dose-related ways.

Low is good

Low dosages of aspirin (81 mg/day) appear to inhibit clot formation by blocking the synthesis of prostaglandin, which in turn prevents formation of the platelet-aggregating substance thromboxane A_2. Dipyridamole may inhibit platelet aggregation.

Anticlumping

Clopidogrel inhibits platelet aggregation by blocking adenosine diphosphate receptors on platelets, thereby preventing the clumping of platelets.

Once does it

Sulfinpyrazone appears to inhibit several platelet functions. At dosages of 400 to 800 mg/day, it lengthens platelet survival; dosages of more than 600 mg/day prolong the patency of arteriovenous shunts used for hemodialysis. A single dose rapidly inhibits platelet aggregation.

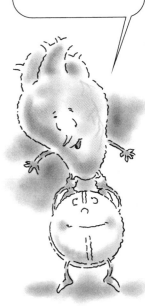

A little aspirin a day keeps the blood clots away!

Understanding anticoagulants

Anticoagulants reduce the blood's ability to clot and are included in the treatment plans for many patients with cardiovascular disorders. Use this table to learn about the indications and adverse reactions associated with these drugs.

Drugs	Indications	Adverse reactions
Heparins		
heparin and low-molecular-weight heparins, such as dalteparin (Fragmin) and enoxaparin (Lovenox)	• Deep vein thrombosis • Disseminated intravascular coagulation • Embolism prophylaxis • Prevention of complications after myocardial infarction (MI)	• Bleeding
Oral anticoagulants		
warfarin (Coumadin)	• Atrial arrhythmias • Deep vein thrombosis prophylaxis • Prevention of complications of prosthetic heart valves or diseased mitral valves	• Bleeding (may be severe)
Antiplatelet drugs		
aspirin, dipyridamole (Persatine), sulfinpyrazone (Anturane), ticlopidine (Ticlid), and clopidogrel (Plavix)	• Decreases the risk of death after MI • Patients at risk for ischemic events (clopidogrel) • Patients with acute coronary syndrome (clopidogrel) • Prevention of complications of prosthetic heart valves	• Bleeding • GI distress • Headache (clopidogrel)

Broken bindings

Ticlopidine inhibits the binding of fibrinogen to platelets during the first stage of the clotting cascade.

Heparin

Heparin, prepared commercially from animal tissue, is used to prevent clot formation. Low-molecular-weight heparin, such as dalteparin and enoxaparin, prevents deep vein thrombosis (a blood clot in the deep veins, usually of the legs) in surgical patients. Be aware, however, that a patient placed on any form of heparin is at risk for developing heparin-induced thrombocytopenia. While the risk of severe adverse effects is low, you must monitor the patient's platelet count. A decrease in platelet count is cause for alarm and should be addressed and closely monitored.

No new clots

Because it doesn't affect the synthesis of clotting factors, heparin can't dissolve already formed clots. It does prevent the formation of new thrombi. Here's how it works:
• Heparin inhibits the formation of thrombin and fibrin by activating antithrombin III.
• Antithrombin III then inactivates factors IXa, Xa, XIa, and XIIa in the intrinsic and common pathways. The end result is prevention of a stable fibrin clot.
• In low doses, heparin increases the activity of antithrombin III against factor Xa and thrombin and inhibits clot formation. Much larger doses are necessary to inhibit fibrin formation after a clot has formed. This relationship between dose and effect is the rationale for using low-dose heparin to prevent clotting.
• Whole blood-clotting time, thrombin time, and partial thromboplastin time are prolonged during heparin therapy. However, these times may be only slightly prolonged with low or ultra-low preventive doses.

Circulate freely

Heparin can be used to prevent clotting when a patient's blood must circulate outside the body through a machine, such as a cardiopulmonary bypass machine or hemodialysis machine.

Oral anticoagulants

Oral anticoagulants alter the ability of the liver to synthesize vitamin K–dependent clotting factors, including prothrombin and factors VII, IX, and X. Clotting factors already in the bloodstream continue to coagulate blood until they become depleted, so anticoagulation doesn't begin immediately.

Warfarin vs. coagulation

The major oral anticoagulant used in the United States is warfarin.

Antihypertensives

Antihypertensive drugs act to reduce blood pressure. They're used to treat patients with hypertension, a disorder characterized by high systolic blood pressure, high diastolic blood pressure, or both.

Like its name suggests, warfarin "fares" well in the "war" against blood coagulation.

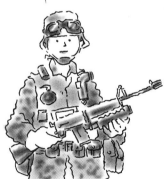

Know the program

Although treatment for hypertension begins with beta-adrenergic blockers and diuretics, antihypertensives are used if those drugs aren't effective. Antihypertensive therapy includes the use of sympatholytics (other than beta-adrenergic blockers), vasodilators, angiotensin-converting enzyme (ACE) inhibitors, and angiotensin receptor blockers alone or in combination. (See *Understanding antihypertensives*, page 138.)

Sympatholytics

Sympatholytic drugs include several different types of drugs. However, all of these drugs work by inhibiting or blocking the sympathetic nervous system, which causes dilation of the peripheral blood vessels or decreases cardiac output, thereby reducing blood pressure.

Where and how

Sympatholytic drugs are classified by their site or mechanism of action and include:
• central-acting sympathetic nervous system inhibitors, such as clonidine, guanabenz, guanfacine, and methyldopa
• alpha blockers, such as doxazosin, prazosin, and terazosin
• mixed alpha- and beta-adrenergic blockers such as labetalol
• norepinephrine depletors, such as guanadrel and guanethidine.

Vasodilators

The two types of vasodilating drugs include calcium channel blockers and direct vasodilators. These drugs decrease systolic and diastolic blood pressure.

Calcium stoppers

Calcium channel blockers produce arteriolar relaxation by preventing the entry of calcium into the cells. This relaxation prevents the contraction of vascular smooth muscle.

Direct dial

Direct vasodilators act on arteries, veins, or both. They work by relaxing peripheral vascular smooth muscles, causing the blood vessels to dilate. This dilation decreases blood pressure by increasing the diameter of the blood vessels, reducing total peripheral resistance.

Hydralazine and minoxidil are usually used to treat patients with resistant or refractory hypertension. Diazoxide and nitroprusside are reserved for use in hypertensive crisis.

Understanding antihypertensives

Antihypertensives are prescribed to reduce blood pressure in patients with hypertension. Use this table to learn about the indications and adverse reactions associated with these drugs.

Drugs	Indications	Adverse reactions
Sympatholytic drugs		
Central-acting sympathetic nervous system inhibitors clonidine (Catapres), guanabenz (Wytensin), guanfacine (Tenex), and methyldopa (Aldomet) **Alpha blockers** doxazosin (Cardura), phentolamine, prazosin (Minipress), and terazosin (Hytrin) **Mixed alpha- and beta-adrenergic blockers** labetalol (Normodyne) **Norepinephrine depletors** guanadrel (Hylorel) and guanethidine (Ismelin)	• Hypertension	• Depression • Drowsiness • Edema • Hypotension (alpha blockers) • Vertigo (central-acting drugs)
Vasodilators		
hydralazine (Apresoline), minoxidil (Rogaine), and nitroprusside (Nitropress)	• Used in combination with other drugs to treat moderate to severe hypertension	• Angina • Breast tenderness • Edema • Fatigue • Headache • Palpitations • Rash • Severe pericardial effusion • Tachycardia • Vasoconstriction
Angiotensin-converting enzyme inhibitors		
benazepril (Lotensin), captopril (Capoten), enalapril (Vasotec), fosinopril (Monopril), lisinopril (Zestril), quinapril (Accupril), and ramipril (Altace)	• Heart failure • Hypertension	• Angioedema • Fatigue • Headache • Increased serum potassium concentrations • Persistent cough

ACE inhibitors

ACE inhibitors reduce blood pressure by interrupting the renin-angiotensin-aldosterone system.

Without ACE inhibition

Here's how the renin-angiotensin-aldosterone system works:
• Normally, the kidneys maintain blood pressure by releasing the hormone renin.
• Renin acts on the plasma protein angiotensinogen to form angiotensin I.
• Angiotensin I is then converted to angiotensin II.
• Angiotensin II, a potent vasoconstrictor, increases peripheral resistance and promotes the excretion of aldosterone.
• Aldosterone, in turn, promotes the retention of sodium and water, increasing the volume of blood the heart needs to pump.

With ACE inhibition

ACE inhibitors work by preventing the conversion of angiotensin I to angiotensin II. As angiotensin II is reduced, arterioles dilate, reducing peripheral vascular resistance.

Less water, less work

By reducing aldosterone secretion, ACE inhibitors promote the excretion of sodium and water. Less sodium and water reduces the amount of blood the heart needs to pump, resulting in lower blood pressure.

Angiotensin II receptor antagonists

Unlike ACE inhibitors, which prevent production of angiotensin, angiotensin II receptor antagonists block the action of angiotensin II, a major culprit in the development of hypertension, by attaching to tissue-binding receptor sites.

Cardiac glycosides and PDE inhibitors

Cardiac glycosides and PDE inhibitors increase the force of the heart's contractions. Increasing the force of contractions is known as a *positive inotropic effect,* so these drugs are also called *inotropic agents* (effecting the force or energy of muscular contractions). (See *Understanding cardiac glycosides and PDE inhibitors,* page 140.)

Slower rate

Cardiac glycosides, such as digoxin, also slow the heart rate (called a *negative chronotropic effect*) and slow electrical impulse conduction through the AV node (called a *negative dromotropic effect*).

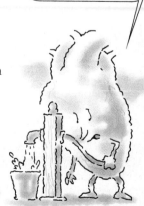

The more water and sodium excreted thanks to ACE inhibitors, the less blood I need to pump. Thank goodness—my arm is killing me!

Understanding cardiac glycosides and PDE inhibitors

Cardiac glycosides and phosphodiesterase (PDE) inhibitors have a positive inotropic effect on the heart, meaning they increase the force of contraction. Use this table to learn about the indications and adverse reactions associated with these drugs.

Drugs	Indications	Adverse reactions
Cardiac glycoside		
digoxin (Lanoxin)	• Heart failure, supraventricular arrhythmias	• Digoxin toxicity (abdominal pain, arrhythmias, depression, headache, insomnia, irritability, nausea, vision disturbances)
PDE inhibitors		
inamrinone (Inocor) and milrinone (Primacor)	• Heart failure refractory to digoxin, diuretics, and vasodilators	• Arrhythmias • Chest pain • Fever • Headache • Hypokalemia • Mild increase in heart rate • Nausea • Thrombocytopenia • Vomiting

The short and long of it

PDE inhibitors, such as inamrinone and milrinone, are typically used for short-term management of heart failure or long-term management in patients awaiting heart transplant surgery.

Boosting output

PDE inhibitors improve cardiac output by strengthening contractions. These drugs are thought to help move calcium into the cardiac cell or to increase calcium storage in the sarcoplasmic reticulum. By directly relaxing vascular smooth muscle, they also decrease peripheral vascular resistance (afterload) and the amount of blood returning to the heart (preload).

Diuretics

Diuretics are used to promote the excretion of water and electrolytes by the kidneys. By doing so, diuretics play a major role in

Understanding diuretics

Diuretics are used to treat patients with various cardiovascular conditions. They work by promoting the excretion of water and electrolytes by the kidneys. Use this table to learn about the indications and adverse reactions associated with these drugs.

Drugs	Indications	Adverse reactions
Thiazide and thiazide-like diuretics		
bendroflumethiazide (Naturetin), chlorthalidone (Hygroton), hydrochlorothiazide (HydroDIURIL), hydroflumethiazide, and indapamide (Lozol)	• Edema • Hypertension	• Hypokalemia • Hyponatremia • Orthostatic hypotension
Loop diuretics		
bumetanide (Bumex), ethacrynate sodium (Edecrin sodium), ethacrynic acid (Edecrin), and furosemide (Lasix)	• Edema • Heart failure • Hypertension	• Dehydration • Hyperuricemia • Hypocalcemia • Hypochloremia • Hypokalemia • Hypomagnesemia • Hyponatremia • Orthostatic hypotension
Potassium-sparing diuretics		
amiloride (Midamor), spironolactone (Aldactone), and triamterene (Dyrenium)	• Cirrhosis • Diuretic-induced hypokalemia in patients with heart failure • Edema • Hypertension • Nephrotic syndrome	• Hyperkalemia

treating hypertension and other cardiovascular conditions. (See *Understanding diuretics.*)

The major diuretics used as cardiovascular drugs include:
• loop diuretics
• potassium-sparing diuretics
• thiazide and thiazide-like diuretics.

Loop diuretics

Loop (high-ceiling) diuretics are highly potent drugs.

High potency, big risk

Loop diuretics are the most potent diuretics available, producing the greatest volume of diuresis (urine production). They also carry a high potential for causing severe adverse reactions.

In the loop

Loop diuretics receive their name because they act primarily on the thick ascending loop of Henle (the part of the nephron responsible for concentrating urine) to increase the secretion of sodium, chloride, and water. These drugs may also inhibit sodium, chloride, and water reabsorption.

Potassium-sparing diuretics

Potassium-sparing diuretics have weaker diuretic and antihypertensive effects than other diuretics, but they have the advantage of conserving potassium.

Potassium-sparing effects

The direct action of the potassium-sparing diuretics on the distal tubule of the kidneys produces:
- increased urinary excretion of sodium and water
- increased excretion of chloride and calcium ions
- decreased excretion of potassium and hydrogen ions.
    These effects lead to reduced blood pressure and increased serum potassium levels.

Thiazide and thiazide-like diuretics

Thiazide and thiazide-like diuretics are sulfonamide derivatives.

Sodium stoppers

Thiazide and thiazide-like diuretics work by preventing sodium from being reabsorbed in the kidney. As sodium is excreted, it pulls water along with it. Thiazide and thiazide-like diuretics also increase the excretion of chloride, potassium, and bicarbonate, which can result in electrolyte imbalances.

Stability with time

Initially, these drugs decrease circulating blood volume, leading to a reduced cardiac output. However, if therapy is maintained, cardiac output stabilizes but plasma fluid volume decreases.

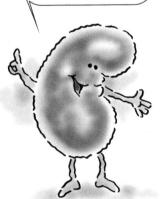

Sodium once, shame on you; sodium twice, shame on me! Thiazide diuretics prevent me from reabsorbing the stuff.

Thrombolytics

Thrombolytic drugs are used to dissolve a preexisting clot or thrombus and are commonly used in an acute or emergency situation. They work by converting plasminogen to plasmin, which ly-

Understanding thrombolytics

Sometimes called *clot busters,* thrombolytic drugs are prescribed to dissolve a preexisting clot or thrombus. These drugs are typically used in acute or emergency situations. Use this table to learn about the indications and adverse reactions associated with these drugs.

Drugs	Indications	Adverse reactions
alteplase (Activase), reteplase (Retavase), and streptokinase (Streptase)	• Acute ischemic stroke • Acute myocardial infarction • Arterial thrombosis • Catheter occlusion • Pulmonary embolus	• Allergic reaction • Bleeding

ses (dissolves) thrombi, fibrinogen, and other plasma proteins. (See *Understanding thrombolytics.*)

Some commonly used thrombolytic drugs include:
- reteplase
- alteplase
- streptokinase.

Surgery

Types of surgery used to treat cardiovascular system disorders include coronary artery bypass graft (CABG), vascular repair, and insertion of a ventricular assist device (VAD).

Coronary artery bypass graft

CABG circumvents an occluded coronary artery with an autogenous graft (usually a segment of the saphenous vein from the leg or internal mammary artery), thereby restoring blood flow to the myocardium. CABG is one of the most commonly performed surgeries because it's done to prevent MI in a patient with acute or chronic myocardial ischemia. The need for CABG is determined by the results of cardiac catheterization and patient symptoms.

Why bypass?

If successful, CABG can relieve anginal pain, improve cardiac function and, possibly, enhance the patient's quality of life.

CABG varieties

CABG techniques vary according to the patient's condition and the number of arteries being bypassed. Newer surgical techniques, such as the mini-CABG and direct coronary artery bypass, can reduce the risk of cerebral complications and accelerate recovery for patients requiring grafts of only one or two arteries. In some patients, it's possible to perform the CABG procedure without using a heart-lung bypass machine, which increases recovery time but decreases complications.

Nursing considerations

When caring for a patient who's undergoing CABG, your major roles include patient instruction and caring for the patient's changing cardiovascular needs:

I think if I take the coronary artery bypass instead of the freeway, I can avoid anginal pain AND make good time.

- Check and record vital signs and hemodynamic parameters frequently, possibly every 5 to 15 minutes depending on the patient's condition.
- Administer medications and titrate according to the patient's response as ordered.
- Monitor ECGs continuously for disturbances in heart rate and rhythm.
- Reinforce the practitioner's explanation of the surgery.
- Explain the complex equipment and procedures used in the critical care unit (CCU) or postanesthesia care unit (PACU).
- Explain to the patient that he'll awaken from surgery with an endotracheal (ET) tube in place and connected to a mechanical ventilator. He'll also be connected to a cardiac monitor and have in place a nasogastric tube, a chest tube, an indwelling urinary catheter, arterial lines, epicardial pacing wires and, possibly, a PA catheter. Tell him that discomfort is minimal and that the equipment is removed as soon as possible.
- Make sure that the patient or a responsible family member has signed a consent form.
- Assist with PA catheterization and insertion of arterial lines. Some facilities insert PA catheters and arterial lines in the operating room before surgery.

Vascular repair

Vascular repair may be needed to treat patients with:
- vessels damaged by arteriosclerotic or thromboembolic disorders, trauma, infections, or congenital defects
- vascular obstructions that severely compromise circulation
- vascular disease that doesn't respond to drug therapy or nonsurgical treatments such as balloon catheterization
- life-threatening dissecting or ruptured aortic aneurysms
- limb-threatening acute arterial occlusion.

Repair review

Vascular repair methods include aneurysm resection, grafting, embolectomy, vena caval filtering, and endarterectomy. The surgery used depends on the type, location, and extent of vascular occlusion or damage.

Nursing considerations

• Make sure the patient and his family understand the practitioner's explanation of the surgery and possible complications.
• Tell the patient that he'll receive a general anesthetic and will awaken from the anesthetic in the CCU or PACU. Explain that he'll have an I.V. line in place, ECG electrodes for continuous cardiac monitoring and, possibly, an arterial line or a PA catheter to provide continuous pressure monitoring. He may also have a urinary catheter in place to allow accurate output measurement. If appropriate, explain that he'll be intubated and placed on mechanical ventilation.
• Before surgery, perform a complete vascular assessment. Take vital signs to provide a baseline. Evaluate the strength and sound of the blood flow and the symmetry of the pulses, and note bruits. Record the temperature of the extremities, their sensitivity to motor and sensory stimuli, and pallor, cyanosis, or redness. Rate peripheral pulse volume and strength on a scale of 0 (pulse absent) to 4 (bounding and strong pulse). Check capillary refill time by blanching the fingernail or toenail; normal refill time is less than 3 seconds.
• Auscultate heart, breath, and bowel sounds and report abnormal findings. Monitor the ECG for abnormalities in heart rate or rhythm. Also monitor other pressure readings and carefully record intake and output.
• Withhold food according to the surgeon's orders and facility policy.
• If the patient is awaiting surgery for aortic aneurysm repair, be on guard for signs and symptoms of acute dissection or rupture. Notify the practitioner immediately if the patient experiences especially sudden severe pain in the chest, abdomen, or lower back; severe weakness; diaphoresis; tachycardia; or a precipitous drop in blood pressure.

PTCA

Percutaneous transluminal coronary angioplasty (PTCA) is a nonsurgical way to open coronary vessels narrowed by arteriosclerosis. It's usually used with cardiac catheterization to assess the stenosis and efficacy of angioplasty. It can also be used as a visual tool to direct the balloon-tipped catheter through a vessel's area of stenosis.

PTCA for pain

In PTCA, a balloon-tipped catheter is inserted into a narrowed coronary artery. This procedure, performed in the cardiac catheterization laboratory under local anesthesia, relieves pain caused by angina and myocardial ischemia.

Through one artery and into another

After coronary angiography confirms the presence and location of the occlusion, the practitioner threads a guide catheter through the patient's femoral artery and into the coronary artery under fluoroscopic guidance.

Plaque, meet Balloon

When the guide catheter's position at the occlusion site is confirmed by angiography, the practitioner carefully introduces a double-lumen balloon into the catheter and through the lesion, where a marked increase in the pressure gradient is obvious. The practitioner alternately inflates and deflates the balloon until arteriography verifies successful arterial dilation and a decrease in the pressure gradient. With balloon inflation, the plaque is compressed against the vessel wall, allowing coronary blood to flow more freely.

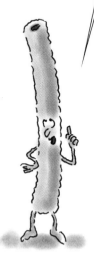

PTCA can help widen me up after arteriosclerosis.

Nursing considerations
• Describe the procedure to the patient and his family, and tell them the procedure takes 1 to 4 hours to complete.
• Explain that a catheter will be inserted into an artery or a vein in the patient's groin and that he may feel pressure as the catheter moves along the vessel.
• Reassure the patient that although he'll be awake during the procedure, he'll be given a sedative. Instruct him to report angina during the procedure.
• Explain that the practitioner injects a contrast medium to outline the lesion's location. Warn the patient that he may feel a hot, flushing sensation or transient nausea during the injection.
• Check the patient's history for allergies; if he has had allergic reactions to shellfish, iodine, or contrast media, notify the practitioner.

Take two aspirin and call me...

• Give 650 mg of aspirin before the procedure, as ordered, to prevent platelet aggregation.
• Make sure the patient signs an informed consent form.
• Restrict food and fluids before the procedure.

• Make sure that the results of coagulation studies, complete blood count (CBC), serum electrolyte studies, blood typing and crossmatching, blood urea nitrogen (BUN), and serum creatinine are available.
• Obtain baseline vital signs and assess peripheral pulses; continue to assess the patient's vital signs and oxygen saturation frequently.
• Apply ECG electrodes and insert an I.V. line if not already in place. Monitor I.V. infusions as indicated.
• Administer oxygen through a nasal cannula.
• Give the patient a sedative as ordered.

Other treatments

Other treatments for cardiovascular disorders include synchronized cardioversion, defibrillation, and pacemaker insertion.

Synchronized cardioversion

Synchronized cardioversion (synchronized countershock) is an elective or emergency procedure used to treat unstable tachyarrhythmias (such as atrial flutter, atrial fibrillation, and supraventricular tachycardia and ventricular tachycardia). It's also the treatment of choice for patients with arrhythmias that don't respond to drug therapy.

Electrifying experience

In synchronized cardioversion, an electric current is delivered to the heart to correct an arrhythmia. Compared with defibrillation, it uses much lower energy levels and is synchronized to deliver an electric charge to the myocardium at the peak R wave.

The procedure causes immediate depolarization, interrupting reentry circuits (abnormal impulse conduction resulting when cardiac tissue is activated two or more times, causing reentry arrhythmias) and allowing the SA node to resume control.

Synchronizing the electrical charge with the R wave ensures that the current won't be delivered on the vulnerable T wave and disrupt repolarization. Thus, it reduces the risk that the current will strike during the relative refractory period of a cardiac cycle and induce ventricular fibrillation.

Nursing considerations
• Describe this elective procedure to the patient and make sure an informed consent is obtained.
• Obtain a baseline 12-lead ECG.
• Withhold food beginning as soon as possible.

Stay on the ball

Choosing the correct cardioversion energy level

When choosing an energy level for cardioversion, try the lowest energy level first. If the arrhythmia isn't corrected, repeat the procedure using the next energy level. Repeat this procedure until the arrhythmia is corrected or until the highest energy level is reached. The recommended energy doses used for cardioversion are:
• 50, 100 joules for unstable supraventricular tachycardia
• 100, 200 joules (with a monophasic waveform) for atrial fibrillation
• 100, 120 joules (with a biphasic waveform) for unstable atrial flutter.

• Give a sedative as ordered.
• Apply conductive gel to the paddles or attach defibrillation pads to the chest wall; position the pads so that one pad is to the right of the sternum, just below the clavicle, and the other is at the fifth or sixth intercostal space in the left anterior axillary line.
• Turn on the defibrillator and select the ordered energy level, usually between 50 and 100 joules. (See *Choosing the correct cardioversion energy level.*)
• Activate the synchronized mode by depressing the synchronizer switch.
• Check that the machine is sensing the R wave correctly.
• Place the paddles on the chest and apply firm pressure.
• Charge the paddles.
• Instruct other personnel to stand clear of the patient and the bed to avoid the risk of an electric shock by stating "all clear."
• Discharge the current by pushing both paddles' DISCHARGE buttons simultaneously.

Repeat, repeat, and repeat again

• If cardioversion is unsuccessful, repeat the procedure two or three times as ordered, gradually increasing the energy with each additional countershock.
• If normal rhythm is restored, continue to monitor the patient and provide supplemental ventilation as long as needed.
• If the patient's cardiac rhythm changes to ventricular fibrillation, switch the mode from SYNCHRONIZED to DEFIBRILLATE and defibrillate the patient immediately after charging the machine.
• When using handheld paddles, continue to hold the paddles on the patient's chest until the energy is delivered.

In sync

• Remember to reset the SYNC MODE on the defibrillator after each synchronized cardioversion. Resetting this switch is necessary because most defibrillators automatically reset to an unsynchronized mode.

• Document the use of synchronized cardioversion, the rhythm before and after cardioversion, the amperage used, and how the patient tolerated the procedure.

Defibrillation

In defibrillation, electrode paddles are used to direct an electric current through the patient's heart. The current causes the myocardium to depolarize, which in turn encourages the SA node to resume control of the heart's electrical activity.

The electrode paddles delivering the current may be placed on the patient's chest or, during cardiac surgery, directly on the myocardium.

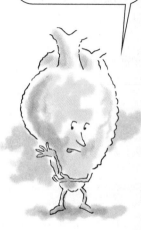

Resetting the SYNC MODE defibrillator switch after each cardioversion ensures that the machine stays synchronized.

One or both

Defibrillators can be monophasic or biphasic. *Monophasic defibrillators* deliver a single current of electricity that travels in one direction between the two pads or paddles on the patient's chest. A large amount of electrical current is needed for effective monophasic defibrillation.

Positively speaking

A *biphasic defibrillator* delivers the electrical current in a positive direction for a specified duration and then reverses and flows in a negative direction for the remaining time of the electrical discharge. The biphasic defibrillator delivers two currents of electricity and lowers the defibrillation threshold of the heart muscle, making it possible to successfully defibrillate ventricular fibrillation with smaller amounts of energy. For example, instead of using 200 joules, an initial shock of 150 joules is commonly effective.

Adjustable

Additionally, the biphasic defibrillator is able to adjust for differences in impedance or the resistance of the current through the chest, thereby reducing the number of shocks needed to terminate ventricular fibrillation. Also, damage to the myocardial muscle is reduced because of the lower energy levels used and fewer shocks needed.

Act early and quickly

Because some arrhythmias, such as ventricular fibrillation, can cause death if not corrected, the success of defibrillation depends on early recognition and quick treatment. In addition to treating ventricular fibrillation, defibrillation may also be used to treat ventricular tachycardia that doesn't produce a pulse.

Nursing considerations

• Assess the patient to determine if he lacks a pulse. If so, call for help and perform cardiopulmonary resuscitation (CPR) until the defibrillator and other emergency equipment arrive.
• Connect the monitoring leads of the defibrillator to the patient, and assess his cardiac rhythm in two leads.
• Expose the patient's chest and apply conductive pads at the paddle placement positions. (See *Defibrillator paddle placement.*)
• Turn on the defibrillator and, if performing external defibrillation, set the energy level at 360 joules for an adult patient.

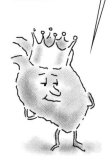

Having jewels would be nice, but I'd rather have 360 joules when it comes to external defibrillation.

Charge!!

• Charge the paddles by pressing the CHARGE buttons, which are located on the machine or paddles.
• Place the paddles over the conductive pads and press firmly against the patient's chest, using 25 lb (11.3 kg) of pressure.
• Reassess the patient's cardiac rhythm in two leads.
• If the patient remains in ventricular fibrillation or pulseless ventricular tachycardia, instruct all personnel to stand clear of the patient and the bed. Also, make a visual check to make sure everyone is clear of the patient and the bed.

And discharge!

• Discharge the current by pressing both paddle DISCHARGE buttons simultaneously.
• Reassess the patient's pulse, and give 2 minutes of CPR. Reassess his cardiac rhythm.
• If necessary, prepare to defibrillate a second time at 360 joules. Announce that you're preparing to defibrillate, and follow the procedure described above.
• Reassess the patient and continue CPR.
• If the patient still has no pulse after the first two cycles of defibrillation and CPR, give supplemental oxygen, and begin administering appropriate medications such as epinephrine. Also, consider possible causes for failure of the patient's rhythm to convert, such as acidosis and hypoxia.

Rhythm restoration

• If defibrillation restores a normal rhythm, assess the patient. Obtain baseline ABG levels and a 12-lead ECG. Provide supple-

Stay on the ball

Defibrillator paddle placement

Here's a guide to correct paddle placement for defibrillation.

Anterolateral placement

For anterolateral placement, place one paddle to the right of the upper sternum, just below the right clavicle. Place the other over the fifth or sixth intercostal space at the left anterior axillary line.

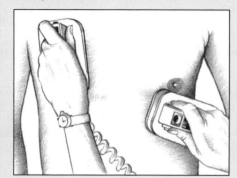

Anteroposterior placement

For anteroposterior placement, place the anterior paddle directly over the heart at the precordium, to the left of the lower sternal border. Place the flat posterior paddle under the patient's body beneath the heart and immediately below the scapula (but not under the vertebral column).

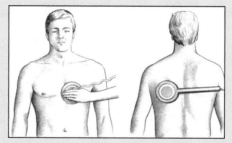

mental oxygen, ventilation, and medications as needed. Prepare the defibrillator for immediate reuse.
• Document the procedure, including the patient's ECG rhythms before and after defibrillation; the number of times defibrillation was performed; the voltage used during each attempt; whether a pulse returned; the dosage, route, and time of drugs administered; whether CPR was used; how the airway was maintained; and the patient's outcome.
• Prepare the patient for possible insertion of an implantable cardioverter-defibrillator.

Transcutaneous pacemaker

A transcutaneous pacemaker, also referred to as *external* or *non-invasive pacing*, is a temporary pacemaker that's used in an emergency. The device consists of an external, battery-powered pulse generator and a lead or electrode system.

Dire straits

In a life-threatening situation, a transcutaneous pacemaker works by sending an electrical impulse from the pulse generator to the patient's heart by way of two electrodes that are placed on the front and back of the patient's chest.

Transcutaneous pacing is quick and effective, but it's used only until the practitioner can institute transvenous pacing.

Nursing considerations

• Attach monitoring electrodes to the patient in the lead I, II, or III position. Do so even if the patient is already on telemetry monitoring, because you must connect the electrodes to the pacemaker. If you select the lead II position, adjust the left leg (LL) electrode placement to accommodate the anterior pacing electrode and the patient's anatomy.
• Plug the patient cable into the ECG input connection on the front of the pacing generator. Set the selector switch to the MONITOR ON position.
• You should see the ECG waveform on the monitor. Adjust the R-wave beeper volume to a suitable level and activate the alarm by pressing the ALARM ON button. Set the alarm for 10 to 20 beats lower and 20 to 30 beats higher than the intrinsic rate.
• Press the START/STOP button for a printout of the waveform.
• Now you're ready to apply the two pacing electrodes.

Proper placement

• First, make sure the patient's skin is clean and dry to ensure good skin contact.
• Pull off the protective strip from the posterior electrode (marked BACK) and apply the electrode on the left side of the back, just below the scapula and to the left of the spine.
• The anterior pacing electrode (marked FRONT) has two protective strips—one covering the jellied area and one covering the outer ring. Expose the jellied area and apply it to the skin in the anterior position—to the left of the precordium in the usual V_2 to V_5 position. Move this electrode around to get the best waveform. Then expose the electrode's outer rim and firmly press it to the skin. (See *Proper electrode placement.*)

Now to pacing

• After making sure the energy output in milliamperes (mA) is on, connect the electrode cable to the monitor output cable.
• Check the waveform, looking for a tall QRS complex in lead II.

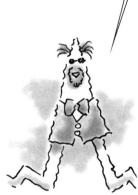

I'll never be dark or handsome, but as long as I'm tall you can turn on the transcutaneous pacemaker.

Proper electrode placement

Place the two pacing electrodes for a transcutaneous pacemaker at heart level on the patient's chest and back (as shown). This placement ensures that the electrical stimulus must travel only a short distance to the heart.

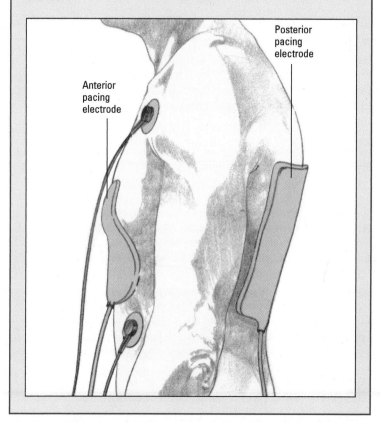

Posterior pacing electrode

Anterior pacing electrode

• Next, turn the selector switch to PACER ON. Tell the patient that he may feel a thumping or twitching sensation. Reassure him that you'll give him medication if he can't tolerate the discomfort.

Set the beat

• Now set the rate dial to 10 to 20 beats higher than the patient's intrinsic rate. Look for pacer artifact or spikes, which will appear as you increase the rate. If the patient doesn't have an intrinsic rhythm, set the rate at 60.
• Slowly increase the amount of energy delivered to the heart by adjusting the OUTPUT MA dial. Do so until capture is achieved; you'll see a pacer spike followed by a widened QRS complex that

resembles a permanent ventricular contraction. This setting is the pacing threshold. To ensure consistent capture, increase output by 10%. Don't go higher because you could cause the patient needless discomfort.
• With full capture, the patient's heart rate should be approximately the same as the pacemaker rate set on the machine. The usual pacing threshold is between 40 and 60 mA.

Them bones, them bones

• Don't place the electrodes over a bony area because bone conducts current poorly. For female patients, place the anterior electrode under the patient's breast but not over her diaphragm. If the practitioner inserts the electrode through the brachial or femoral vein, immobilize the patient's arm or leg to avoid putting stress on the pacing wires.

Check back with the vitals

• After placement of a transcutaneous pacemaker, assess the patient's vital signs, skin color, LOC, and peripheral pulses to determine the effectiveness of the paced rhythm. Perform a 12-lead ECG to serve as a baseline, and then perform additional ECGs daily or with clinical changes. If possible, also obtain a rhythm strip before, during, and after pacemaker placement; any time that pacemaker settings are changed; and whenever the patient receives treatment because of a complication due to the pacemaker.
• Continuously monitor the ECG reading, noting capture, sensing, rate, intrinsic beats, and competition of paced and intrinsic rhythms. If the pacemaker is sensing correctly, the sense indicator on the pulse generator should flash with each beat.

Common disorders

In the ED, you're likely to encounter patients with common cardiac emergencies, especially acute coronary syndrome, aortic aneurysm, cardiac arrest, cardiac arrhythmias, cardiac contusion, cardiac tamponade, heart failure, and hypertensive crisis. Regardless of the disorder, the priorities are always to ensure vital functioning—that is, airway, breathing, and circulation.

Acute coronary syndrome

Patients with acute coronary syndrome have some degree of coronary artery occlusion. The degree of occlusion defines whether the acute coronary syndrome is:
• unstable angina

- non-ST-segment elevation MI (non-STEMI)
- ST-segment elevation MI (STEMI).

Plaque's place

The development of acute coronary syndrome begins with a rupture or erosion of plaque, an unstable and lipid-rich substance. The rupture results in platelet adhesions, fibrin clot formation, and thrombin activation.

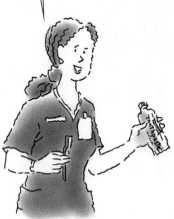

Plaque erosion on the teeth may be welcome, but not around the heart.

What causes it

Patients with certain risk factors appear to face a greater likelihood of developing acute coronary syndrome. These factors include:
- diabetes
- family history of heart disease
- hypertension
- obesity
- high-fat, high-carbohydrate diet
- sedentary lifestyle
- menopause
- hyperlipoproteinemia
- smoking
- stress.

How it happens

Acute coronary syndrome most commonly results when a thrombus progresses and occludes blood flow. (An early thrombus doesn't necessarily block blood flow.) The effect is an imbalance in myocardial oxygen supply and demand.

Degree and duration

The degree and duration of blockage dictate the type of infarct:
- If the patient has *unstable angina,* a thrombus partially occludes a coronary vessel. This thrombus is full of platelets. The partially occluded vessel may have distal microthrombi that cause necrosis in some myocytes.
- If smaller vessels infarct, the patient is at higher risk for MI, which may progress to a *non-STEMI.* Usually, only the innermost layer of the heart is damaged.
- *STEMI* results when reduced blood flow through one of the coronary arteries causes myocardial ischemia, injury, and necrosis. The damage extends through all myocardial layers.

What to look for

A patient with angina typically experiences:

Identifying symptoms of MI

The cardinal symptom of a myocardial infarction (MI) is persistent, intense substernal pain that may radiate to the left arm, jaw, neck, or shoulder blades. This pain is unrelieved by rest or nitroglycerin and may last several hours. Some patients with an MI, such as elderly patients and those with diabetes, may not experience pain at all. Other patients experience only mild pain; for example, female patients who experience atypical chest pain with an MI may present with complaints of indigestion and fatigue. Any patient may experience atypical chest pain, but it's more common in women.

- burning
- squeezing
- crushing tightness in the substernal or precordial chest that may radiate to the left arm, neck, jaw, or shoulder blade. (See *Identifying symptoms of MI.*)

It hurts when I do this

Angina most commonly follows physical exertion but may also follow emotional excitement, cold exposure, or a large meal. Angina is commonly relieved by nitroglycerin. It's less severe and shorter-lived than the pain of acute MI.

Angina has four major forms:

stable—predictable pain, in frequency and duration, which can be relieved with nitrates and rest

unstable—increased pain, which is easily induced

Prinzmetal's or a variant—pain from unpredictable coronary artery spasm

microvascular—angina-like chest pain due to impairment of vasodilator reserve in a patient with normal coronary arteries.

My, my, MI pain

A patient with MI experiences severe, persistent chest pain that isn't relieved by rest or nitroglycerin. He may describe pain as crushing or squeezing. The pain is usually substernal but may radiate to the left arm, jaw, neck, or shoulder blades.

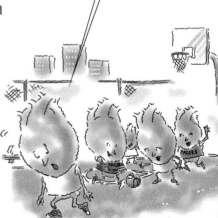

Patients with angina often experience a burning or squeezing sensation after physical exertion. I think I'll sit this one out!

And many more

Other signs and symptoms of MI inclu[de]
- anxiety
- feeling of impending doom
- nausea and vomiting
- perspiration
- shortness of breath
- cool extremities
- fatigue
- hypotension or hypertension
- muffled heart sounds
- palpable precordial pulse.

Pinpointing infarction

The site of myocardial infarc[tion]
- Occlusion of the myocardial infarc[tion]
- Occlusion of the circum[flex]
- Occlusion of the ante[rior]
  infarction.
- True posterior [or]
  artery or one [of]
- Right ven[tricular]
  ny inferi[or]
- In a[
- ST[

What tests tell you

These tests are used to diagnose CAD:
- ECG during an anginal episode shows ischemia. Serial 12-lead ECGs may be normal or inconclusive during the first few hours after an MI. Abnormalities include non-STEMI and STEMI. (See *Pinpointing infarction*, page 158.)
- Coronary angiography reveals coronary artery stenosis or obstruction and collateral circulation and shows the condition of the arteries beyond the narrowing.
- Myocardial perfusion imaging with thallium-201 during treadmill exercise discloses ischemic areas of the myocardium, visualized as "cold spots."
- With MI, serial serum cardiac marker measurements show elevated CK, especially the CK-MB isoenzyme (the cardiac muscle fraction of CK), troponin T and I, and myoglobin.
- With a Q-wave MI, echocardiography shows ventricular wall dyskinesia.

How it's treated

For patients with angina, the goal of treatment is to reduce myocardial oxygen demand or increase oxygen supply. These treatments are used to manage angina:
- Nitrates reduce myocardial oxygen consumption.
- Beta-adrenergic blockers may be administered to reduce the workload and oxygen demands of the heart.
- If angina is caused by coronary artery spasm, calcium channel blockers may be given.
- Antiplatelet drugs minimize platelet aggregation and the danger of coronary occlusion.
- Antilipemic drugs can reduce elevated serum cholesterol or triglyceride levels.

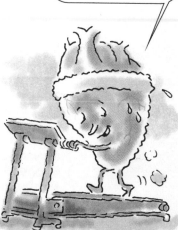

Myocardial perfusion imaging during treadmill exercise reveals the myocardium's ischemic areas.

...ion (MI) depends on the vessels involved:

...flex branch of the left coronary artery causes a lateral wall infarction.

...ior descending branch of the left coronary artery leads to an anterior wall

...r inferior wall infarctions generally result from occlusion of the right coronary

... its branches.

...ricular infarctions can also result from right coronary artery occlusion, can accompa-

...r infarctions, and may cause right-sided heart failure.

... ST-segment elevation MI, tissue damage extends through all myocardial layers; in a non-

...segment elevation MI, damage occurs only in the innermost layer.

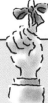
• Obstructive lesions may necessitate CABG or PTCA. Other alternatives include laser angioplasty, minimally invasive surgery, rotational atherectomy, or stent placement.

MI relief

The goals of treatment for MI are to relieve pain, stabilize heart rhythm, revascularize the coronary artery, preserve myocardial tissue, and reduce cardiac workload. Here are some guidelines for treatment:

• Thrombolytic therapy should be started within 3 hours of the onset of symptoms (unless contraindications exist). Thrombolytic therapy involves administration of streptokinase, alteplase, or reteplase.

• PTCA is an option for opening blocked or narrowed arteries.

• Oxygen is administered to increase oxygenation of the blood.

• Nitroglycerin is administered sublingually to relieve chest pain, unless systolic blood pressure is less than 90 mm Hg or heart rate is less than 50 or greater than 100 beats/minute.

• Morphine is administered as analgesia because pain stimulates the sympathetic nervous system, leading to an increase in heart rate and vasoconstriction.

• Aspirin is administered to inhibit platelet aggregation.

Patency protection

• I.V. heparin is given to patients who have received tissue plasminogen activator to increase the chances of patency in the affected coronary artery.

• Lidocaine, transcutaneous pacing patches (or a transvenous pacemaker), defibrillation, or epinephrine may be used if arrhythmias are present.

• Physical activity is limited for the first 12 hours to reduce cardiac workload, thereby limiting the area of necrosis.
• I.V. nitroglycerin is administered for 24 to 48 hours in patients without hypotension, bradycardia, or excessive tachycardia, to reduce afterload and preload and to relieve chest pain.
• Glycoprotein IIb/IIIa inhibitors (such as abciximab [ReoPro]) are administered to patients with continued unstable angina, with acute chest pain, or following invasive cardiac procedures to reduce platelet aggregation.
• I.V. beta-adrenergic blocker is administered early to patients with evolving acute MI; it's followed by oral therapy to reduce heart rate and contractibility and to reduce myocardial oxygen requirements.
• ACE inhibitors are administered to those with evolving MI with ST-segment elevation or left bundle-branch block, to reduce afterload and preload and to prevent remodeling.
• Laser angioplasty, atherectomy, stent placement, or transmyocardial revascularization may be initiated.
• Lipid-lowering drugs are administered to patients with elevated low-density lipoprotein and cholesterol levels.

What to do

• On admission, monitor and record the patient's ECG, blood pressure, temperature, and heart and breath sounds. Also, assess and record the severity, location, type, and duration of pain. (See *Acute coronary syndrome algorithm*, pages 160 and 161.)
• Obtain a 12-lead ECG and assess heart rate and blood pressure when the patient experiences acute chest pain.
• Monitor the patient's hemodynamic status closely. Be alert for indicators suggesting decreased cardiac output, such as decreased blood pressure, increased heart rate, increased PAP, increased PAWP, decreased cardiac output measurements, and decreased right atrial pressure.
• Assess urine output hourly.
• Monitor the patient's oxygen saturation levels, and notify the practitioner if oxygen saturation falls below 90%.
• Check the patient's blood pressure after giving nitroglycerin, especially the first dose.
• During episodes of chest pain, monitor ECG, blood pressure, and PA catheter readings (if applicable) to determine changes.
• Frequently monitor ECG rhythm strips to detect heart rate changes and arrhythmias.
• Obtain serial measurements of cardiac enzyme levels as ordered.
• Watch for crackles, cough, tachypnea, and edema, which may indicate impending left-sided heart failure. Carefully monitor

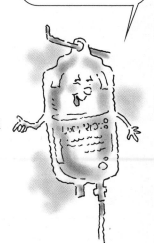

I.V. heparin, nitroglycerin, and beta-adrenergic blocker can help patients with MI.

(Text continues on page 162.)

Acute coronary syndrome algorithm

The algorithm below shows the American Heart Association's guidelines for treating a patient with acute coronary syndrome.

Chest discomfort suggestive of ischemia

EMS assessment and care and hospital preparation
• Monitor and support airway, breathing, and circulation (ABCs). Be prepared to provide CPR and defibrillation.
• Administer oxygen, **aspirin, nitroglycerin,** and **morphine** if needed.
• If available, obtain 12-lead ECG. If ST-segment elevation:
– Notify receiving hospital with transmission or interpretation.
– Begin fibrinolytic checklist.
• Notified hospital should mobilize hospital resources to respond to ST-segment elevation myocardial infarction (STEMI).

Immediate ED assessment (< 10 min)
• Check vital signs; evaluate oxygen saturation.
• Establish I.V. access.
• Obtain and review 12-lead ECG.
• Perform brief, targeted history and physical examination.
• Review or complete fibrinolytic checklist; check contraindications.
• Obtain initial cardiac marker levels and initial electrolyte and coagulation studies.
• Obtain portable chest X-ray (< 30 min).

Immediate ED general treatment
• Start oxygen at 4 L/minute; maintain O_2 sat > 90%.
• **Aspirin** 160 to 325 mg (if not given by EMS)
• **Nitroglycerin** sublingual, spray, or I.V.
• **Morphine** I.V. if pain isn't relieved by nitroglycerin

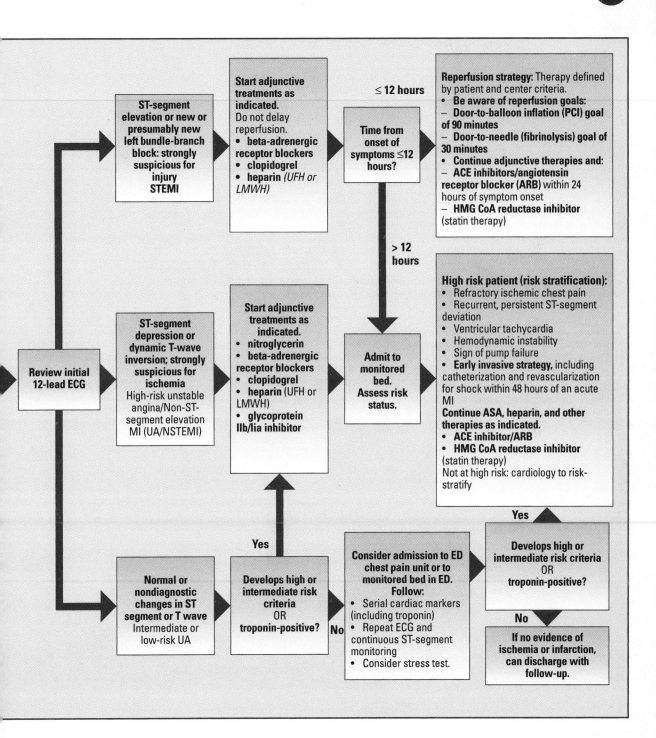

Review initial 12-lead ECG

ST-segment elevation or new or presumably new left bundle-branch block: strongly suspicious for injury STEMI

Start adjunctive treatments as indicated. Do not delay reperfusion.
• beta-adrenergic receptor blockers
• clopidogrel
• heparin *(UFH or LMWH)*

Time from onset of symptoms ≤12 hours?

≤ 12 hours

Reperfusion strategy: Therapy defined by patient and center criteria.
• **Be aware of reperfusion goals:**
– **Door-to-balloon inflation (PCI) goal of 90 minutes**
– **Door-to-needle (fibrinolysis) goal of 30 minutes**
• **Continue adjunctive therapies and:**
– **ACE inhibitors/angiotensin receptor blocker (ARB)** within 24 hours of symptom onset
– **HMG CoA reductase inhibitor** (statin therapy)

> 12 hours

ST-segment depression or dynamic T-wave inversion; strongly suspicious for ischemia High-risk unstable angina/Non-ST-segment elevation MI (UA/NSTEMI)

Start adjunctive treatments as indicated.
• nitroglycerin
• beta-adrenergic receptor blockers
• clopidogrel
• heparin (UFH or LMWH)
• glycoprotein IIb/IIa inhibitor

Admit to monitored bed. Assess risk status.

High risk patient (risk stratification):
• Refractory ischemic chest pain
• Recurrent, persistent ST-segment deviation
• Ventricular tachycardia
• Hemodynamic instability
• Sign of pump failure
• **Early invasive strategy,** including catheterization and revascularization for shock within 48 hours of an acute MI
Continue ASA, heparin, and other therapies as indicated.
• **ACE inhibitor/ARB**
• **HMG CoA reductase inhibitor** (statin therapy)
Not at high risk: cardiology to risk-stratify

Yes

Yes

Normal or nondiagnostic changes in ST segment or T wave Intermediate or low-risk UA

Develops high or intermediate risk criteria OR troponin-positive?

No

Consider admission to ED chest pain unit or to monitored bed in ED. Follow:
• Serial cardiac markers (including troponin)
• Repeat ECG and continuous ST-segment monitoring
• Consider stress test.

Develops high or intermediate risk criteria OR troponin-positive?

No

If no evidence of ischemia or infarction, can discharge with follow-up.

weight, intake and output, respiratory rate, serum enzyme levels, ECG waveforms, and blood pressure. Auscultate for S_3 or S_4 gallops.
• Prepare the patient for reperfusion therapy as indicated.
• Administer and titrate medications as ordered. Avoid giving I.M. injections; I.V. administration provides more rapid symptom relief.
• Organize patient care and activities to allow rest periods. If the patient is immobilized, turn him often and use intermittent compression devices. Gradually increase the patient's activity level as tolerated.

Aortic aneurysm

An aortic aneurysm is a localized outpouching or an abnormal dilation in a weakened arterial wall. Aortic aneurysm is typically found in the aorta between the renal arteries and the iliac branches, but the abdominal, thoracic, or ascending arch of the aorta may be affected.

What causes it

The exact cause of an aortic aneurysm is unclear, but several factors place a person at risk, including:
• pregnancy
• Marfan syndrome
• long-standing history of systemic hypertension and a preexisting aneurysm (in advanced age)
• trauma.

How it happens

Aneurysms arise from a defect in the middle layer of the arterial wall (*tunica media*, or medial layer). When the elastic fibers and collagen in the middle layer are damaged, stretching and segmental dilation occur. As a result, the medial layer loses some of its elasticity and it fragments. Smooth-muscle cells are lost and the wall thins.

Thin and thinner

The thinned wall may contain calcium deposits and atherosclerotic plaque, making the wall brittle. As a person ages, the elastin in the wall decreases, further weakening the vessel. If hypertension is present, blood flow slows, resulting in ischemia and additional weakening.

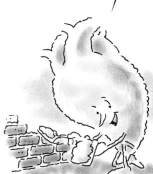

I wish my arterial walls were made of stuff this sturdy. I'd never have to worry about aneurysms again!

Wide vessel, slow flow

When an aneurysm begins to develop, lateral pressure increases, causing the vessel lumen to widen and blood flow to slow. Over time, mechanical stressors contribute to elongation of the aneurysm.

Blood forces

Hemodynamic forces may also play a role, causing pulsatile stresses on the weakened wall and pressing on the small vessels that supply nutrients to the arterial wall. In aortic aneurysms, this stress and pressure causes the aorta to become bowed and tortuous.

What to look for

Most patients with aortic aneurysms are asymptomatic until the aneurysms enlarge and compress surrounding tissue. A large aneurysm may produce signs and symptoms that mimic those of an MI, renal calculi, lumbar disk disease, or duodenal compression.

When symptoms arise

Usually, the patient exhibits symptoms if rupture, expansion, embolization, thrombosis, or pressure from the mass on surrounding structures exists. Rupture is more common if the patient also has hypertension or if the aneurysm is larger than 6 cm. If the patient has a suspected thoracic aortic aneurysm, assess for:
• difficulty breathing
• complaints of sudden, excruciating, tearing pain that moves from the anterior to the posterior
• hoarseness or coughing
• nausea and vomiting
• diaphoresis
• hematemesis
• dysphagia
• aortic insufficiency murmur
• hemoptysis
• palpable pulsations at the left sternoclavicular joint
• tachycardia
• unequal blood pressure and pulse when measured in both arms.

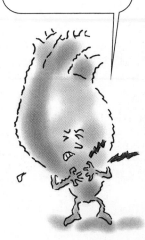

A sudden, tearing pain that moves from the anterior to the posterior is a sure sign of aortic aneurysm.

Acute expansion

When there's an acute expansion of a thoracic aortic aneurysm, assess for:
• severe hypertension
• neurologic changes
• jugular vein distention

- new murmur of aortic sufficiency
- right sternoclavicular lift
- tracheal deviation.

What tests tell you

No specific laboratory test diagnoses an aortic aneurysm; however, several other tests may be helpful:
- If blood is leaking from the aneurysm, leukocytosis and a decrease in hemoglobin and hematocrit may be noted.
- TEE allows visualization of the thoracic aorta. It's commonly combined with Doppler flow studies to provide information about blood flow.
- Abdominal ultrasonography or echocardiography can be used to determine the size, shape, length, and location of the aneurysm.
- Anteroposterior and lateral X-rays of the chest or abdomen can be used to detect aortic calcification and widened areas of the aorta.
- Computed tomography (CT) scan and magnetic resonance imaging (MRI) can disclose the aneurysm's size and effect on nearby organs.
- Serial ultrasonography at 6-month intervals reveals growth of small aneurysms.
- Aortography is used to determine the aneurysm's approximate size and the patency of visceral vessels.

How it's treated

Aneurysm treatment usually involves surgery and appropriate drug therapy. Aortic aneurysms usually require resection and replacement of the aortic section using a vascular or Dacron graft. However, keep these points in mind:
- If the aneurysm is small and produces no symptoms, surgery may be delayed, with regular physical examination and ultrasonography performed to monitor its progression.
- Large or symptomatic aneurysms are at risk for rupture and need immediate repair.
- Endovascular grafting may be an option for a patient with an abdominal aortic aneurysm. This procedure, which can be done using local or regional anesthesia, is a minimally invasive procedure whereby the walls of the aorta are reinforced to prevent expansion and rupture of the aneurysm.
- Medications to control blood pressure, relieve anxiety, and control pain are also prescribed.

Emergency measures

Rupture of an aortic aneurysm is a medical emergency requiring prompt treatment, including:
• resuscitation with fluid and blood replacement
• I.V. propranolol to reduce myocardial contractility
• I.V. nitroprusside to reduce blood pressure and maintain it at 90 to 100 mm Hg systolic
• analgesics to relieve pain
• arterial line and indwelling urinary catheter to monitor the patient's condition preoperatively.

What to do

• Assess the patient's vital signs, especially blood pressure, every 2 to 4 hours or more frequently, depending on the severity of his condition. Monitor blood pressure and pulse in extremities, and compare findings bilaterally. If the difference in systolic blood pressure exceeds 10 mm Hg, notify the practitioner immediately.
• Assess cardiovascular status frequently, including heart rate, rhythm, ECG, and cardiac enzyme levels. MI can appear if an aneurysm ruptures along the coronary arteries.
• Obtain blood samples to evaluate kidney function by assessing BUN, creatinine, and electrolyte levels. Measure intake and output, hourly if necessary, depending on the patient's condition.
• Monitor CBC for evidence of blood loss, including decreased hemoglobin, hematocrit, and red blood cell (RBC) count.

ABGs and arterial lines

• Obtain an arterial sample for ABG analysis, as ordered, and monitor cardiac rhythm. Assist with arterial line insertion to allow for continuous blood pressure monitoring. Assist with insertion of a PA catheter to assess hemodynamic balance.
• Administer beta blockers to decrease blood pressure, heart rate, and left ventricular contractility.
• Administer I.V. morphine as ordered, to relieve pain if present.
• Administer nitroprusside (Nipride) I.V. only after beta blockers have been initiated because the heart rate can increase and potentially extend the dissection.
• Observe the patient for signs of rupture, which may be immediately fatal. Watch closely for signs of acute blood loss, such as decreasing blood pressure, increasing pulse and respiratory rates, restlessness, decreased LOC, and cool, clammy skin.

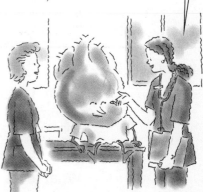

Pay close attention to blood pressure in an aortic aneurysm patient. Check it every 2 to 4 hours or more.

Rupture response

- If rupture does take place, insert a large-bore I.V. catheter, begin fluid resuscitation, and administer nitroprusside I.V. as ordered, usually to maintain a mean arterial pressure (MAP) of 70 to 80 mm Hg. Also administer propranolol I.V. (to reduce left ventricular ejection velocity), as ordered, until the heart rate ranges from 60 to 80 beats/minute. Expect to administer additional doses every 4 to 6 hours until oral medications can be used.
- If the patient is experiencing acute pain, administer morphine I.V. as ordered.
- Prepare the patient for emergency surgery.
- Inform the patient and his family of possible transfer to the CCU after surgery.

Cardiac arrest

Cardiac arrest is the absence of mechanical functioning of the heart muscle. The heart stops beating or beats abnormally and doesn't pump effectively. If blood circulation isn't restored within minutes, cardiac arrest can lead to the loss of arterial blood pressure, brain damage, and death. (See *Adult BLS cardiac arrest algorithm*. See also *ACLS pulseless arrest algorithm*, pages 168 and 169.)

What causes it

Cardiac arrest can be caused by a wide variety of conditions, including acute MI, ventricular fibrillation, ventricular tachycardia, severe trauma, hypovolemia, metabolic disorders, brain injury, respiratory arrest, drowning, or drug overdose.

How it happens

In cardiac arrest, myocardial contractility stops, resulting in a lack of cardiac output. An imbalance in myocardial oxygen supply and demand follows, leading to myocardial ischemia, tissue necrosis, and death.

What to look for

The patient experiencing a cardiac arrest suddenly loses consciousness. Spontaneous respirations are absent, and the patient has no palpable pulse.

What tests tell you

No specific diagnostic tests are used to confirm a cardiac arrest. However, cardiac monitoring or ECG may reveal an underlying cardiac arrhythmia, such as ventricular fibrillation or asystole.

Adult BLS cardiac arrest algorithm

This algorithm shows the basic life support (BLS) steps to follow when you suspect cardiac arrest in an adult patient.

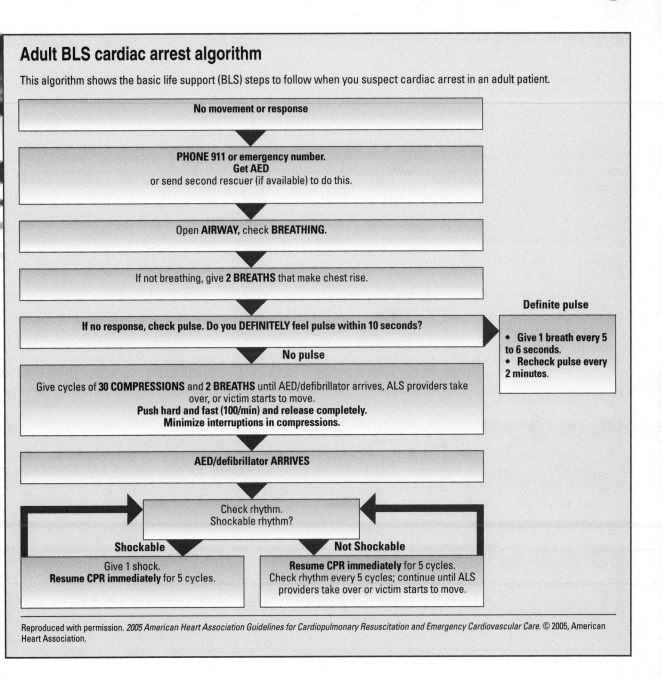

No movement or response

PHONE 911 or emergency number.
Get AED
or send second rescuer (if available) to do this.

Open **AIRWAY,** check **BREATHING.**

If not breathing, give **2 BREATHS** that make chest rise.

If no response, check pulse. Do you **DEFINITELY** feel pulse within 10 seconds?

Definite pulse

- **Give 1 breath every 5 to 6 seconds.**
- **Recheck pulse every 2 minutes.**

No pulse

Give cycles of **30 COMPRESSIONS** and **2 BREATHS** until AED/defibrillator arrives, ALS providers take over, or victim starts to move.
Push hard and fast (100/min) and release completely.
Minimize interruptions in compressions.

AED/defibrillator ARRIVES

Check rhythm.
Shockable rhythm?

Shockable

Give 1 shock.
Resume CPR immediately for 5 cycles.

Not Shockable

Resume CPR immediately for 5 cycles.
Check rhythm every 5 cycles; continue until ALS providers take over or victim starts to move.

Reproduced with permission. *2005 American Heart Association Guidelines for Cardiopulmonary Resuscitation and Emergency Cardiovascular Care.* © 2005, American Heart Association.

How it's treated

Treatment of cardiac arrest involves basic and advanced cardiac life support measures in conjunction with treating the underlying

(Text continues on page 170.)

ACLS pulseless arrest algorithm

This algorithm shows the American Heart Association's guidelines for treating a patient in pulseless cardiac arrest.

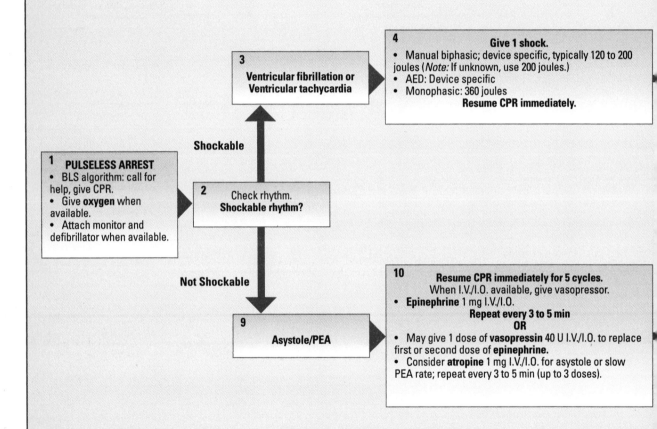

1 PULSELESS ARREST
- BLS algorithm: call for help, give CPR.
- Give **oxygen** when available.
- Attach monitor and defibrillator when available.

2 Check rhythm.
Shockable rhythm?

Shockable

3 Ventricular fibrillation or Ventricular tachycardia

4 Give 1 shock.
- Manual biphasic; device specific, typically 120 to 200 joules (*Note:* If unknown, use 200 joules.)
- AED: Device specific
- Monophasic: 360 joules
  Resume CPR immediately.

Not Shockable

9 Asystole/PEA

10 Resume CPR immediately for 5 cycles.
When I.V./I.O. available, give vasopressor.
- **Epinephrine** 1 mg I.V./I.O.
  Repeat every 3 to 5 min
  OR
- May give 1 dose of **vasopressin** 40 U I.V./I.O. to replace first or second dose of **epinephrine.**
- Consider **atropine** 1 mg I.V./I.O. for asystole or slow PEA rate; repeat every 3 to 5 min (up to 3 doses).

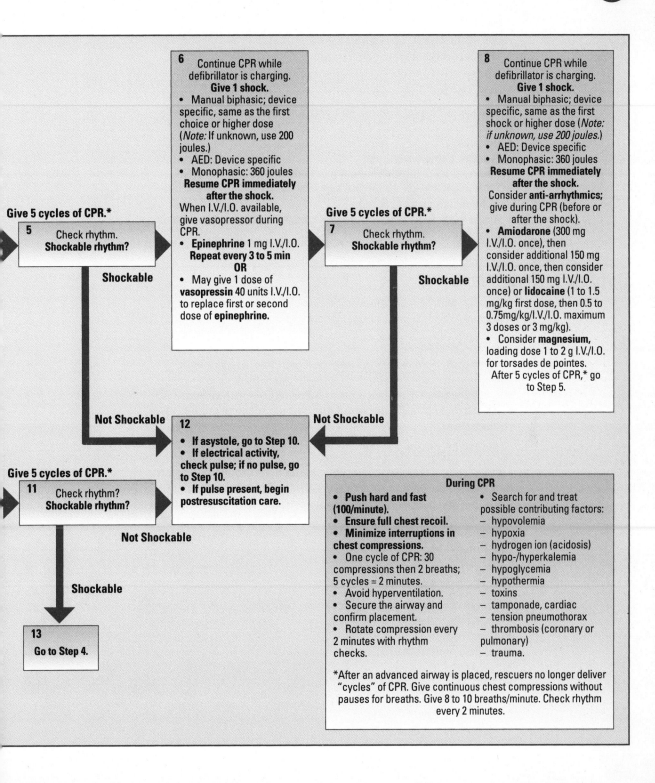

Give 5 cycles of CPR.*

5 Check rhythm. **Shockable rhythm?**

Shockable

6 Continue CPR while defibrillator is charging. **Give 1 shock.**
• Manual biphasic; device specific, same as the first choice or higher dose (*Note:* If unknown, use 200 joules.)
• AED: Device specific
• Monophasic: 360 joules
Resume CPR immediately after the shock.
When I.V./I.O. available, give vasopressor during CPR.
• **Epinephrine** 1 mg I.V./I.O. **Repeat every 3 to 5 min OR**
• May give 1 dose of **vasopressin** 40 units I.V./I.O. to replace first or second dose of **epinephrine.**

Give 5 cycles of CPR.*

7 Check rhythm. **Shockable rhythm?**

Shockable

8 Continue CPR while defibrillator is charging. **Give 1 shock.**
• Manual biphasic; device specific, same as the first shock or higher dose (*Note: if unknown, use 200 joules.*)
• AED: Device specific
• Monophasic: 360 joules
Resume CPR immediately after the shock.
Consider **anti-arrhythmics**; give during CPR (before or after the shock).
• **Amiodarone** (300 mg I.V./I.O. once), then consider additional 150 mg I.V./I.O. once, then consider additional 150 mg I.V./I.O. once) or **lidocaine** (1 to 1.5 mg/kg first dose, then 0.5 to 0.75mg/kg/I.V./I.O. maximum 3 doses or 3 mg/kg).
• Consider **magnesium**, loading dose 1 to 2 g I.V./I.O. for torsades de pointes.
After 5 cycles of CPR,* go to Step 5.

Not Shockable

Not Shockable

12
• **If asystole, go to Step 10.**
• **If electrical activity, check pulse; if no pulse, go to Step 10.**
• **If pulse present, begin postresuscitation care.**

Give 5 cycles of CPR.*

11 Check rhythm? **Shockable rhythm?**

Not Shockable

Shockable

13 Go to Step 4.

During CPR
• **Push hard and fast (100/minute).**
• **Ensure full chest recoil.**
• **Minimize interruptions in chest compressions.**
• One cycle of CPR: 30 compressions then 2 breaths; 5 cycles = 2 minutes.
• Avoid hyperventilation.
• Secure the airway and confirm placement.
• Rotate compression every 2 minutes with rhythm checks.

• Search for and treat possible contributing factors:
– hypovolemia
– hypoxia
– hydrogen ion (acidosis)
– hypo-/hyperkalemia
– hypoglycemia
– hypothermia
– toxins
– tamponade, cardiac
– tension pneumothorax
– thrombosis (coronary or pulmonary)
– trauma.

*After an advanced airway is placed, rescuers no longer deliver "cycles" of CPR. Give continuous chest compressions without pauses for breaths. Give 8 to 10 breaths/minute. Check rhythm every 2 minutes.

cause of the arrest. The ultimate goal of treatment is to restore the patient's cardiac rhythm and function.

What to do

• Determine responsiveness and notify the practitioner and resuscitation team.
• Initiate CPR.
• Monitor cardiac rhythm.
• Assist with ET intubation and mechanical ventilation.
• Follow advanced cardiac life support (ACLS) protocols; administer medications as ordered.
• Assist with defibrillation for ventricular fibrillation or pulseless ventricular tachycardia.

Cardiac arrhythmias

In cardiac arrhythmia, abnormal electrical conduction or automaticity changes heart rate and rhythm.

Asymptomatic to catastrophic

Cardiac arrhythmias vary in severity, from those that are mild, asymptomatic, and require no treatment (such as sinus arrhythmia, in which heart rate increases and decreases with respiration) to catastrophic ventricular fibrillation, which requires immediate resuscitation.

Organized by origin and effects

Cardiac arrhythmias are generally classified according to their origin (ventricular or supraventricular). Their effect on cardiac output and blood pressure, partially influenced by the site of origin, determines their clinical significance. Lethal arrhythmias, such as ventricular tachycardia and ventricular fibrillation, are a major cause of sudden cardiac death.

What causes it

Common causes of cardiac arrhythmias include:
• emotional stress
• drug toxicity
• congenital defects
• acid-base imbalances
• electrolyte imbalances
• cellular hypoxia
• connective tissue disorders

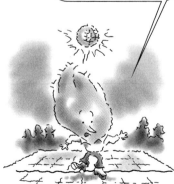

Boy, having this cardiac arrhythmia change my rhythm sure does make it harder to dance.

- degeneration of the conductive tissue
- hypertrophy of the heart muscle
- myocardial ischemia or infarction
- organic heart disease.

How it happens

Cardiac arrhythmias may result from:
- abnormal electrical conduction
- escape beats (additional abnormal heart beats resulting from a very slow heart rate)
- enhanced automaticity
- reentry.

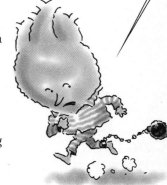

Look out! Escape beats are a major cause of arrhythmias!

What to look for

When a patient presents with a history of symptoms suggesting cardiac arrhythmias or has been treated for a cardiac arrhythmia, be alert for:
- reports of precipitating factors, such as exercise, smoking, sleep patterns, emotional stress, exposure to heat or cold, caffeine intake, position changes, or recent illnesses
- attempts to alleviate the symptoms, such as coughing, rest, medications, or deep breathing
- reports of sensing the heart's rhythm, such as palpitations, irregular beating, skipped beats, or rapid or slow heart rate.

A matter of degree

Physical examination findings vary depending on the arrhythmia and the degree of hemodynamic compromise. Circulatory failure, along with an absence of pulse and respirations, is found with asystole, ventricular fibrillation and, sometimes, ventricular tachycardia.

That's not all

Additional findings may include:
- dizziness
- weakness
- chest pains
- cold and clammy extremities
- hypotension
- dyspnea
- pallor
- reduced urine output
- syncope (with severely impaired cerebral circulation).

What tests tell you

• A 12-lead ECG is the standard test for identifying cardiac arrhythmias. A 15-lead ECG (in which additional leads are applied to the right side of the chest) or an 18-lead ECG (in which additional leads are also added to the posterior scapular area) may be done to provide more definitive information about the patient's right ventricle and posterior wall of the left ventricle. (See *Understanding cardiac arrhythmias*, pages 174 to 181.)
• Laboratory testing may reveal electrolyte abnormalities, hypoxemia or acid-base abnormalities (with ABG analysis), or drug toxicities as the cause of arrhythmias.
• Electrophysiologic testing may be used to identify the mechanism of an arrhythmia and location of accessory pathways and to assess the effectiveness of antiarrhythmic drugs.

How it's treated

The goals of treatment for cardiac arrhythmias are to return pacer function to the sinus node, increase or decrease ventricular rate to normal, regain AV synchrony, and maintain normal sinus rhythm. Treatments to correct abnormal rhythms include therapy with:
• antiarrhythmic drugs
• electrical conversion with defibrillation and cardioversion
• management of the underlying disorder, such as correction of hypoxia
• temporary or permanent placement of a pacemaker to maintain heart rate
• Valsalva's maneuver
• implantable cardioverter-defibrillator (ICD), if indicated
• surgical removal or cryotherapy of an irritable ectopic focus to prevent recurring arrhythmias.

What to do

• Evaluate the patient's ECG frequently for arrhythmia and assess hemodynamic parameters as indicated. Document arrhythmias and notify the practitioner immediately.
• When life-threatening arrhythmias develop, rapidly assess the patient's LOC, pulse and respiratory rates, and hemodynamic parameters. Monitor his ECG continuously. Be prepared to initiate CPR, if indicated. Follow ACLS protocol to treat specific life-threatening arrhythmias.
• Assess the patient for predisposing factors, such as fluid and electrolyte imbalance, and signs of drug toxicity, especially with digoxin.
• Administer medications as ordered, monitor for adverse effects, and monitor vital signs, hemodynamic parameters (as appropri-

ate), and appropriate laboratory studies. Prepare to assist with or perform cardioversion or defibrillation, if indicated.
• If you suspect drug toxicity, report it to the practitioner immediately and withhold the next dose.
• Prepare the patient for transcutaneous or transvenous pacing, if appropriate.
• Prepare the patient for cardioversion, electrophysiology studies, an angiogram, internal cardiac defibrillator placement, or pacemaker placement as indicated.
• If a temporary pacemaker must be inserted, monitor the patient's pulse rate regularly after insertion and watch for signs of pacemaker failure and decreased cardiac output.

Cardiac contusion

Cardiac contusion refers to the bruising of the myocardium. It's the most common type of injury sustained from blunt trauma to the chest.

> Another contusion? We're going to have to buy you a helmet soon!

What causes it

A cardiac contusion typically results from blunt trauma. This trauma can be related to vehicular collisions or falls. The right ventricle is the most common site of injury because it's located directly behind the sternum.

How it happens

During deceleration injuries, the myocardium strikes the sternum when the heart and aorta move forward. In addition, the aorta may be lacerated by shearing forces. Direct force may also be applied to the sternum, causing injury. Crushing and compressive forces may result in contusion as the heart is compressed between the sternum and vertebral column.

What to look for

Cardiac contusion should be suspected after any blow to the chest. Be alert for these signs and symptoms of trauma:
• shortness of breath
• bruising on the chest
• murmurs
• bradycardia or tachycardia
• precordial chest pain.

And also...

Keep these signals in mind as well:

(Text continues on page 180.)

Understanding cardiac arrhythmias

Here's an outline of many common cardiac arrhythmias and their features, causes, and treatments. Use a normal electrocardiogram strip, if available, to compare normal cardiac rhythm configurations with the rhythm strips shown here. Characteristics of normal sinus rhythm include:

- ventricular and atrial rates of 60 to 100 beats/minute
- regular and uniform QRS complexes and P waves
- PR interval of 0.12 to 0.20 second
- QRS duration < 0.12 second
- identical atrial and ventricular rates, with constant PR intervals.

Arrhythmia and features

Sinus tachycardia

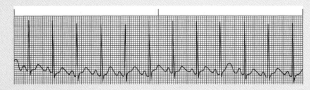

- Atrial and ventricular rhythms regular
- Rate > 100 beats/minute; rarely, > 160 beats/minute
- Normal P waves preceding each QRS complex

Sinus bradycardia

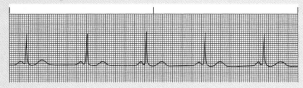

- Atrial and ventricular rhythms regular
- Rate < 60 beats/minute
- Normal P waves preceding each QRS complex

Paroxysmal supraventricular tachycardia

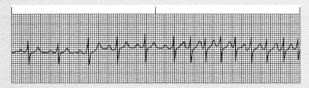

- Atrial and ventricular rhythms regular
- Heart rate > 160 beats/minute; rarely exceeds 250 beats/minute
- P waves regular but aberrant; difficult to differentiate from preceding T waves
- P waves preceding each QRS complex
- Sudden onset and termination of arrhythmia

Atrial flutter

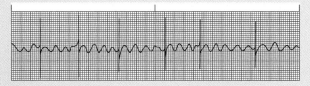

- Atrial rhythm regular; rate 250 to 400 beats/minute
- Ventricular rate variable, depending on degree of AV block (usually 60 to 100 beats/minute)
- No P waves; atrial activity appears as flutter waves (F waves); saw-tooth configuration common in lead II
- QRS complexes are uniform in shape but commonly irregular in rhythm

Causes	Treatment
• Normal physiologic response to fever, exercise, anxiety, pain, dehydration; may also accompany shock, left-sided heart failure, cardiac tamponade, hyperthyroidism, anemia, hypovolemia, pulmonary embolism (PE), and anterior wall myocardial infarction (MI) • May also occur with atropine, epinephrine, isoproterenol, quinidine, caffeine, alcohol, cocaine, amphetamine, and nicotine use	• Correction of underlying cause • Beta-adrenergic blockers or calcium channel blocker
• Normal in a well-conditioned heart, as in an athlete • Increased intracranial pressure; increased vagal tone due to straining during defecation, vomiting, intubation, or mechanical ventilation; sick sinus syndrome (SSS); hypothyroidism; and inferior-wall MI • May also occur with anticholinesterase, beta-adrenergic blocker, digoxin, and morphine use	• Correction of underlying cause • For low cardiac output, dizziness, weakness, altered level of consciousness, or low blood pressure, advanced cardiac life support (ACLS) protocol for administration of atropine • Transcutaneous or permanent pacemaker • Dopamine or epinephrine infusion
• Intrinsic abnormality of atrioventricular (AV) conduction system • Physical or psychological stress, hypoxia, hypokalemia, cardiomyopathy, congenital heart disease, MI, valvular disease, Wolff-Parkinson-White syndrome, cor pulmonale, hyperthyroidism, and systemic hypertension • Digoxin toxicity; use of caffeine, marijuana, or central nervous system stimulants	• If patient is unstable, immediate cardioversion • If QRS complex is narrow and regular and patient is stable, perform vagal maneuvers or administer adenosine • If QRS complex is narrow and irregular, control the rate using calcium channel blockers or beta-adrenergic blockers • If QRS complex is wide and irregular, administer antiarrhythmics such as amiodarone; if ineffective, then magnesium
• Heart failure, tricuspid or mitral valve disease, PE, cor pulmonale, inferior-wall MI, and pericarditis • Digoxin toxicity	• If patient is unstable with a ventricular rate > 150 beats/minute, immediate cardioversion • If patient is stable, follow ACLS protocol for cardioversion and drug therapy, which may include calcium channel blockers, beta-adrenergic blockers, amiodarone, or digoxin • Anticoagulation therapy possibly also needed • Radiofrequency ablation to control rhythm

(continued)

Understanding cardiac arrhythmias (continued)

Arrhythmia and features

Atrial fibrillation

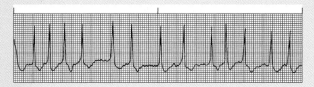

- Atrial rhythm grossly irregular; rate > 400 beats/minute
- Ventricular rhythm grossly irregular
- QRS complexes of uniform configuration and duration
- PR interval indiscernible
- No P waves; atrial activity appears as erratic, irregular, baseline fibrillatory waves (F waves)

Junctional rhythm

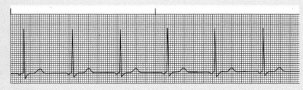

- Atrial and ventricular rhythms regular; atrial rate 40 to 60 beats/minute; ventricular rate usually 40 to 60 beats/minute (60 to 100 beats/minute is accelerated junctional rhythm)
- P waves preceding, hidden within (absent), or after QRS complex; usually inverted if visible
- PR interval (when present) < 0.12 second
- QRS complex configuration and duration normal, except in aberrant conduction

First-degree AV block

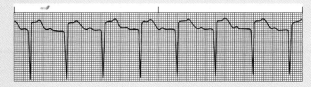

- Atrial and ventricular rhythms regular
- PR interval > 0.20 second
- P wave precedes QRS complex
- QRS complex normal

Second-degree AV block Mobitz I (Wenckebach)

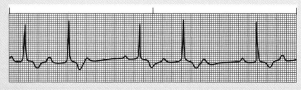

- Atrial rhythm regular
- Ventricular rhythm irregular
- Atrial rate exceeds ventricular rate
- PR interval progressively longer with each cycle until QRS complex disappears (dropped beat); PR interval shorter after dropped beat

Second-degree AV block Mobitz II

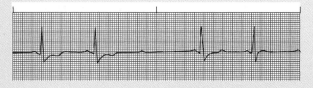

- Atrial rhythm regular
- Ventricular rhythm regular or irregular, with varying degree of block
- PR interval constant for conducted beats
- P waves normal size and shape, but some aren't followed by a QRS complex

Causes	Treatment
• Heart failure, chronic obstructive pulmonary disease, thyrotoxicosis, constrictive pericarditis, ischemic heart disease, sepsis, PE, rheumatic heart disease, hypertension, mitral stenosis, atrial irritation, or complication of coronary bypass or valve replacement surgery • Nifedipine and digoxin use	• If patient is unstable with a ventricular rate > 150 beats/minute, immediate cardioversion • If patient is stable, follow ACLS protocol and drug therapy, which may include calcium channel blockers, beta-adrenergic blockers, amiodarone, or digoxin • Anticoagulation therapy possibly also needed • In some patients with refractory atrial fibrillation uncontrolled by drugs, radiofrequency catheter ablation
• Inferior-wall MI or ischemia, hypoxia, vagal stimulation, and SSS • Acute rheumatic fever • Valve surgery • Digoxin toxicity	• Correction of underlying cause • Atropine for symptomatic slow rate • Pacemaker insertion if patient doesn't respond to drugs • Discontinuation of digoxin, if appropriate
• Possible in healthy persons • Inferior-wall MI or ischemia, hypothyroidism, hypokalemia, and hyperkalemia • Digoxin toxicity; use of quinidine, procainamide, beta-adrenergic blockers, calcium channel blockers, or amiodarone	• Correction of underlying cause • Possibly atropine if severe symptomatic bradycardia develops • Cautious use of digoxin, calcium channel blockers, and beta-adrenergic blockers
• Inferior-wall MI, cardiac surgery, acute rheumatic fever, and vagal stimulation • Digoxin toxicity; use of propranolol, quinidine, or procainamide	• Treatment of underlying cause • Atropine or transcutaneous pacemaker for symptomatic bradycardia • Discontinuation of digoxin, if appropriate
• Severe coronary artery disease (CAD), anterior-wall MI, and acute myocarditis • Digoxin toxicity	• Temporary or permanent pacemaker • Atropine, dopamine, or epinephrine for symptomatic bradycardia • Discontinuation of digoxin, if appropriate

(continued)

Understanding cardiac arrhythmias *(continued)*

Arrhythmia and features

Third-degree AV block (complete heart block)

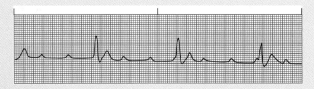

- Atrial rhythm regular
- Ventricular rhythm regular and rate slower than atrial rate
- No relation between P waves and QRS complexes
- No constant PR interval
- QRS duration normal (junctional pacemaker) or wide and bizarre (ventricular pacemaker)

Premature ventricular contraction (PVC)

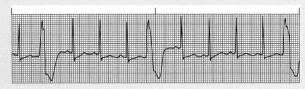

- Atrial rhythm regular
- Ventricular rhythm irregular
- QRS complex premature, usually followed by a complete compensatory pause
- QRS complex wide and distorted, usually > 0.12 second
- Premature QRS complexes occurring alone, in pairs, or in threes, alternating with normal beats; focus from one or more sites
- Ominous when clustered, multifocal, with R-wave-on-T pattern

Ventricular tachycardia

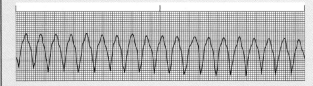

- Ventricular rate 100 to 220 beats/minute; rhythm usually regular
- QRS complexes wide, bizarre, and independent of P waves
- P waves not discernible
- May start and stop suddenly

Causes	Treatment
• Inferior- or anterior-wall MI, congenital abnormality, rheumatic fever, hypoxia, postoperative complication of mitral valve replacement, post-procedure complication of radiofrequency ablation in or near AV nodal tissue, Lev's disease (fibrosis and calcification that spreads from cardiac structures to the conductive tissue), and Lenégre's disease (conductive tissue fibrosis) • Digoxin toxicity	• Atropine, dopamine, or epinephrine for symptomatic bradycardia • Transcutaneous or permanent pacemaker
• Heart failure; old or acute MI, ischemia, or contusion; myocardial irritation by ventricular catheter or a pacemaker; hypercapnia; hypokalemia; hypocalcemia; and hypomagnesemia • Drug toxicity (digoxin, aminophylline, tricyclic antidepressants, beta-adrenergic blockers, isoproterenol, or dopamine) • Caffeine, tobacco, or alcohol use • Psychological stress, anxiety, pain, or exercise	• If warranted, procainamide, amiodarone, or lidocaine I.V. • Treatment of underlying cause • Discontinuation of drug causing toxicity • Potassium chloride I.V. if PVC induced by hypokalemia • Magnesium sulfate I.V. if PVC induced by hypomagnesemia
• Myocardial ischemia, MI, or aneurysm; CAD; rheumatic heart disease; mitral valve prolapse; heart failure; cardiomyopathy; ventricular catheters; hypokalemia; hypercalcemia; hypomagnesemia; and PE • Digoxin, procainamide, epinephrine, or quinidine toxicity • Anxiety	• If regular QRS rhythm (monomorphic), administer amiodarone (follow ACLS protocol); if drug is unsucessful, cardioversion • If irregular QRS rhythm (polymorphic) and QT interval is prolonged, stop medications that may prolong QT interval; correct electrolyte imbalance; administer magnesium; if ineffective, cardioversion • If irregular QRS rhythm (polymorphic) and QT interval is normal, stop medications that may prolong QT interval; correct electrolyte balance; administer amiodarone; if ineffective, cardioversion • If the patient with monomorphic or polymorphic QRS complexes becomes unstable, immediate defibrillation • If pulseless, initiate CPR; follow ACLS protocol for defibrillation, endotracheal (ET) intubation, and administration of epinephrine or vasopressin, followed by amiodarone or lidocaine and, if ineffective, magnesium sulfate or procainamide • Implantable cardioverter-defibrillator (ICD) if recurrent ventricular tachycardia

(continued)

Understanding cardiac arrhythmias (continued)

Arrhythmia and features

Ventricular fibrillation

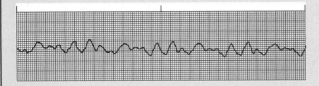

- Ventricular rhythm and rate chaotic and rapid
- QRS complexes wide and irregular; no visible P waves

Asystole

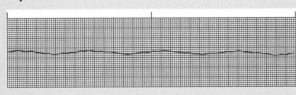

- No atrial or ventricular rate or rhythm
- No discernible P waves, QRS complexes, or T waves

- arrhythmias due to ventricular irritability
- cardiac tamponade
- hemodynamic instability
- pericardial friction rub.

What tests tell you

- ECG will reveal rhythm disturbances, such as premature ventricular contractions, premature atrial contractions, ventricular tachycardia, atrial tachycardia, and ventricular fibrillation, along with nonspecific ST-segment or T-wave changes occurring within 24 to 48 hours after the injury.
- Echocardiogram will show evidence of abnormal ventricular wall movement and decreased ejection fraction.
- Multiple-gated acquisition scan will show decreased ability of effective heart pumping.
- Cardiac enzyme levels will show elevations of CK-MB to greater than 8% of total CK within 3 to 4 hours after the injury.
- Cardiac troponin I levels may be elevated 24 hours after the injury.

How it's treated

Maintaining hemodynamic stability and adequate cardiac output are key. I.V. fluid therapy may be necessary. Continuous ECG mon-

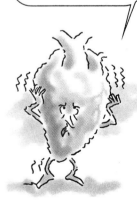

Ventricular irritability is a sure sign of cardiac contusion.

Causes	Treatment
• Myocardial ischemia, MI, untreated ventricular tachycardia, R-on-T phenomenon, hypokalemia, hyperkalemia, hypercalcemia, hypoxemia, alkalosis, electric shock, and hypothermia • Digoxin, epinephrine, or quinidine toxicity	• CPR; follow ACLS protocol for defibrillation, ET intubation, and administration of epinephrine or vasopressin, amiodarone, or lidocaine and, if ineffective, magnesium sulfate or procainamide • ICD if risk of recurrent ventricular fibrillation
• Myocardial ischemia, MI, aortic valve disease, heart failure, hypoxia, hypokalemia, severe acidosis, electric shock, ventricular arrhythmia, AV block, PE, heart rupture, cardiac tamponade, hyperkalemia, and electromechanical dissociation • Cocaine overdose	• Continue CPR; follow ACLS protocol for ET intubation, temporary pacing, and administration of epinephrine or vasopressin and atropine

itoring is used to detect arrhythmias. Lidocaine may be administered to treat ventricular arrhythmias, and digoxin may be given to treat pump failure. Inotropic agents maybe used to assist with improving cardiac output and ejection fraction.

Close watch

The patient with a cardiac contusion must be monitored closely for signs and symptoms of cardiopulmonary compromise because trauma leading to cardiac contusion is commonly associated with pulmonary trauma. Supplemental oxygen therapy may be necessary. If the extent of pulmonary trauma is great, ET intubation and mechanical ventilation may be necessary.

No if hypo

I.V. morphine may be used to treat severe pain, unless the patient is hypotensive. In the latter case, other, less potent analgesics may be used.

What to do

• Assess the patient's cardiopulmonary status at least hourly, or more frequently if indicated, to detect signs and symptoms of possible injury.
• Auscultate breath sounds at least hourly, reporting signs of congestion or fluid accumulation. Evaluate peripheral pulses and capillary refill to detect decreased peripheral tissue perfusion.

- Monitor heart rate and rhythm, heart sounds, and blood pressure every hour for changes; institute hemodynamic monitoring, including central venous pressure, PAWP, and cardiac output as indicated, at least every 1 to 2 hours.
- Administer fluid replacement therapy, including blood component therapy as prescribed, typically to maintain systolic blood pressure above 90 mm Hg.
- Monitor urine output every hour, notifying the practitioner if output is less than 30 ml/hour.
- Institute continuous cardiac monitoring to detect arrhythmias or conduction defects. If arrhythmias appear, administer antiarrhythmic agents as ordered.
- Assess the patient's degree of pain and administer analgesic therapy as ordered, monitoring him for effectiveness. Position the patient comfortably, usually with the head of the bed elevated 30 to 45 degrees.
- Prepare the patient and his family for surgery, if indicated.
- Anticipate transfer of the patient to a critical care unit when appropriate.

Cardiac tamponade

Cardiac tamponade is a rapid, unchecked increase in pressure in the pericardial sac. This increased pressure compresses the heart, impairs diastolic filling, and reduces cardiac output.

Pericardial pressure

The increase in pressure usually results from blood or fluid accumulation in the pericardial sac. Even a small amount of fluid (50 to 100 ml) can cause a serious tamponade if it accumulates rapidly.

If fluid accumulates rapidly, cardiac tamponade requires emergency lifesaving measures to prevent death. A slow accumulation and increase in pressure may not produce immediate symptoms because the fibrous wall of the pericardial sac can gradually stretch to accommodate as much as 1 to 2 L of fluid. (See *Understanding cardiac tamponade.*)

What causes it

Cardiac tamponade may result from:
- viral or postirradiation pericarditis
- acute MI
- chronic renal failure requiring dialysis

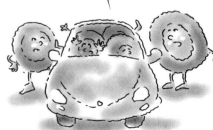

Good thing they aren't in a pericardial sac—too much blood accumulation there can lead to cardiac tamponade.

Understanding cardiac tamponade

The pericardial sac, which surrounds and protects the heart, is composed of several layers:
• The fibrous pericardium is the tough, outermost membrane.
• The inner membrane, called the *serous membrane*, consists of the visceral and parietal layers.
• The visceral layer of the heart, also known as the *epicardial layer*, clings to the heart.
• The parietal layer lies between the visceral layer and the fibrous pericardium.

• The pericardial space—between the visceral and parietal layers—contains 10 to 30 ml of pericardial fluid. This fluid lubricates the layers and minimizes friction when the heart contracts.

In cardiac tamponade (shown below right), blood or fluid fills the pericardial space, compressing the heart chambers, increasing intracardiac pressure, and obstructing venous return. As blood flow into the ventricles decreases, so does cardiac output. Without prompt treatment, low cardiac output can be fatal.

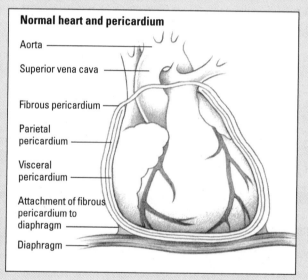

Normal heart and pericardium

Aorta

Superior vena cava

Fibrous pericardium

Parietal pericardium

Visceral pericardium

Attachment of fibrous pericardium to diaphragm

Diaphragm

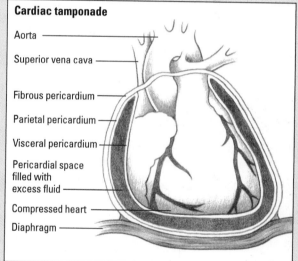

Cardiac tamponade

Aorta

Superior vena cava

Fibrous pericardium

Parietal pericardium

Visceral pericardium

Pericardial space filled with excess fluid

Compressed heart

Diaphragm

• connective tissue disorders (such as rheumatoid arthritis, systemic lupus erythematosus, rheumatic fever, vasculitis, and scleroderma)
• effusion (from cancer, bacterial infections, tuberculosis and, rarely, acute rheumatic fever)
• hemorrhage due to nontraumatic causes (such as anticoagulant therapy in patients with pericarditis or rupture of the heart or great vessels)
• hemorrhage due to trauma (such as gunshot or stab wounds of the chest)
• idiopathic causes (such as Dressler's syndrome)
• drug reaction from procainamide (Procanbid), hydralazine (Apresoline), minoxidil (Rogaine), isoniazid (Nydrazid), penicillin (Bicillin), or daunorubicin (DaunoXome).

How it happens

In cardiac tamponade, accumulation of fluid in the pericardial sac causes compression of the heart chambers. This compression obstructs blood flow into the ventricles and reduces the amount of blood that can be pumped out of the heart with each contraction.

What to look for

Cardiac tamponade has three classic features known as *Beck's triad:*

 elevated CVP with jugular vein distention

 muffled heart sounds

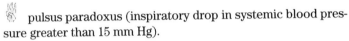 pulsus paradoxus (inspiratory drop in systemic blood pressure greater than 15 mm Hg).

That's not all

Other signs include:
- restlessness
- anxiety
- cold, clammy skin
- cyanosis
- diaphoresis
- orthopnea
- decreased arterial pressure, decreased systolic blood pressure, and narrow pulse pressure
- tachycardia and a weak, thready pulse.

What tests tell you

- Chest X-ray shows a slightly widened mediastinum and an enlarged cardiac silhouette.
- ECG may show a low-amplitude QRS complex and electrical alternans, or an alternating beat-to-beat change in amplitude of the P wave, QRS complex, and T wave. Generalized ST-segment elevation is noted in all leads. An ECG is used to rule out other cardiac disorders; it may reveal changes produced by acute pericarditis.
- PA catheterization discloses increased right atrial pressure, right ventricular diastolic pressure, and CVP.
- Echocardiography may reveal pericardial effusion with signs of right ventricular and atrial compression.
- CT scan or MRI may be used to identify pericardial effusions or pericardial thickening caused by constrictive pericarditis.

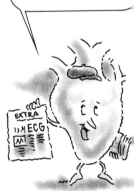

Read all about it! QRS complex amplitude at an all-time low!

How it's treated

The goal of treatment is to relieve intrapericardial pressure and cardiac compression by removing accumulated blood or fluid, which can be done three different ways:

👆 pericardiocentesis (needle aspiration of the pericardial cavity)

✌️ insertion of a drain into the pericardial sac to drain the effusion

🖐️ surgical creation of an opening, called a *pericardial window*.

When pressure is low

If the patient is hypotensive, trial volume loading with crystalloids, such as I.V. normal saline solution, may be used to maintain systolic blood pressure. An inotropic drug, such as dopamine, may be necessary to improve myocardial contractility until fluid in the pericardial sac can be removed.

Additional treatments

Additional treatment may necessary, depending on the cause. Examples of such causes and treatments are:
• heparin-induced tamponade—administration of the heparin antagonist protamine sulfate
• traumatic injury—blood transfusion or a thoracotomy to drain reaccumulating fluid or repair bleeding sites
• warfarin-induced tamponade—vitamin K administration.

What to do

• Monitor the patient's cardiovascular status frequently, at least every hour, noting the extent of jugular vein distention, quality of heart sounds, and blood pressure.
• Assess hemodynamic status, including CVP, right atrial pressure, and PAP, and determine cardiac output.
• Monitor for pulsus paradoxus.
• Be alert for ST-segment and T-wave changes on the ECG. Note rate and rhythm, and report evidence of arrhythmias.

Keep an eye on the increase

• Watch closely for signs of increasing tamponade, increasing dyspnea, and arrhythmias; report them immediately.
• Infuse I.V. solutions and inotropic drugs, such as dopamine, as ordered to maintain the patient's blood pressure.

• Administer oxygen therapy as needed and assess oxygen saturation levels. Monitor the patient's respiratory status for signs of respiratory distress, such as severe tachypnea and changes in the patient's LOC. Anticipate the need for ET intubation and mechanical ventilation if the patient's respiratory status deteriorates.

• Prepare the patient for pericardiocentesis or thoracotomy.

• If the patient has trauma-induced tamponade, assess for other signs of trauma and institute appropriate care, including the use of colloids, crystalloids, and blood component therapy under pressure or by rapid volume infuser if massive fluid replacement is needed; administration of protamine sulfate for heparin-induced tamponade; and vitamin K administration for warfarin-induced tamponade.

• Assess renal function status closely, monitoring urine output every hour and notifying the practitioner if output is less than 0.5 mg/kg/hour.

• Monitor capillary refill time, LOC, peripheral pulses, and skin temperature for evidence of diminished tissue perfusion.

• Anticipate transfer of the patient to a CCU when appropriate.

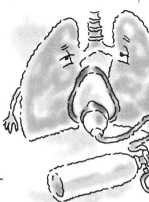

Oxygen therapy is just one aspect of cardiac tamponade treatment.

Heart failure

Heart failure results when the heart can't pump enough blood to meet the metabolic needs of the body. It results in intravascular and interstitial volume overload and poor tissue perfusion. An individual with heart failure experiences reduced exercise tolerance, a reduced quality of life, and a shortened life span.

What causes it

The most common cause of heart failure is CAD, but it also occurs in infants, children, and adults with congenital and acquired heart defects.

How it happens

Heart failure may be classified into four general categories:

 left-sided heart failure

 right-sided heart failure

 systolic dysfunction

 diastolic dysfunction.

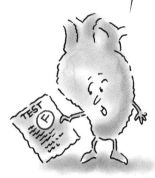

I can't believe failure was an option. I'm in real trouble!

When the left loses its faculties

Left-sided heart failure is a result of ineffective left ventricular contractile function. As the pumping ability of the left ventricle fails, cardiac output drops. Blood is no longer effectively pumped out into the body; it backs up into the left atrium and then into the lungs, causing pulmonary congestion, dyspnea, and activity intolerance. If the condition persists, pulmonary edema and right-sided heart failure may result. Common causes include:
• hypertension
• aortic and mitral valve stenosis
• left ventricular infarction.

When right goes wrong

Right-sided heart failure results from ineffective right ventricular contractile function. When blood isn't pumped effectively through the right ventricle to the lungs, blood backs up into the right atrium and into the peripheral circulation. The patient gains weight and develops peripheral edema and engorgement of the kidney and other organs.

Blame it on the left

Right-sided heart failure may be due to an acute right ventricular infarction or a pulmonary embolus. However, the most common cause is profound backward flow due to left-sided heart failure.

Just can't pump enough

Systolic dysfunction results when the left ventricle can't pump enough blood out to the systemic circulation during systole and the ejection fraction falls. Consequently, blood backs up into the pulmonary circulation and pressure increases in the pulmonary venous system. Cardiac output decreases; weakness, fatigue, and shortness of breath may occur. Causes of systolic dysfunction include MI and dilated cardiomyopathy.

It all goes to swell from here

Diastolic dysfunction results when the ability of the left ventricle to relax and fill during diastole is reduced and the stroke volume falls. Therefore, higher volumes are needed in the ventricles to maintain cardiac output. Consequently, pulmonary congestion and peripheral edema develop. Diastolic dysfunction may occur as a result of left ventricular hypertrophy, hypertension, or restrictive cardiomyopathy. This type of heart failure is less common than heart failure resulting from systolic dysfunction, and treatment isn't as clear.

Compensatory mechanisms

All types of heart failure eventually lead to reduced cardiac output, which triggers compensatory mechanisms that improve cardiac output at the expense of increased ventricular work. These compensatory mechanisms include:

- increased sympathetic activity
- activation of the renin-angiotensin-aldosterone system
- ventricular dilation
- ventricular hypertrophy.

Increased sympathetic activity

Increased sympathetic activity—a response to decreased cardiac output and blood pressure—enhances peripheral vascular resistance, contractility, heart rate, and venous return. Signs of increased sympathetic activity, such as cool extremities and clamminess, may indicate impending heart failure.

Renin-angiotensin-aldosterone system

Increased sympathetic activity also restricts blood flow to the kidneys, causing them to secrete renin, which in turn converts angiotensinogen to angiotensin I. Angiotensin I then becomes angiotensin II—a potent vasoconstrictor. Angiotensin causes the adrenal cortex to release aldosterone, leading to sodium and water retention and an increase in circulating blood volume.

This renal mechanism is helpful; however, if it persists unchecked, it can aggravate heart failure as the heart struggles to pump against the increased volume.

Ventricular dilation

In ventricular dilation, an increase in end-diastolic ventricular volume (preload) causes increased stroke work and stroke volume during contraction. This increased volume stretches cardiac muscle fibers so that the ventricle can accept the increased volume. Eventually, the muscle becomes stretched beyond optimal limits and contractility declines.

Ventricular hypertrophy

In ventricular hypertrophy, an increase in ventricular muscle mass allows the heart to pump against increased resistance to the outflow of blood, improving cardiac output. However, this increased muscle mass also increases the myocardial oxygen requirements.

Compromising situation

An increase in the ventricular diastolic pressure necessary to fill the enlarged ventricle may compromise diastolic coronary blood flow, limiting the oxygen supply to the ventricle and causing ischemia and impaired muscle contractility.

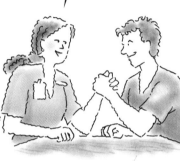

Check extremities for signs of sympathetic activity. Cold hands could mean impending heart failure.

Counterregulatory substances

In heart failure, counterregulatory substances—prostaglandins and atrial natriuretic factor—are produced in an attempt to reduce the negative effects of volume overload and vasoconstriction caused by the compensatory mechanisms.

Kidneys' contributions

The kidneys release the prostaglandins prostacyclin and prostaglandin E_2, which are potent vasodilators. These vasodilators also act to reduce volume overload produced by the renin-angiotensin-aldosterone system by inhibiting sodium and water reabsorption by the kidneys.

Counteracting hormone

Atrial natriuretic factor is a hormone that's secreted mainly by the atria in response to stimulation of the stretch receptors in the atria caused by excess fluid volume. Atrial natriuretic factor works to counteract the negative effects of sympathetic nervous system stimulation and the renin-angiotensin-aldosterone system by producing vasodilation and diuresis.

What to look for

Early signs and symptoms of left-sided heart failure include:
- fatigue
- nonproductive cough
- orthopnea
- dyspnea
- paroxysmal nocturnal dyspnea.

Later, on the left

Later clinical manifestations of left-sided heart failure may include:
- cool, pale skin
- restlessness and confusion
- displacement of the PMI toward the left anterior axillary line
- hemoptysis
- crackles on auscultation
- S_3 heart sound
- S_4 heart sound
- tachycardia.

On the right side

Clinical manifestations of right-sided heart failure include:
- weight gain
- anorexia, fullness, and nausea
- edema

- ascites or anasarca
- hepatojugular reflux and hepatomegaly
- jugular vein distention
- nocturia
- right upper quadrant pain.

What tests tell you

- Chest X-ray shows increased pulmonary vascular markings, interstitial edema, or pleural effusion and cardiomegaly.
- ECG may indicate hypertrophy, ischemic changes, or infarction and may also reveal tachycardia and extrasystoles.
- Laboratory testing may reveal abnormal liver function and elevated BUN and creatinine levels.
- ABG analysis may reveal hypoxemia from impaired gas exchange and respiratory alkalosis because the patient blows off more carbon dioxide as the respiratory rate increases in compensation.
- Echocardiography may reveal left ventricular hypertrophy, dilation, and abnormal contractility.
- Pulmonary artery monitoring typically demonstrates elevated PAP and PAWP, left ventricular end-diastolic pressure in left-sided heart failure, and elevated right atrial pressure or CVP in right-sided heart failure.
- Radionuclide ventriculography may reveal an ejection fraction less than 40%; in diastolic dysfunction, the ejection fraction may be normal.

How it's treated

The goal of therapy is to improve pump function. Correction of heart failure may involve:
- ACE inhibitors for patients with left ventricular dysfunction to reduce production of angiotensin II, resulting in preload and afterload reduction
- beta-adrenergic blockers to prevent remodeling in patients with mild to moderate heart failure caused by left ventricular systolic dysfunction
- CABG surgery or angioplasty for patients with heart failure due to CAD
- digoxin (Lanoxin) for patients with heart failure due to left ventricular systolic dysfunction to increase myocardial contractility, improve cardiac output, reduce the volume of the ventricle, and decrease ventricular stretch
- diuretics to reduce fluid volume overload, venous return, and preload

• diuretics, nitrates, morphine, and oxygen to treat pulmonary edema
• heart transplantation in patients receiving aggressive medical treatment but still experiencing limitations or repeated hospitalizations
• lifestyle modifications, such as weight loss (if obese), limited sodium (to 2 g/day) and alcohol intake, reduced fat intake, smoking cessation, stress reduction, and development of an exercise program to reduce symptoms
• other surgery or invasive procedures, such as cardiomyoplasty, insertion of an intra-aortic balloon pump (IABP), partial left ventriculectomy, use of a mechanical VAD, and implantation of an ICD or a biventricular pacemaker
• treatment of the underlying cause, if known.

What to do

• Place the patient in Fowler's position to maximize chest expansion and give supplemental oxygen, as ordered, to ease his breathing. Monitor oxygen saturation levels and ABGs as indicated. If respiratory status deteriorates, anticipate the need for ET intubation and mechanical ventilation.
• Institute continuous cardiac monitoring and notify the practitioner of changes in rhythm and rate. If the patient develops tachycardia, administer beta-adrenergic blockers as ordered; if atrial fibrillation is present, administer anticoagulants or antiplatelet agents, as ordered, to prevent thrombus formation.
• If the patient develops a new arrhythmia, obtain a 12-lead ECG immediately.
• Monitor hemodynamic status, including cardiac output, cardiac index, and pulmonary and systemic vascular pressures, at least hourly, noting trends.
• Administer medications as ordered. Check the apical heart rate before administering digoxin.

Pump up the potassium

• Expect to administer electrolyte replacement therapy (especially potassium) after the administration of diuretics to prevent such imbalances as hypokalemia and the arrhythmias that they may cause.
• Assess respiratory status frequently—at least every hour. Auscultate lungs for abnormal breath sounds, such as crackles, wheezes, and rhonchi. Encourage coughing and deep breathing.
• Obtain a baseline weight and observe for peripheral edema.
• Assess hourly urine output. Also, monitor fluid intake, including I.V. fluids.

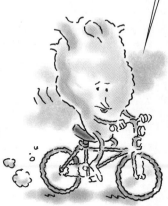

Developing an exercise program is just one lifestyle modification that can reduce symptoms of heart failure.

Education edge

Teaching about heart failure

For a patient with heart failure, education about the disorder and treatments is essential to prevent complications and minimize the effects of this condition on quality of life. Additionally, a thorough understanding of the condition may help prevent future admission to the emergency department (ED).

Although admission to the ED is commonly filled with activity, it's an opportune time to begin your teaching. Consider these points:

• Explain underlying problems associated with the patient's heart failure and typical signs and symptoms.

• Review the medications prescribed to treat heart failure.

• Review suggested lifestyle changes, including diet and energy conservation measures.

• Teach the patient about avoiding foods high in sodium, and provide him with a list of foods and their sodium content, indicating which to avoid and which to include in his diet.

• Instruct how to replace potassium lost through diuretic therapy (if appropriate) by taking prescribed potassium supplements or eating potassium-rich foods, such as bananas and apricots, and drinking orange juice.

• Encourage the patient to weigh himself daily and keep a record of his weights; urge the patient to report a weight gain or loss of 2 lb (0.9 kg) or more in 3 or 4 days.

• Stress the importance of taking medications as prescribed; instruct the patient in possible adverse effects and signs and symptoms of toxicity.

• Instruct the patient on how to monitor pulse rate; advise him to report a pulse rate that's unusually irregular or less than 60 beats/minute.

• Review the danger signs and symptoms to report to his practitioner, such as dizziness, blurred vision, shortness of breath, persistent dry cough, palpitations, increased fatigue, swelling of the ankles, and decreased urine output.

• Encourage adherence to medical follow-up, including checkups and periodic blood tests.

• Organize all activities to provide maximum rest periods. Assess for signs of activity intolerance, such as increased shortness of breath, chest pain, increased arrhythmias, heart rate greater than 120 beats/minute, and ST-segment changes, and have the patient stop activity.

• Prepare the patient for surgical intervention or insertion of an IABP or ICD, or transfer to the critical care unit if indicated.

• Begin patient teaching related to heart failure and measures to reduce the risk of complications. (See *Teaching about heart failure.*)

Hypertensive crisis

A hypertensive emergency, commonly called *hypertensive crisis*, refers to the abrupt, acute, marked increase in blood pressure from the patient's baseline that ultimately leads to acute and rapidly progressing end-organ damage.

Rapid rise

Typically, in a hypertensive crisis, the patient's diastolic blood pressure is greater than 120 mm Hg. The increased blood pressure value, although important, is probably less important than how rapidly the blood pressure increases.

What causes it

Most patients who develop hypertensive crisis have long histories of chronic, poorly controlled, or untreated primary hypertension. Conditions that cause secondary hypertension, such as pheochromocytoma or Cushing's syndrome, may also be responsible.

How it happens

Arterial blood pressure is a product of total peripheral resistance and cardiac output:
• Cardiac output is increased by conditions that increase heart rate, stroke volume, or both.
• Peripheral resistance is increased by factors that increase blood viscosity or reduce the lumen size of vessels, especially the arterioles.

Faulty mechanisms

Hypertension may result from a disturbance in one of the body's intrinsic mechanisms, including:
• sympathetic nervous system
• antidiuretic hormone
• autoregulation
• renin-angiotensin system.

Up with pressure

The renin-angiotensin system increases blood pressure in several ways.
• Sodium depletion, reduced blood pressure, and dehydration stimulate renin release.
• Renin reacts with angiotensinogen, a liver enzyme, and converts it to angiotensin I, which increases preload and afterload.
• Angiotensin I converts to angiotensin II in the lungs; angiotensin II is a potent vasoconstrictor that targets the arterioles.

• Circulating angiotensin II increases preload and afterload by stimulating the adrenal cortex to secrete aldosterone. This secretion increases blood volume by conserving sodium and water.

Maintaining flow

In autoregulation, several intrinsic mechanisms together change an artery's diameter to maintain tissue and organ perfusion despite fluctuations in systemic blood pressure. These mechanisms include:
• stress relaxation, in which blood vessels gradually dilate when blood pressure increases, reducing peripheral resistance
• capillary fluid shift, in which plasma moves between vessels and extravascular spaces to maintain intravascular volume.

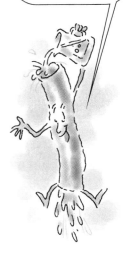

Capillary fluid shift is part of autoregulation.

Taking control

Sympathetic nervous system mechanisms control blood pressure. When blood pressure decreases, baroreceptors in the aortic arch and carotid sinuses decrease their inhibition of the medulla's vasomotor center.

Consequent increases in sympathetic stimulation of the heart by norepinephrine increases cardiac output by:
• strengthening the contractile force
• raising the heart rate
• augmenting peripheral resistance by vasoconstriction.

Regulating reabsorption

Stress can also stimulate the sympathetic nervous system to increase cardiac output and peripheral vascular resistance. The release of antidiuretic hormone can regulate hypotension by increasing reabsorption of water by the kidney. In reabsorption, blood plasma volume increases, thus raising blood pressure. In hypertensive crisis, one or more of these regulating mechanisms is disrupted. (See *What happens in hypertensive crisis.*)

Strain for the brain

In hypertensive crisis, the blood pressure–regulating mechanism is disturbed, causing cerebral vasodilation. Blood flow increases, causing an increase in pressure and subsequent cerebral edema. This increase in pressure damages the intimal and medial lining of the arterioles.

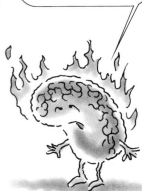

Bad for the heart, bad for the head. Hypertensive crisis can lead to cerebral edema.

What to look for

Your assessment of a patient in hypertensive crisis almost always reveals a history of hypertension that's poorly controlled or hasn't been treated. Signs and symptoms may include:
• dizziness

What happens in hypertensive crisis

Hypertensive crisis is a severe rise in arterial blood pressure caused by a disturbance in one or more of the regulating mechanisms. If untreated, hypertensive crisis may result in renal, cardiac, or cerebral complications and, possibly, death. This flowchart outlines the process.

Causes of hypertensive crisis

- Abnormal renal function
- Eclampsia
- Hypertensive encephalopathy
- Intracerebral hemorrhage
- Monoamine oxidase inhibitor interactions
- Myocardial ischemia
- Pheochromocytoma
- Withdrawal of antihypertensive drugs (abrupt)

↓

Prolonged hypertension

↓

Inflammation and necrosis of arterioles

↓

Narrowing of blood vessels

↓

Restriction of blood flow to major organs

↓

Organ damage

↓

Renal
- Decreased renal perfusion
- Progressive deterioration of nephrons
- Decreased ability to concentrate urine
- Increased serum creatinine and blood urea nitrogen
- Increased renal tubule permeability with protein leakage into tubules
- Renal insufficiency
- Uremia
- Renal failure

Cardiac
- Decreased cardiac perfusion
- Coronary artery disease
- Angina or myocardial infarction
- Increased cardiac workload
- Left ventricular hypertrophy
- Heart failure

Cerebral
- Decreased cerebral perfusion
- Increased stress on vessel wall
- Arterial spasm
- Ischemia
- Transient ischemic attacks
- Weakening of vessel intima
- Aneurysm formation
- Intracranial hemorrhage

- confusion, somnolence, or stupor
- irritability
- nausea
- vomiting
- anorexia
- edema
- acute retinopathy and hemorrhage, retinal exudates, and papilledema
- angina
- dyspnea on exertion, orthopnea, or paroxysmal nocturnal dyspnea
- possible left ventricular heave palpated at the mitral valve area
- severe, throbbing headache in the back of the head
- S_4 heart sound
- vision loss, blurred vision, or diplopia.

Check the head

If the patient has hypertensive encephalopathy, you may note:
- disorientation
- decreased LOC
- seizures.

Kidney-related consequences

If the hypertensive emergency has affected the kidneys, you may note reduced urine output as well as elevated BUN and creatinine levels.

What tests tell you

- Blood pressure measurement—when obtained several times at an interval of at least 2 minutes, revealing an elevated diastolic pressure greater than 120 mm Hg—confirms the diagnosis of hypertensive crisis.
- RBC count may be decreased secondary to hematuria if the kidneys are involved.
- If the kidneys are involved, BUN may be greater than 20 mg/dl and the serum creatinine level may be greater than 1.3 mg/dl.
- ECG may reveal ischemic changes or left ventricular hypertrophy. ST-segment depression and T-wave inversion suggest repolarization problems from endocardial fibrosis associated with left ventricular hypertrophy.
- Echocardiography may reveal increased wall thickness with or without an increase in left ventricle size.
- Chest X-ray may reveal enlargement of the cardiac silhouette with left ventricular dilation, or pulmonary congestion and pleural effusions with heart failure.

• Urinalysis results may be normal unless renal impairment occurs; then specific gravity is low (less than 1.010), and hematuria, casts, and proteinuria may also be found. If the patient's condition is due to a disease condition such as pheochromocytoma, a 24-hour urine test reveals increases in vanillylmandelic acid and urinary catecholamines.

How it's treated

Treatment of hypertensive crisis immediately focuses on reducing the patient's blood pressure with I.V. antihypertensive therapy. However, you must take care not to reduce the patient's blood pressure too rapidly because his autoregulatory control is impaired.

Slow pressure cuts

The current recommendation is to reduce blood pressure by no more than 25% of the MAP over the first 2 hours. The next several days should bring further reductions. Here are some additional guidelines:

• Sodium nitroprusside, given as an I.V. infusion and titrated according to the patient's response, is the drug of choice. It has a rapid onset of action, and its effects cease within 1 to 5 minutes of stopping the drug. Thus, if the patient's blood pressure drops too low, stopping the drug enables the blood pressure to increase almost immediately.

• Other agents that may be used include labetalol (Normodyne), nitroglycerin (Nitro-Bid) (the drug of choice for treating hypertensive crisis when myocardial ischemia, acute MI, or pulmonary edema is present), and hydralazine (Apresoline) (specifically indicated for treating hypertension in pregnant women with preeclampsia).

• Lifestyle changes may include weight reduction, smoking cessation, exercise, and dietary changes.

• After the acute episode is controlled, maintenance pharmacotherapy to control blood pressure plays a key role.

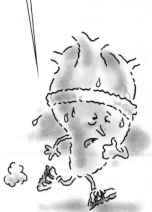

When it comes to reducing blood pressure with I.V. antihypertensive therapy, slow and steady wins the race: no more than 25% of the MAP over the first 2 hours.

What to do

• Immediately obtain the patient's blood pressure.

• Institute continuous cardiac and arterial pressure monitoring to assess blood pressure directly; determine the patient's MAP.

• Assess ABGs. Monitor the patient's oxygen saturation level using pulse oximetry; if you're monitoring the patient hemodynamically, assess mixed venous oxygen saturation. Administer supplemental oxygen, as ordered, based on the findings.

- Administer I.V. antihypertensive therapy as ordered; titrate I.V. antihypertensive medications according to the desired response and parameters set by the practitioner.
- If using nitroprusside (Nipride), wrap the container in foil to protect it from the light and titrate the dose based on specified target ranges for systolic and diastolic pressures. Immediately stop the drug if the patient's blood pressure drops below the target range.
- If the patient is receiving nitroprusside (Nitropress) therapy, assess for signs and symptoms of thiocyanate toxicity, such as fatigue, nausea, tinnitus, blurred vision, and delirium. Nitroprusside is metabolized to thiocyanate, which is excreted by the kidneys. If signs are present, obtain a serum thiocyanate level; if it's greater than 10 mg/dl, notify the practitioner.

Much monitoring

- Monitor blood pressure every 1 to 5 minutes while titrating drug therapy, then every 15 minutes to 1 hour as the patient's condition stabilizes.
- Continuously monitor ECG and institute treatment as indicated if you find arrhythmias. Auscultate the patient's heart, noting signs of heart failure such as S_3 or S_4 heart sounds.
- Assess the patient's neurologic status frequently—every 15 to 30 minutes initially and then every hour, based on the patient's response to therapy.

Check in on output

- Monitor urine output every hour, and notify the practitioner if output is less than 0.5 ml/kg/hour. Evaluate BUN and serum creatinine levels for changes, and monitor daily weights.
- Administer other antihypertensives as ordered. If the patient is experiencing fluid overload, administer diuretics as ordered.
- Assess the patient's vision and report changes, such as increased blurred vision, diplopia, or loss of vision.
- Administer analgesics as ordered for headache; keep your patient's environment quiet, with low lighting.
- Anticipate transfer of the patient to the CCU as indicated.
- Provide support to the patient and his family; begin patient teaching related to the condition and measures to reduce the risk of complications as the patient's condition begins to stabilize. (See *Teaching about hypertensive crisis.*)

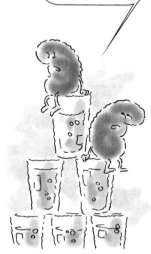

Stay in the know about your patient's urine flow! Less than 0.5 ml/kg/hour means there's a problem.

Education edge

Teaching about hypertensive crisis

Hypertensive crisis is an emergency situation that most commonly results from inadequately controlled hypertension or untreated hypertension. As a result, you need to educate the patient about measures to control his hypertension to reduce the risk of complications and a recurrence of the crisis. As the patient's condition begins to stabilize and time permits, begin your teaching. Consider these points:

• Explain the underlying events associated with the patient's current crisis.

• Review the medications being used to treat this acute condition.

• Reinforce all aspects of blood pressure control, such as diet, medications, and lifestyle changes.

• Stress the need for adherence to medication therapy and frequent medical follow up.

• Explain the prescribed medication regimen, including dosage, frequency, adverse effects, and when to notify the practitioner.

• Reinforce necessary lifestyle changes and the need for regular exercise.

• Instruct the patient in signs and symptoms associated with possible complications, such as changes in levels of alertness, headache, vision changes, reduced urine output, and weight gain, along with the need to notify the practitioner if any occur.

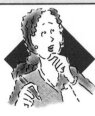

Quick quiz

1. Which sign or symptom would the nurse expect to assess in a patient who's admitted to the ED with a diagnosis of cardiac tamponade?

    A.   Shortness of breath
    B.   Pulsus paradoxus
    C.   Holosystolic murmur
    D.   Bounding peripheral pulse

Answer: B. Pulsus paradoxus (inspiratory drop in systemic blood pressure greater than 15 mm Hg) is one of the three classic signs of cardiac tamponade. The other classic signs are elevated CVP with jugular vein distention and muffled heart sounds.

2. A patient receiving I.V. nitroprusside for treatment of hypertensive crisis develops blurred vision and tinnitus. The nurse also notes that his LOC has decreased. Which action is most appropriate?

    A. Increase the rate of nitroprusside infusion.
    B. Obtain an order for an antiarrhythmic.
    C. Obtain a serum thiocyanate level.
    D. Increase the flow rate of supplemental oxygen.

Answer: C. The patient is exhibiting signs and symptoms of thiocyanate toxicity, which include fatigue, nausea, tinnitus, blurred vision, and delirium. Therefore, the nurse must obtain a serum thiocyanate level and notify the practitioner if the level is greater than 10 mg/dl.

3. Which assessment finding would the nurse expect to find elevated in a client admitted with right-sided heart failure?

    A. CVP
    B. Left-ventricular end-diastolic pressure
    C. PAWP
    D. Cardiac output

Answer: A. CVP is elevated in right-sided heart failure.

4. When performing synchronized cardioversion, the nurse understands that the electrical charge is delivered at which point?

    A. Initiation of the QRS complex
    B. During the ST segment
    C. At the peak of the R wave
    D. Just before the onset of the P wave

Answer: C. Synchronized cardioversion delivers an electrical charge to the myocardium at the peak of the R wave.

Scoring

☆☆☆ If you answered all four questions correctly, let your heart swell with pride. You're tops when it comes to cardiac emergencies!

☆☆ If you answered three questions correctly, congratulations on all your "heart" work. You're a member of the cardiac emergency team!

☆ If you answered fewer than three questions correctly, don't be heartbroken. Just go back and review the chapter!

Respiratory emergencies

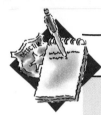

Just the facts

In this chapter, you'll learn:

♦ assessment of the respiratory system

♦ respiratory disorders and treatments

♦ diagnostic tests and procedures for respiratory emergencies.

Understanding respiratory emergencies

Respiratory emergencies can be caused by obstructions, infections, or injury of the respiratory system. Any trauma that alters the integrity of the respiratory system can alter gas exchange. Respiratory emergencies can be life-threatening and require your expert assessment techniques and prompt interventions.

Assessment

Respiratory assessment is a critical nursing responsibility in the emergency department (ED). Conduct a thorough assessment to detect subtle and obvious respiratory changes.

History

Build your patient's health history by asking short, open-ended questions. Conduct the interview in several short sessions if you have to, depending on the severity of your patient's condition. Ask his family to provide information if he can't.

I know respiratory emergencies can be life-threatening, but don't panic! This chapter helps you deal with them.

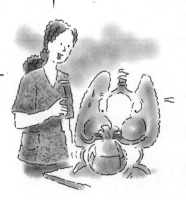

Cover all the bases

Respiratory disorders may be caused or exacerbated by obesity, smoking, and workplace conditions, so be sure to ask about these factors.

Current health status

Begin by asking why your patient is seeking care. Because many respiratory disorders are chronic, ask how his latest acute episode compares with the previous episode and which relief measures are helpful and not helpful. Patients with respiratory disorders commonly report such complaints as:

- chest pain
- cough
- shortness of breath
- sleep disturbance
- sputum production
- wheezing.

Chest pain

If the patient has chest pain, ask: Where's the pain? What does it feel like? Is it sharp, stabbing, burning, or aching? Does it move to another area? How long does it last? What causes it? What makes it better?

Pain provocations

Chest pain due to a respiratory problem is usually the result of pleural inflammation, inflammation of the costochondral junctions, soreness of chest muscles because of coughing, or indigestion. Less common causes of pain include rib or vertebral fractures caused by coughing or osteoporosis.

Cough

Ask the patient with a cough: At what time of day do you cough most often? Is the cough productive? If the cough is a chronic problem, has it changed recently? If so, how? What makes the cough better? What makes it worse?

Shortness of breath

Assess your patient's shortness of breath by asking him to rate his usual level of dyspnea on a scale of 1 to 10, in which 1 means no dyspnea and 10 means the worst he has experienced. Then ask him to rate the level that day. Other scales grade dyspnea as it relates to activity, such as climbing a set of stairs or walking a city block. (See *Grading dyspnea*.)

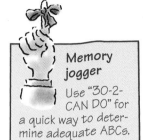

Memory jogger

Use "30-2-CAN DO" for a quick way to determine adequate ABCs.

The adult patient has adequate oxygenation and perfusion or circulation if the patient:

- has fewer than 30 respirations per minute (30)
- is oriented to person and situation (2)
- obeys simple verbal requests (CAN DO).

Pillow talk

A patient with orthopnea (shortness of breath when lying down) tends to sleep with his upper body elevated. Ask the patient how many pillows he uses; the answer reflects the severity of the orthopnea. For instance, a patient who uses three pillows can be said to have *three-pillow orthopnea*.

Don't forget to ask

In addition to using a severity scale, ask: What do you do to relieve the shortness of breath? How well does it usually work?

Sleep disturbance

Sleep disturbances may be related to obstructive sleep apnea or another sleep disorder requiring additional evaluation.

Daytime drowsiness

If the patient complains of being drowsy or irritable in the daytime, ask: How many hours of continuous sleep do you get at night? Do you wake up often during the night? Does your family complain about your snoring or restlessness?

Sputum production

If a patient produces sputum, ask him to estimate—in teaspoons or some other common measurement—the amount produced. Also ask: What's the color and consistency of the sputum? If sputum is a chronic problem, has it changed recently? If so, how? Do you cough up blood? If so, how much and how often?

Wheezing

If a patient wheezes, ask: When do you wheeze? What makes you wheeze? Do you wheeze loudly enough for others to hear it? What helps stop your wheezing?

Previous health status

Look at the patient's health history, being especially watchful for:
• allergies
• respiratory diseases, such as pneumonia and tuberculosis (TB)
• smoking habit
• exposure to secondhand smoke
• previous operations.

   Ask about current immunizations, such as a flu shot or pneumococcal vaccine. Also determine whether the patient uses respiratory equipment, such as oxygen and nebulizers, at home.

Grading dyspnea

To assess dyspnea as objectively as possible, ask your patient to briefly describe how various activities affect his breathing. Then document his response using this grading system:
• *Grade 0*—not troubled by breathlessness except with strenuous exercise
• *Grade 1*—troubled by shortness of breath when hurrying on a level path or walking up a slight hill
• *Grade 2*—walks more slowly than people of the same age on a level path because of breathlessness, or has to stop to breathe when walking on a level path at his own pace
• *Grade 3*—stops to breathe after walking about 100 yards (91 m) on a level path
• *Grade 4*—too breathless to leave the house, or breathless when dressing or undressing.

Family history

Ask the patient whether he has a family history of cancer, sickle cell anemia, heart disease, or chronic illness, such as asthma and emphysema. Determine if he lives with anyone who has an infectious disease, such as TB or influenza.

Lifestyle patterns

Ask about the patient's workplace, because some jobs, such as coal mining and construction work, expose workers to substances that can cause lung disease.

Also ask about the patient's home, community, and other environmental factors that may influence how he deals with his respiratory problems. For example, you may ask questions about interpersonal relationships, stress management, and coping methods. Ask about the patient's sex habits or drug use, which may be connected with acquired immunodeficiency syndrome–related pulmonary disorders.

Physical examination

In most cases, you should begin the physical examination after you take the patient's history. However, you may not be able to take a complete history if the patient develops an ominous sign such as acute respiratory distress. If your patient is in respiratory distress, establish the priorities of your nursing assessment, progressing from the most critical factors (airway, breathing, and circulation) to less critical factors. (See *Emergency respiratory assessment.*)

Four steps

Use a systematic approach to detect subtle and obvious respiratory changes. The four steps for conducting a physical examination of the respiratory system are:

- inspection
- palpation
- percussion
- auscultation.

Back, then front

Examine the back of the chest first, using inspection, palpation, percussion, and auscultation. Always compare one side with the other. Then examine the front of the chest using the same sequence. The patient can lie back when you examine the front of the chest if that's more comfortable for him.

Stay on the ball

Emergency respiratory assessment

If your patient is in acute respiratory distress, immediately assess the ABCs—airway, breathing, and circulation. If these are absent, call for help and start cardiopulmonary resuscitation.

Next, quickly check for these signs of impending crisis:
• Is the patient having trouble breathing?
• Is the patient using accessory muscles to breathe? If chest excursion is less than the normal 1⅛" to 2⅜" (3 to 6 cm), look for evidence that the patient is using accessory muscles when he breathes, including shoulder elevation, intercostal muscle retraction, and use of scalene and sternocleidomastoid muscles.
• Has the patient's level of consciousness diminished?
• Is he confused, anxious, or agitated?

• Does he change his body position to ease breathing?
• Does his skin look pale, diaphoretic, or cyanotic?

Setting priorities
If your patient is in respiratory distress, establish priorities for your nursing assessment. Don't assume the obvious. Note positive and negative factors, starting with the most critical factors (the ABCs) and progressing to less critical factors.

If you don't have time to go through each step of the nursing process, make sure you gather enough data to answer vital questions. A single sign or symptom has many possible meanings, so gather a group of findings to assess the patient and develop interventions.

Inspection

Make a few observations about the patient as soon as you enter the patient care area and include these observations in your assessment. Note the patient's position on the stretcher. Does he appear comfortable? Is he sitting up, lying quietly, or shifting about? Does he appear anxious? Is he having trouble breathing? Does he require oxygen?

Chest inspection

Inspect the patient's chest configuration, tracheal position, chest symmetry, skin condition, nostrils (for flaring), and accessory muscle use.

Beauty in symmetry

Look for chest wall symmetry. Both sides of the chest should be equal at rest and expand equally as the patient inhales. The diameter of the chest, from front to back, should be about one-half of the width of the chest.

A new angle

Also, look at the costal angle (the angle between the ribs and the sternum at the point immediately above the xiphoid process). This angle should be less than 90 degrees in an adult. The angle is larger if the chest wall is chronically expanded because of an enlargement of the intercostal muscles, as can happen with chronic obstructive pulmonary disease (COPD).

Muscles in motion

When the patient inhales, his diaphragm should descend and the intercostal muscles should contract. This dual motion causes the abdomen to push out and the lower ribs to expand laterally.

When the patient exhales, his abdomen and ribs return to their resting positions. The upper chest shouldn't move much. Accessory muscles may hypertrophy, indicating frequent use. This may be normal in some athletes, but for most patients it indicates a respiratory problem, especially when the patient purses his lips and flares his nostrils when breathing.

Chest wall abnormalities

Inspect for chest wall abnormalities, keeping in mind that a patient with a deformity of the chest wall might have completely normal lungs that could be cramped in the chest. The patient may have a smaller-than-normal lung capacity and limited exercise tolerance.

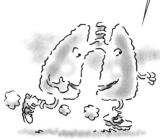

Hypertrophy in accessory muscles can be normal in some athletes, but in most patients it signals respiratory problems.

Raising a red flag

Watch for paradoxical (uneven) movement of the patient's chest wall. Paradoxical movement may appear as an abnormal collapse of part of the chest wall when the patient inhales or an abnormal expansion when the patient exhales. In either case, such uneven movement indicates a loss of normal chest wall function.

Breathing rate and pattern

Assess your patient's respiratory function by determining the rate, rhythm, and quality of respirations.

Count on it

The respiratory pattern should be even, coordinated, and regular, with occasional sighs. The normal ratio of inspiration to expiration (ratio I:E) is about 1:2.

Abnormal respiratory patterns

Cheyne-Stokes

Cheyne-Stokes respirations are initially shallow but gradually become deeper and deeper; then a period of apnea follows, lasting up to 20 seconds, and the cycle starts again. This respiratory pattern is seen in patients with heart failure, kidney failure, or central nervous system (CNS) damage. Cheyne-Stokes respirations can be a normal breathing pattern during sleep in elderly patients.

Biot's respirations
Biot's respirations involve rapid, deep breaths that alternate with abrupt periods of apnea. It's an ominous sign of severe CNS damage.

Inspecting related structures
Inspect the patient's skin for cyanosis or clubbing.

Don't be blue

Skin color varies considerably among patients, but a patient with a bluish tint to his skin, nail beds, and mucous membranes is considered cyanotic. Cyanosis, which results when oxygenation to the tissues is poor, is a late sign of hypoxemia.

Finger findings

When you inspect the fingers, assess for clubbing, a sign of long-standing respiratory or cardiac disease. The fingernail normally enters the skin at an angle of less than 180 degrees. In clubbed fingers, the angle is greater than or equal to 180 degrees.

Palpation

Palpation of the chest provides some important information about the respiratory system and the processes involved in breathing.

Leaky lungs

The chest wall should feel smooth, warm, and dry. Crepitus, which feels like puffed-rice cereal crackling under the skin, indicates that air is leaking from the airways or lungs.

Probing palpation pain

Gentle palpation shouldn't cause the patient pain. If the patient complains of chest pain, try to find a painful area on the chest wall. Here's a guide to assessing some types of chest pain:
• Painful costochondral joints are typically located at the mid-clavicular line or next to the sternum.
• A rib or vertebral fracture is quite painful over the fracture.
• Protracted coughing may cause sore muscles.
• A collapsed lung can cause pain in addition to dyspnea.

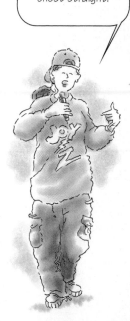

Don't hate me cuz I palpate; I'm only tryin' to get the pain in your chest straight!

Feeling for fremitus

Palpate for tactile fremitus (palpable vibrations caused by the transmission of air through the bronchopulmonary system). Fremitus decreases over areas where pleural fluid collects, when the patient speaks softly, and with pneumothorax, atelectasis, and emphysema.

Fremitus is increased normally over the large bronchial tubes and abnormally over areas in which alveoli are filled with fluid or exudates, as happens in pneumonia. (See *Checking for tactile fremitus.*)

Evaluating symmetry

To evaluate your patient's chest wall symmetry and expansion, place your hands on the front of the chest wall with your thumbs touching each other at the second intercostal space. As the patient inhales deeply, watch your thumbs. They should separate simultaneously and equally to a distance several centimeters away from the sternum. Repeat the measurement at the fifth intercostal space. You may make the same measurement on the back of the chest near the 10th rib.

Warning signs

The patient's chest may expand asymmetrically if he has:
• pneumonia
• atelectasis
• pleural effusion
• pneumothorax.

Chest expansion may be decreased at the level of the diaphragm if the patient has:
• respiratory depression
• emphysema
• obesity
• ascites
• atelectasis
• diaphragm paralysis.

Percussion

Percuss the chest to:
• find the boundaries of the lungs
• determine whether the lungs are filled with air, fluid, or solid material
• evaluate the distance the diaphragm travels between the patient's inhalation and exhalation.

> Percuss the chest to determine whether lungs are filled with air, fluid, or solid material.

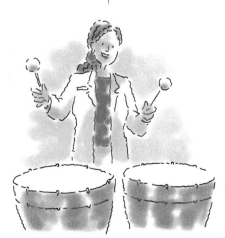

Checking for tactile fremitus

When you check the back of the thorax for tactile fremitus, ask the patient to fold his arms across his chest, as shown here. This movement shifts the scapulae out of the way.

What to do
Check for tactile fremitus by lightly placing your open palms on both sides of the patient's back without touching his back with your fingers, as shown here. Ask the patient to repeat the phrase "ninety-nine" loudly enough to produce palpable vibrations. Then palpate the front of the chest using the same hand positions.

What the results mean
Vibrations that feel more intense on one side than on the other indicate tissue consolidation on that side. Less intense vibrations may indicate emphysema, pneumothorax, or pleural effusion. Faint or no vibrations in the upper posterior thorax may indicate bronchial obstruction or a fluid-filled pleural space.

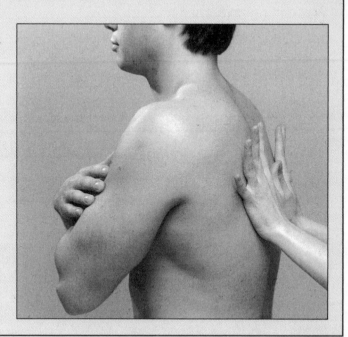

Sites and sounds

Listen for normal, resonant sounds over most of the chest. In the left front chest wall from the third or fourth intercostal space at the sternum to the third or fourth intercostal space at the midclavicular line, listen for a dull sound because that's the space occupied by the heart. With careful percussion, you can identify the borders of the heart when lung tissue is normal. Resonance resumes at the sixth intercostal space. The sequence of sounds in the back is slightly different. (See *Percussion sequences*, page 210.)

Warning sounds

When you hear hyperresonance during percussion, it means you've found an area of increased air in the lung or pleural space. Expect to hear hyperresonance in patients with:
• acute asthma
• pneumothorax
• bullous emphysema (large holes in the lungs from alveolar destruction).

When you hear abnormal dullness, it means you've found areas of decreased air in the lungs. Expect abnormal dullness in the presence of:

Percussion sequences

Follow these percussion sequences to distinguish between normal and abnormal sounds in the patient's lungs. Compare sound variations from one side with the other as you proceed. Carefully describe abnormal sounds you hear and note their locations. (Follow the same sequence for auscultation.)

Anterior

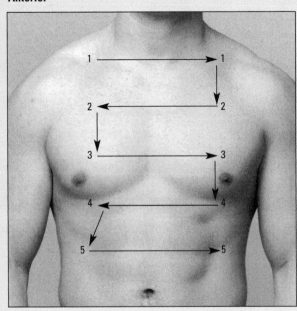

Posterior

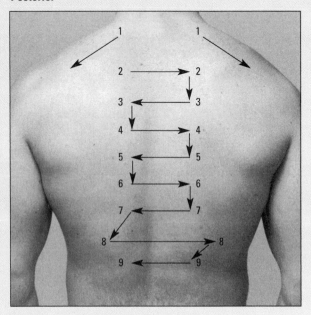

- pleural fluid
- consolidation atelectasis
- tumor.

Detecting diaphragm movement

Percussion also allows you to assess how much the diaphragm moves during inspiration and expiration. The normal diaphragm descends $1^{1}/_{8}''$ to $1^{7}/_{8}''$ (3 to 5 cm) when the patient inhales. The diaphragm doesn't move as far in patients with emphysema, respiratory depression, diaphragm paralysis, atelectasis, obesity, or ascites.

Auscultation

As air moves through the bronchi, it creates sound waves that travel to the chest wall. The sound produced by breathing changes as air moves from larger to smaller airways. Sounds also change if they pass through fluid, mucus, or narrowed airways.

Auscultation preparation

Auscultation sites are the same as percussion sites. Using the diaphragm of the stethoscope, listen to a full cycle of inspiration and expiration at each site. Ask the patient to breathe through his mouth if it doesn't cause discomfort; nose breathing alters the pitch of breath sounds.

Be firm

To auscultate for breath sounds, press the diaphragm side of the stethoscope firmly against the skin. Remember that, if you listen through clothing or chest hair, breath sounds won't be heard clearly and you may hear unusual and deceptive sounds.

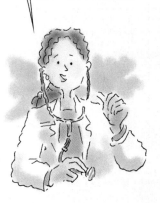

Normally I'd say that breathing through one's mouth is rude, but when you're auscultating, I say the mouth the merrier!

Interpreting breath sounds

Classify each breath sound you auscultate by its intensity, pitch, duration, characteristic, and location. Note whether it occurs during inspiration, expiration, or both.

Normal breath sounds

During auscultation, listen for four types of breath sounds over normal lungs. (See *Locations of normal breath sounds*, page 212.) Here's a rundown of the normal breath sounds and their characteristics:
• Tracheal breath sounds, heard over the trachea, are harsh and discontinuous. They're present when the patient inhales or exhales.
• Bronchial breath sounds, usually heard next to the trachea just above or below the clavicle, are loud, high-pitched, and discontinuous. They're loudest when the patient exhales.
• Bronchovesicular sounds are medium-pitched and continuous. They're best heard over the upper third of the sternum and between the scapulae when the patient inhales or exhales.
• Vesicular sounds, heard over the rest of the lungs, are soft and low-pitched. They're prolonged during inhalation and shortened during exhalation. (See *Qualities of normal breath sounds*, page 212.)

Abnormal breath sounds

Because solid tissue transmits sound better than air or fluid, breath sounds (as well as spoken or whispered words) are louder than normal over areas of consolidation. If pus, fluid, or air fills the pleural space, breath sounds are quieter than normal. If a for-

Qualities of normal breath sounds

Use this chart as a quick reference for the qualities of normal breath sounds.

Breath sound	Quality	Inspiration-expiration ratio	Location
Tracheal	Harsh, high-pitched	I < E	Over trachea
Bronchial	Loud, high-pitched	I > E	Next to trachea
Bronchovesicular	Medium in loudness and pitch	I = E	Next to sternum, between scapula
Vesicular	Soft, low-pitched	I > E	Remainder of lungs

Locations of normal breath sounds

These photographs show the normal locations of different types of breath sounds.

Anterior thorax

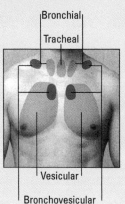

Posterior thorax

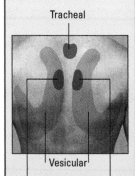

eign body or secretions obstruct a bronchus, breath sounds are diminished or absent over lung tissue distal to the obstruction.

Detect the unexpected

Breath sounds heard in an unexpected area are also abnormal. For instance, if you hear bronchial sounds where you expect to hear vesicular sounds, the area you're auscultating might be filled with fluid or exudates, as in pneumonia. The vesicular sounds you expect to hear in those areas are absent because no air is moving through the small airways. Some common abnormal breath sounds are vocal fremitus and adventitious breath sounds.

Vocal fremitus

Vocal fremitus is the sound produced by chest vibrations as the patient speaks. Voice sounds can transmit abnormally over consolidated areas because sound travels well through fluid. There are three common abnormal voice sounds:

Bronchophony—Ask the patient to say "ninety-nine" or "blue moon." Over normal tissue, the words sound muffled, but over consolidated areas, the words sound unusually loud.

Egophony—Ask the patient to say "E." Over normal lung tissue, the sound is muffled, but over consolidated areas, it sounds like the letter A.

Whispered pectoriloquy—Ask the patient to whisper "1, 2, 3." Over normal lung tissue, the numbers are almost indistinguishable. Over consolidated tissue, the numbers sound loud and clear.

Abnormal breath sounds

Here's a quick guide to assessing abnormal breath sounds.

Crackles

Crackles are intermittent, nonmusical, crackling sounds heard during inspiration. They're classified as *fine* or *coarse* and are common in elderly people when small sections of the alveoli don't fully aerate and secretions accumulate during sleep. Alveoli reexpand or pop open when the patient takes deep breaths upon awakening. Fine crackles sound like strands of hair being rubbed between the fingers. Coarse crackles sound like bubbling or gurgling as air moves through secretions in larger airways.

Wheezes

Wheezes are high-pitched sounds caused by blocked airflow and are heard on exhalation, or also on inspection as the block increases.

Patients may wheeze as a result of asthma, infection, or airway obstruction from a tumor or foreign body.

Rhonchi

Rhonchi are low-pitched, snoring or rattling sounds heard primarily on exhalation, and usually change with coughing.

Stridor

Stridor is a loud, high-pitched sound heard during inspiration.

Pleural friction rub

Pleural friction rub is a low-pitched, grating sound heard during inspiration and expiration and is accompanied by pain.

Adventitious sounds

Adventitious sounds are abnormal no matter where you hear them in the lungs. (See *Abnormal breath sounds*.) There are five types of adventitious breath sounds:

 crackles

 wheezes

 rhonchi

 stridor

 pleural friction rub.

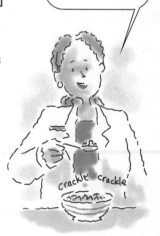

Crackles aren't just for breakfast—they also signal problems with alveoli.

Diagnostic tests

If your patient's history and the physical examination findings reveal evidence of pulmonary dysfunction, diagnostic tests can identify and evaluate the dysfunction. These tests include:
• bedside testing procedures
• blood and sputum studies

- endoscopy and imaging
- pulmonary angiography.

Pulse oximetry

Pulse oximetry is a relatively simple procedure used to monitor arterial oxygen saturation noninvasively. It's performed intermittently or continuously.

Shedding light on the subject

In this procedure, two diodes send red and infrared light through a pulsating arterial vascular bed such as the one in the fingertip. A photodetector (also called a *sensor* or *transducer*) slipped over the finger measures the transmitted light as it passes through the vascular bed, detects the relative amount of color absorbed by arterial blood, and calculates the saturation without interference from the venous blood, skin, or connective tissue. The percentage expressed is the ratio of oxygen to hemoglobin. (See *A closer look at pulse oximetry.*)

Note denotation

In pulse oximetry, arterial oxygen saturation values are usually denoted with the symbol Spo_2. Arterial oxygen saturation values that are measured invasively using arterial blood gas (ABG) analysis are denoted by the symbol Sao_2.

Practice pointers

- Place the sensor over the finger or other site—such as the toe, bridge of the nose, or earlobe—so that the light beams and sensors are opposite each other.
- Protect the sensor from exposure to strong light, such as fluorescent lighting, because it interferes with results. Check the sensor site frequently to make sure the device is in place, and examine the skin for abrasion and circulatory impairment.
- The pulse oximeter displays the patient's pulse rate and oxygen saturation reading. The pulse rate on the oximeter must correspond to the patient's actual pulse. If the rates don't correspond, the saturation reading can't be considered accurate. You may need to reposition the sensor to obtain an accurate reading.
- Rotate the sensor site at least every 4 hours, following the manufacturer's instructions and your facility's policy for site rotation, to avoid skin irritation and circulatory impairment.
- If oximetry is done properly, the oxygen saturation readings are usually within 2% of ABG values. A normal reading is 95% to 100%.

A closer look at pulse oximetry

Oximetry may be intermittent or continuous and is used to monitor arterial oxygen saturation. Normal oxygen saturation levels are 95% to 100% for adults. Lower levels may indicate hypoxemia and warrant intervention.

Interfering factors

Certain factors can interfere with the accuracy of oximetry readings. For example, an elevated bilirubin level may falsely lower oxygen saturation readings, whereas elevated carboxyhemoglobin or methemoglobin levels can falsely elevate oxygen saturation readings.

Certain intravascular substances, such as lipid emulsions and dyes, can also prevent accurate readings. Other interfering factors include excessive light (such as from phototherapy or direct sunlight), excessive patient movement, excessive ear pigment, hypothermia, hypotension, and vasoconstriction.

Some acrylic nails and certain colors of nail polish (blue, green, black, and brown-red) may also interfere with readings.

Poisoning precludes pulse oximetry

- Pulse oximetry isn't used when carbon monoxide poisoning is suspected because the oximeter doesn't differentiate between oxygen and carbon monoxide bound to hemoglobin. An ABG analysis should be performed in such cases.

End-tidal carbon dioxide monitoring

End-tidal carbon dioxide monitoring ($ETCO_2$) is used to measure the carbon dioxide concentration at end expiration. An $ETCO_2$ monitor may be a separate monitor or part of the patient's bedside hemodynamic monitoring system.

Indications for $ETCO_2$ monitoring include:
- monitoring apnea, respiratory function, and patency of the airway in acute airway obstruction
- early detection of hypercapnia, hyperthermia, and changes in carbon dioxide production and elimination with hyperventilation therapy
- assessing effectiveness of such interventions as mechanical ventilation, neuromuscular blockade used with mechanical ventilation, and prone positioning.

n-lightened

In $ETCO_2$ monitoring, a photodetector measures the amount of infrared light absorbed by the airway during inspiration and expiration. (Light absorption increases along with carbon dioxide concentration.) The monitor converts these data to a carbon dioxide value and a corresponding waveform or capnogram, if capnography is used.

Crunching the numbers

Values are obtained by monitoring samples of expired gas from an endotracheal (ET) tube or an oral or nasopharyngeal airway. Although the values are similar, the $ETCO_2$ values are usually 2 to 5 mm Hg lower than the partial pressure of arterial carbon dioxide ($PaCO_2$) value. End exhalation contains the highest carbon dioxide concentration. Normal $ETCO_2$ is 35 to 45 mm Hg.

Capnograms and $ETCO_2$ monitoring reduce the need for frequent ABG sampling.

Practice pointers

- Explain the procedure to the patient and his family.
- Assess the patient's respiratory status, vital signs, oxygen saturation, and $ETCO_2$ readings.
- Observe waveform quality and trends of $ETCO_2$ readings, and observe for sudden increases (which may indicate hypoventilation, partial airway obstruction, or respiratory depressant effects from drugs) or decreases (due to complete airway obstruction, a dislodged ET tube, or ventilator malfunction). Notify the practitioner of a 10% increase or decrease in readings.

ABG analysis

ABG analysis enables evaluation of gas exchange in the lungs by measuring the partial pressures of gases dissolved in arterial blood.

ABCs of ABGs

Arterial blood is measured because it reflects how much oxygen is available to peripheral tissues. Together, ABG values tell the story of how well a patient is oxygenated and whether he's developing acidosis or alkalosis.

Here's a summary of commonly assessed ABG values and what the findings indicate:
- pH measurement of the hydrogen ion (H^+) concentration is an indication of the blood's acidity or alkalinity.
- $PaCO_2$ reflects the adequacy of ventilation of the lungs.
- Partial pressure of arterial oxygen (PaO_2) reflects the body's ability to pick up oxygen from the lungs.
- Bicarbonate (HCO_3^-) level reflects the activity of the kidneys in retaining or excreting bicarbonate.

- Sao_2 is the ratio of actual hemoglobin oxygen content to potential maximum oxygen carrying capacity of the hemoglobin. (See *Normal ABG values.*)

Valuable values

Here's an interpretation of possible ABG values:
- A Pao_2 value greater than 100 mm Hg reflects more-than-adequate supplemental oxygen administration. A value less than 80 mm Hg indicates hypoxemia.
- An Sao_2 value less than 95% represents decreased saturation and may contribute to a low Pao_2 value.
- A pH value above 7.45 (alkalosis) reflects an H^+ deficit; a value below 7.35 (acidosis) reflects an H^+ excess.

A sample scenario

Suppose you find a pH value greater than 7.45, indicating alkalosis. Investigate further by checking the $Paco_2$ value, which is known as the *respiratory parameter.* This value reflects how efficiently the lungs eliminate carbon dioxide. A $Paco_2$ value below 35 mm Hg indicates respiratory alkalosis and hyperventilation.

Next, check the HCO_3^- value, called the *metabolic parameter.* An HCO_3^- value greater than 26 mEq/L indicates metabolic alkalosis.

Likewise, a pH value below 7.35 indicates acidosis. A $Paco_2$ value above 45 mm Hg indicates respiratory acidosis; an HCO_3^- value below 22 mEq/L indicates metabolic acidosis.

See-saw systems

The respiratory and metabolic systems work together to keep the body's acid-base balance within normal limits. If respiratory acidosis develops, for example, the kidneys compensate by conserving HCO_3^-. That's why you expect to see an above-normal HCO_3^- value.

Similarly, if metabolic acidosis develops, the lungs compensate by increasing the respiratory rate and depth to eliminate carbon dioxide. (See *Understanding acid-base disorders*, page 218.)

Practice pointers

- A practitioner, respiratory therapist, or specially trained emergency nurse draws ABG samples, usually from an arterial line if the patient has one. If a percutaneous puncture must be done, choose the site carefully. The most common site is the radial artery, but the brachial or femoral arteries can be used.

> ## Normal ABG values
>
> Arterial blood gas (ABG) values provide information about the blood's acid-base balance and oxygenation. Normal values are:
> - pH: 7.35 to 7.45
> - $Paco_2$: 35 to 45 mm Hg
> - Pao_2: 80 to 100 mm Hg
> - HCO_3^-: 22 to 26 mEq/L
> - Sao_2: 95% to 100%.

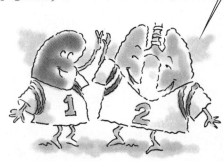

Here's the game plan: If you develop respiratory acidosis, I'll cover you and conserve HCO_3^-. Ready? Break!

Understanding acid-base disorders

This chart provides an overview of selected acid-base disorders.

Disorder and arterial blood gas findings	Possible causes	Signs and symptoms
Respiratory acidosis (excess carbon dioxide retention) pH < 7.35 Bicarbonate (HCO_3^-) > 26 mEq/L (if compensating) Partial pressure of arterial carbon dioxide ($Paco_2$) > 45 mm Hg	• Asphyxia • Central nervous system depression from drugs, injury, or disease • Hypoventilation from pulmonary, cardiac, musculoskeletal, or neuromuscular disease	Diaphoresis, headache, tachycardia, confusion, restlessness, apprehension, flushed face
Respiratory alkalosis (excess carbon dioxide excretion) pH > 7.45 HCO_3^- < 22 mEq/L (if compensating) $Paco_2$ < 35 mm Hg	• Gram-negative bacteremia • Hyperventilation from anxiety, pain, or improper ventilator settings • Respiratory stimulation by drugs, disease, hypoxia, fever, or high room temperature	Rapid, deep respirations; paresthesias; light-headedness; twitching; anxiety; fear
Metabolic acidosis (bicarbonate loss, acid retention) pH < 7.35 HCO_3^- < 22 mEq/L $Paco_2$ < 35 mm Hg (if compensating)	• Bicarbonate depletion from diarrhea • Excessive production of organic acids from hepatic disease, endocrine disorders, shock, or drug intoxication • Inadequate excretion of acids from renal disease	Rapid, deep breathing; fruity breath; fatigue; headache; lethargy; drowsiness; nausea; vomiting; coma (if severe); abdominal pain
Metabolic alkalosis (bicarbonate retention, acid loss) pH > 7.45 HCO_3^- > 26 mEq/L $Paco_2$ > 45 mm Hg (if compensating)	• Excessive alkali ingestion • Loss of hydrochloric acid from prolonged vomiting or gastric suctioning • Loss of potassium from increased renal excretion (as in diuretic therapy) or steroids	Slow, shallow breathing; hypertonic muscles; restlessness; twitching; confusion; irritability; apathy; tetany; seizures; coma (if severe)

• After obtaining the sample, apply pressure to the puncture site for 5 minutes and tape a gauze pad firmly in place. Regularly monitor the site for bleeding and check the arm for signs of complications, such as swelling, discoloration, pain, numbness, and tingling. (See *Obtaining an ABG sample.*)

• Note whether the patient is breathing room air or oxygen. If the patient is on oxygen, document the number of liters. If the patient is receiving mechanical ventilation, document the fraction of inspired oxygen.

• Make sure you remove all air bubbles in the sample syringe because air bubbles also alter results.

• Make sure the sample of arterial blood is kept cold, preferably on ice, and delivered as soon as possible to the laboratory for analysis.

Sputum analysis

Sputum analysis assesses sputum specimens to diagnose respiratory disease, identify the cause of pulmonary infection (including viral and bacterial causes), identify abnormal lung cells, and manage lung disease.

Practice pointers

• When he's ready to expectorate, instruct the patient to take three deep breaths and force a deep cough.
• Before sending the specimen to the laboratory, make sure it's sputum, not saliva. Saliva has a thinner consistency and more bubbles (froth) than sputum.

Bronchoscopy

Bronchoscopy allows direct visualization of the larynx, trachea, and bronchi through a fiber-optic bronchoscope (a slender, flexible tube with mirrors and a light at its distal end). The flexible fiber-optic bronchoscope is preferred to metal because it's smaller, allows a better view of the bronchi, and carries less risk of trauma.

To remove and evaluate

The purpose of a bronchoscopy is to:
• remove foreign bodies, malignant or benign tumors, mucus plugs, or excessive secretions from the tracheobronchial tree and to control massive hemoptysis
• pass brush biopsy forceps or a catheter through the bronchoscope to obtain specimens for cytologic evaluation.

Practice pointers

• The patient may be premedicated with atropine to dry secretions and a mild sedative or antianxiety agent such as midazolam (Versed) to help him relax. Before insertion of the bronchoscope, a topical anesthetic is applied to the oropharynx, nasopharynx, larynx, vocal cords, and trachea to suppress the cough reflex and prevent gagging.
• The practitioner introduces the bronchoscope tube through the patient's nose or mouth into the airway. Various ports on the bron-

Obtaining an ABG sample

Follow these steps to obtain a sample for arterial blood gas (ABG) analysis:
• After performing Allen's test, perform a cutaneous arterial puncture (or, if an arterial line is in place, draw blood from the arterial line).
• Use a heparinized blood gas syringe to draw the sample.
• Eliminate all air from the sample, place it on ice immediately, and transport it for analysis.
• Apply pressure to the puncture site for 3 to 5 minutes. If the patient is receiving anticoagulants or has a coagulopathy, hold the puncture site longer than 5 minutes, if necessary.
• Tape a gauze pad firmly over the puncture site. If the puncture site is on the arm, don't tape the entire circumference because this may restrict circulation.

choscope allow for suctioning, oxygen administration, and biopsies during the procedure. Monitor vital signs, oxygen saturation levels (with pulse oximetry), and heart rhythm throughout the procedure.

• After the procedure, the patient is positioned on his side or may have the head of the bed elevated 30 degrees until the gag reflex returns. Assess respiratory status and monitor vital signs, oxygen saturation levels, and heart rhythm. Report signs and symptoms of respiratory distress, such as dyspnea, laryngospasm, or hypoxemia.

• Monitor cardiac status frequently for changes in heart rate or rhythm. Report any tachycardia or evidence of arrhythmia.

• If the patient isn't intubated, assess for return of the gag, cough, and swallow reflexes.

Chest X-ray

During chest radiography (commonly known as *chest X-ray*), X-ray beams penetrate the chest and react on specially sensitized film. Because normal pulmonary tissue is radiolucent, such abnormalities as infiltrates, foreign bodies, fluid, and tumors appear dense on the film.

More is better

A chest X-ray is most useful when compared with the patient's previous films, allowing the radiologist to detect changes. By themselves, chest X-rays may not provide definitive diagnostic information. For example, they may not reveal mild to moderate obstructive pulmonary disease. However, they can show the location and size of lesions and can also be used to identify structural abnormalities that influence ventilation.

X-ray vision

Examples of abnormalities visible on X-ray include:
• fibrosis
• infiltrates
• atelectasis
• pneumothorax.

Practice pointers

• When a patient in the ED can't be moved, chest X-ray is commonly performed at the bedside.

• Make sure that female patients of childbearing age wear a lead apron. Males should have protection for the testes.

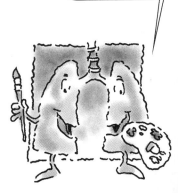

Comparing two chest X-rays can paint a better picture of respiratory change than looking at just one.

Magnetic resonance imaging

Magnetic resonance imaging (MRI) is a noninvasive test that employs a powerful magnet, radio waves, and a computer. It's used to diagnose respiratory disorders by providing high-resolution, cross-sectional images of lung structures and by tracing blood flow.

View that's see-through

The greatest advantage of MRI is that it enables you to "see through" bone and delineate fluid-filled soft tissue in great detail without using ionizing radiation or contrast media. It's used to distinguish tumors from other structures such as blood vessels.

Practice pointers

• All metal objects must be removed from the patient before entering the scanning room. (See *MRI and metals don't mix.*)
• If the patient is claustrophobic, he may be sedated before the test.
• Tell the patient that the test usually takes 15 to 30 minutes. Some facilities can perform open MRIs, which are more tolerable for patients who are claustrophobic.

Thoracic computed tomography scan

Thoracic computed tomography (CT) scan provides cross-sectional views of the chest by passing an X-ray beam from a computerized scanner through the body at different angles and depths. A contrast agent is sometimes used to highlight blood vessels and allow greater visual discrimination.

CT in 3-D

Thoracic CT scan provides a three-dimensional image of the lung, allowing the practitioner to assess abnormalities in the configuration of the trachea or major bronchi and evaluate masses or lesions, such as tumors and abscesses, and abnormal lung shadows.

Practice pointers

• Confirm that the patient isn't allergic to iodine or shellfish. A patient with these allergies may have an adverse reaction to the contrast medium. Diphenhydramine (Benadryl) and prednisone (Deltasone) may be administered, as ordered, before the test to reduce the risk of a reaction to the dye.
• If a contrast medium is used, explain that it's injected into the existing I.V. line or that a new line may be inserted.

MRI and metals don't mix

Before your patient undergoes magnetic resonance imaging (MRI), make sure he doesn't have a pacemaker or surgically implanted joint, pin, clip, valve, or pump containing metal. Such objects could be attracted to the strong MRI magnet.

Ask your patient whether he's ever worked with metals or has metal in his eyes. (Some facilities have a checklist that covers all pertinent questions regarding metals, clips, pins, pacemakers, and other devices). If he has such a device, the test can't be done.

• Explain to the patient that he may feel flushed or notice a metallic or salty taste in his mouth when the contrast medium is injected.
• Explain that the CT scanner circles around the patient for 10 to 30 minutes, depending on the procedure, and that the equipment may make him feel claustrophobic.
• Instruct the patient to lie still during the test.
• Inform the patient that the contrast medium may discolor his urine for 24 hours.
• Encourage oral fluid intake to flush the contrast medium out of the patient's system unless it's contraindicated or the patient is on nothing-by-mouth status. The practitioner may write an order to increase the rate of I.V. fluid infusion.

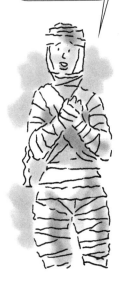

CT scanner and MRI equipment can make some patients feel claustrophobic.

Ventilation-perfusion scan

A ventilation-perfusion ($\dot{V}/\dot{Q}$) scan is used to:
• evaluate $\dot{V}/\dot{Q}$ mismatch
• detect pulmonary embolus
• evaluate pulmonary function, especially in patients with marginal lung reserves.

Although it's less reliable than pulmonary angiography, $\dot{V}/\dot{Q}$ scanning carries fewer risks.

Two-tined test

A $\dot{V}/\dot{Q}$ scan has two parts:

During the ventilation portion of the test, the patient inhales the contrast medium gas; ventilation patterns and adequacy of ventilation are noted on the scan.

During the perfusion scan, the contrast medium is injected I.V. and the pulmonary blood flow to the lungs is visualized.

$\dot{V}/\dot{Q}$ caveat

$\dot{V}/\dot{Q}$ scans aren't commonly used for patients on mechanical ventilators because the ventilation portion of the test is difficult to perform. (Pulmonary angiography is the preferred test for a critically ill patient with a suspected pulmonary embolus.)

Practice pointers

• Explain the test to the patient and his family, telling them who performs the test and where it's done.
• Like pulmonary angiography, a $\dot{V}/\dot{Q}$ scan requires the injection of a contrast medium. Confirm that the patient doesn't have an allergy to the contrast material.

- Explain to the patient that the test has two parts. During the ventilation portion, a mask is placed over his mouth and nose and the patient breathes in the contrast medium gas mixed with air while the scanner takes pictures of his lungs. For the perfusion portion, the patient is placed in a supine position on a movable table as the contrast medium is injected into the I.V. line while the scanner again takes pictures of the lungs.
- After the procedure, maintain bed rest as ordered and monitor the patient's vital signs, oxygen saturation levels, and heart rhythm.
- Monitor for adverse reactions to the contrast medium, which may include restlessness, tachypnea and respiratory distress, tachycardia, urticaria, and nausea and vomiting. Keep emergency equipment nearby in case of a reaction.

Pulmonary angiography

Pulmonary angiography, also called *pulmonary arteriography*, allows radiographic examination of the pulmonary circulation.

After injecting a radioactive contrast dye through a catheter inserted into the pulmonary artery or one of its branches, a series of X-rays is taken to detect blood flow abnormalities, possibly caused by embolus or pulmonary infarction.

More reliable, more risks

Pulmonary angiography yields more reliable results than a $\dot{V}/\dot{Q}$ scan but carries higher risks for certain conditions such as cardiac arrhythmias (especially ventricular arrhythmias caused by myocardial irritation from passage of the catheter through the heart chambers). It may be the practitioner's preferred test to evaluate pulmonary circulation, especially if the patient is on a ventilator.

Practice pointers

- Explain the procedure to the patient and his family and answer their questions. Tell them who performs the test, where it's done, and how long it takes.
- Confirm that the patient isn't allergic to shellfish or iodine. Notify the practitioner if the patient has such an allergy because the patient may have an adverse reaction to the contrast medium. Diphenhydramine (Benadryl) and prednisone (Deltasone) may be administered, as ordered, before the test to reduce the risk of a reaction to the dye.
- Preprocedure testing should include evaluation of renal function (by serum creatinine levels and blood urea nitrogen [BUN] levels) and potential risk of bleeding (by prothrombin time, partial

thromboplastin time, and platelet count). Notify the practitioner of abnormal results.
• Instruct the patient to lie still for the procedure.
• Explain that he'll probably feel a flushed sensation in his face as the dye is injected.

Postprocedure procedures

• Maintain bed rest as ordered, and monitor the patient's vital signs, oxygen saturation levels, and heart rhythm.
• Keep a sandbag or femoral compression device over the injection site as ordered.
• Check the pressure dressing for signs of bleeding. Monitor the patient's peripheral pulse in the arm or leg used for catheter insertion (and mark the site). Check the temperature, color, and sensation of the extremity, and compare with the opposite side.
• Unless contraindicated, encourage the patient to drink more fluids to flush the dye or contrast medium from his system, or increase the I.V. flow rate as ordered.
• Check serum creatinine and BUN levels after the procedure because the contrast medium can cause acute renal failure.
• Monitor for adverse reactions to the contrast medium, which may include restlessness, tachypnea and respiratory distress, tachycardia, facial flushing, urticaria, and nausea and vomiting. Keep emergency equipment nearby in case of a reaction.

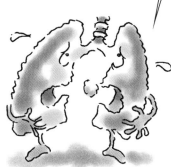

Whew! Is it hot in here, or is it just the dye from my pulmonary angiography?

Treatments

Respiratory disorders interfere with airway clearance, breathing patterns, and gas exchange. If not corrected, they can adversely affect many other body systems and can be life-threatening. Treatments for patients with respiratory disorders include drug therapy, inhalation therapy, and surgery.

Drug therapy

Drugs are used for airway management in patients with such disorders as acute respiratory failure, acute respiratory distress syndrome (ARDS), asthma, emphysema, and chronic bronchitis. Some types of drugs commonly seen in the ED include anti-inflammatory agents, bronchodilators, neuromuscular blocking agents, and sedatives.

Anti-inflammatory agents

Anti-inflammatory agents (corticosteroids) are used to reduce bronchial inflammation.

Reversing obstruction

Corticosteroids are the most effective anti-inflammatory agents used to treat patients with reversible airflow obstruction. They work by suppressing immune responses and reducing inflammation.

Systemic drugs, such as dexamethasone (Decadron), methylprednisolone (Medrol), and prednisone (Deltasone) are given to manage an acute respiratory event, such as acute respiratory failure or exacerbation of COPD. These drugs are initially given I.V.; when the patient stabilizes, the dosage is tapered and oral dosing may be substituted.

Patients with asthma commonly use inhaled steroids, such as beclomethasone (QVAR), budesonide (Pulmicort Turbuhaler), flunisolide (AeroBid), fluticasone (Flovent), salmeterol (Advair), and triamcinolone (Azmacort). These agents also work by suppressing immune response and reducing airway inflammation. (See *Understanding corticosteroids*, page 226.)

Bronchodilators

Bronchodilators relax bronchial smooth muscles and are used to treat patients with bronchospasms. Here's how some types of bronchodilators are used:
• Short-acting inhaled $beta_2$-adrenergic agonists, such as albuterol (Proventil) and pirbuterol (Maxair), are used to relieve acute symptoms in asthma and bronchospasm.
• Epinephrine acts on alpha- and beta-adrenergic receptors. It's used to relieve anaphylactic, allergic, and other hypersensitivity reactions. Its beta-adrenergic effects relax bronchial smooth muscle and relieve bronchospasm.
• Anticholinergic agents, such as ipratropium (Atrovent), act by inhibiting the action of acetylcholine at bronchial smooth-muscle receptor sites and thus produce bronchodilation. (See *Understanding bronchodilators*, page 227.)

Neuromuscular blocking agents

Patients on mechanical ventilation may require neuromuscular blocking agents to eliminate spontaneous breathing efforts that can interfere with the ventilator's

Spontaneous conversations need quick wit; spontaneous breathing efforts need neuromuscular blocking agents if they hamper ventilator function.

Understanding corticosteroids

Use this table to learn about the indications, adverse reactions, and practice pointers associated with corticosteroids.

Drug	Indications	Adverse reactions	Practice pointers
Systemic steroids dexamethasone (Cortastat) methylprednisolone (Solu-Medrol) prednisone (Deltasone)	• Anti-inflammatory for acute respiratory failure, acute respiratory distress syndrome, and chronic obstructive pulmonary disease • Anti-inflammatory and immunosuppressant for asthma	• Arrhythmias • Circulatory collapse • Edema • Heart failure • Pancreatitis • Peptic ulcer • Thromboembolism	• Use cautiously in patients with recent myocardial infarction, hypertension, renal disease, and GI ulcer. • Monitor blood pressure and blood glucose levels.
Inhaled steroids beclomethasone (Beconase) budesonide (Pulmicort) flunisolide (Aerobid) fluticasone (Flonase) triamcinolone (A$_3$macort)	• Long-term asthma control	• Bronchospasm • Dry mouth • Hoarseness • Oral candidiasis • Wheezing	• Don't use for treatment of acute asthma attack. • Use a spacer to reduce adverse effects. • Rinse the patient's mouth after use to prevent oral fungal infection.

function. Neuromuscular blocking agents cause paralysis without altering the patient's level of consciousness (LOC). (See *Understanding neuromuscular blocking agents*, pages 228 and 229.)

Sedatives

Benzodiazepines, such as midazolam and lorazepam (Ativan), are used for conscious sedation and preoperative sedation to reduce anxiety in patients undergoing diagnostic or surgical procedures.

These drugs are also used to relieve anxiety and promote sedation in patients on mechanical ventilators, especially those receiving neuromuscular blocking agents. Such agents cause paralysis without altering the patient's LOC, which—without sedation—is frightening for him. (See *Understanding sedatives*, pages 230 and 231.)

(Text continues on page 231.)

Understanding bronchodilators

Use this table to learn about the indications, adverse reactions, and practice pointers associated with bronchodilators.

Drug	Indications	Adverse reactions	Practice pointers
Beta$_2$-adrenergic agonists			
albuterol (Proventil)	• Short-acting relief of acute symptoms with asthma and bronchospasm	• Hyperactivity • Palpitations • Paradoxical bronchospasm • Tachycardia • Tremor	• Warn the patient about the possibility of paradoxical bronchospasm. If it occurs, stop the drug and seek medical treatment. • An elderly patient may require a lower dose. • Monitor respiratory status, vital signs, and heart rhythm.
epinephrine (Bronkaid Mist)	• Relaxation of bronchial smooth muscle through stimulation of beta$_2$-adrenergic receptors; used for bronchospasm, hypersensitivity reaction, anaphylaxis, and asthma	• Cerebral hemorrhage • Palpitations • Tachycardia • Ventricular fibrillation	• Use cautiously in elderly patients and those with long-standing asthma and emphysema with degenerative heart disease. • Monitor respiratory status, vital signs, and heart rhythm. • This drug is contraindicated in patients with angle-closure glaucoma, coronary insufficiency, and cerebral arteriosclerosis.
pirbuterol (Maxair)	• Relief of acute symptoms with asthma and bronchospasm	• Palpitations • Paradoxical bronchospasm • Tachycardia • Tremor	• Warn the patient about the possibility of paradoxical bronchospasm. If it occurs, stop the drug and seek medical treatment. • An elderly patient may require a lower dose. • Monitor respiratory status, vital signs, and heart rhythm.
Anticholinergic agents			
ipratropium (Atrovent)	• Bronchospasm associated with chronic bronchitis and emphysema	• Bronchospasm • Chest pain • Nervousness • Palpitations	• Because of delayed onset of bronchodilation, this drug isn't recommended for acute respiratory distress. • Use cautiously in patients with angle-closure glaucoma, bladder neck obstruction, and prostatic hypertrophy. • Monitor respiratory status, vital signs, and heart rhythm.

Understanding neuromuscular blocking agents

Use this table to learn about the indications, adverse reactions, and practice pointers associated with neuromuscular blocking agents.

Drug	Indications	Adverse reactions	Practice pointers
Depolarizing			
succinylcholine (Anectine)	• Adjunct to general anesthesia to aid endotracheal (ET) intubation • Induction of skeletal muscle paralysis during surgery or mechanical ventilation	• Bradycardia, arrhythmias, cardiac arrest • Malignant hyperthermia, increased intraocular pressure, flushing • Postoperative muscle pain • Respiratory depression, apnea, bronchoconstriction	• This drug is contraindicated in patients with histories of malignant hyperthermia, myopathies associated with creatinine phosphokinase, acute angle-closure glaucoma, and penetrating eye injuries. • Monitor the patient for histamine release and resulting hypotension and flushing.
Nondepolarizing			
atracurium (Atramed)	• Adjunct to general anesthesia, to facilitate ET intubation, and to provide skeletal muscle relaxation during surgery or mechanical ventilation	• Anaphylaxis • Flushing, bradycardia • Prolonged, dose-related apnea, bronchospasm, laryngospasm	• This drug doesn't affect consciousness or relieve pain. Be sure to keep the patient sedated. Have emergency respiratory support readily available. • This drug has little or no effect on heart rate and doesn't counteract or reverse the bradycardia caused by anesthetics or vagal stimulation. Thus, bradycardia is seen more frequently with atracurium than with other neuromuscular blocking agents. Pretreatment with anticholinergics (atropine or glycopyrrolate) is advised. • Use drug only if ET intubation, administration of oxygen under positive pressure, artificial respiration, and assisted or controlled ventilation are immediately available. • Use a peripheral nerve stimulator to monitor responses during CCU administration; it may be used to detect residual paralysis during recovery and to avoid atracurium overdose.
cisatracurium (Nimbex)	• Adjunct to general anesthesia, to facilitate ET intubation, and to provide skeletal muscle relaxation	• Flushing • Hypotension	• This drug isn't compatible with propofol injection or ketorolac injection for Y-site administration. Drug is acidic and also may not be compatible with an alkaline solution with a pH greater than 8.5, such as barbiturate solutions for Y-site administration. Don't dilute

Understanding neuromuscular blocking agents (continued)

Drug	Indications	Adverse reactions	Practice pointers
Nondepolarizing (continued)			
cisatracurium (Nimbex) (continued)	during surgery or mechanical ventilation in the critical care unit (CCU) • Maintenance of neuromuscular blockade in the CCU		in lactated Ringer's solution because of chemical instability. • This drug isn't recommended for rapid-sequence ET intubation because of its intermediate onset of action. • In patients with neuromuscular disease (myasthenia gravis and myasthenic syndrome), watch for possible prolonged neuromuscular block. • Monitor the patient's acid-base balance and electrolyte levels.
pancuronium (Pavulon)	• Adjunct to anesthesia to induce skeletal muscle relaxation, facilitate intubation and ventilation, and weaken muscle contractions in induced seizures	• Allergic or idiosyncratic hypersensitivity reactions • Prolonged, dose-related respiratory insufficiency or apnea • Residual muscle weakness	• If using succinylcholine, allow its effects to subside before giving pancuronium. • Don't mix in same syringe or give through same needle with barbiturates or other alkaline solutions. • Large doses may increase the frequency and severity of tachycardia.
tubocurarine (Curare)	• Adjunct to general anesthesia to induce skeletal muscle relaxation, facilitate intubation, and reduce fractures and dislocations • Assistance with mechanical ventilation	• Arrhythmias, cardiac arrest, bradycardia • Hypersensitivity reactions • Respiratory depression or apnea; bronchospasm	• The margin of safety between a therapeutic dose and a dose causing respiratory paralysis is small. • Assess baseline tests of renal function and serum electrolyte levels before drug administration. Electrolyte imbalance, particularly of potassium and magnesium, can potentiate the effects of this drug.
vecuronium (Norcuron)	• Adjunct to anesthesia, to facilitate intubation, and to provide skeletal muscle relaxation during surgery or mechanical ventilation	• Prolonged, dose-related respiratory insufficiency or apnea	• Administer by rapid I.V. injection or I.V. infusion. Don't give I.M. • Recovery time may double in patients with cirrhosis or cholestasis. • Assess baseline serum electrolyte levels, acid-base balance, and renal and hepatic function before administration.

Understanding sedatives

Use this table to learn about the indications, adverse reactions, and practice pointers associated with sedatives.

Drug	Indications	Adverse reactions	Practice pointers
lorazepam (Ativan)	• Anxiety, tension, agitation, irritability—especially in anxiety neuroses or organic (especially GI or cardiovascular) disorders • Status epilepticus	• Acute withdrawal syndrome (after sudden discontinuation in physically dependent patients) • Drowsiness, sedation	• This drug is contraindicated in patients with acute angle-closure glaucoma. • Use cautiously in patients with pulmonary, renal, or hepatic impairment and in elderly, acutely ill, or debilitated patients. • Parenteral lorazepam appears to possess potent amnesic effects. • For I.V. administration, dilute lorazepam with an equal volume of a compatible diluent, such as dextrose 5% in water (D_5W), sterile water for injection, or normal saline solution. • Inject the drug directly into a vein or into the tubing of a compatible I.V. infusion, such as normal saline solution or D_5W solution. The rate of lorazepam I.V. injection shouldn't exceed 2 mg/minute. Have emergency resuscitative equipment available when administering I.V. • Monitor liver function studies to prevent cumulative effects and ensure adequate drug metabolism. • Parenteral administration of this drug is more likely to cause apnea, hypotension, bradycardia, and cardiac arrest in elderly patients.
midazolam	• Preoperative sedation (to induce sleepiness or drowsiness and relieve apprehension) • Conscious sedation • Continuous infusion for sedation of intubated and mechanically ventilated patients as a component of anesthesia or during treatment in a critical care setting • Sedation and amnesia before diagnostic, therapeutic, or endoscopic procedures or before induction of anesthesia	• Apnea • Cardiac arrest • Decreased respiratory rate • Hiccups • Nausea • Pain • Respiratory arrest	• This drug is contraindicated in patients with acute angle-closure glaucoma and in those experiencing shock, coma, or acute alcohol intoxication. • Use cautiously in patients with uncompensated acute illnesses, in elderly or debilitated patients, and in patients with myasthenia gravis or neuromuscular disorders and pulmonary disease. • Closely monitor cardiopulmonary function; continuously monitor patients who have received midazolam to detect potentially life-threatening respiratory depression. • Have emergency respiratory equipment readily available. Laryngospasm and bronchospasm, although rare, may occur. • Solutions compatible with midazolam include D_5W, normal saline solution, and lactated Ringer's solution.

Understanding sedatives (continued)

Drug	Indications	Adverse reactions	Practice pointers
propofol (Diprivan)	• Induction and maintenance of sedation in mechanically ventilated patients	• Apnea • Bradycardia • Hyperlipidemia • Hypotension	• This drug is contraindicated in patients hypersensitive to propofol or components of the emulsion, including soybean oil, egg lecithin, and glycerol. Because the drug is administered as an emulsion, administer cautiously to patients with a disorder of lipid metabolism (such as pancreatitis, primary hyperlipoproteinemia, and diabetic hyperlipidemia). Use cautiously if the patient is receiving lipids as part of a total parenteral nutrition infusion; I.V. lipid dose may need to be reduced. • Use cautiously in elderly or debilitated patients and in those with circulatory disorders. • Although the hemodynamic effects of this drug can vary, its major effect in patients maintaining spontaneous ventilation is arterial hypotension (arterial pressure can decrease as much as 30%) with little or no change in heart rate and cardiac output. However, significant depression of cardiac output may occur in patients undergoing assisted or controlled positive pressure ventilation. • Don't mix propofol with other drugs or blood products. If it's to be diluted before infusion, use only D_5W and don't dilute to a concentration of less than 2 mg/ml. After dilution, the drug appears to be more stable in glass containers than in plastic.

Inhalation therapy

Inhalation therapy employs carefully controlled ventilation techniques to help the patient maintain optimal ventilation in the event of respiratory failure. Techniques include aerosol treatments, continuous positive airway pressure (CPAP), ET intubation, mechanical ventilation, and oxygen therapy.

Aerosol treatments

Aerosol therapy is a means of administering medication into the airways. The administration method can use handheld nebulizers or metered-dose inhalers. These devices deliver topical medications to the respiratory tract, producing local and systemic effects.

Using CPAP

This illustration shows the continuous positive airway pressure (CPAP) apparatus used to apply positive pressure to the airway to prevent obstruction during inspiration in patients with sleep apnea.

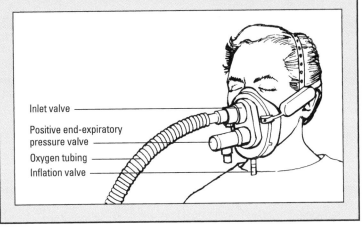

Inlet valve

Positive end-expiratory pressure valve

Oxygen tubing

Inflation valve

The mucosal lining of the respiratory tract absorbs the inhalant almost immediately.

Common inhalants are bronchodilators, used to improve airway patency and facilitate mucus drainage; mucolytics, which attain a high local concentration to liquefy tenacious bronchial secretions; and corticosteroids, used to decrease inflammation.

Nursing considerations
• Monitor the patient's response to the medication.
• Check pulse oximetry after the treatment and document any changes.
• Assess patient's breath sounds and document findings before and after treatment.

Continuous positive airway pressure

As its name suggests, CPAP ventilation maintains positive pressure in the airways throughout the patient's respiratory cycle. Originally delivered only with a ventilator, CPAP may now be delivered to intubated or nonintubated patients through an artificial airway, a mask, or nasal prongs by means of a ventilator or a separate high-flow generating system. (See *Using CPAP.*)

Goes with the flows

CPAP is available as a continuous-flow system and a demand system. In the continuous-flow system, an air-oxygen blend flows through a humidifier and a reservoir bag into a T-piece. In the demand system, a valve opens in response to the patient's inspiratory flow.

Other talents

In addition to treating respiratory distress syndrome, CPAP has been used successfully in pulmonary edema, pulmonary embolus, bronchiolitis, fat embolus, pneumonitis, viral pneumonia, and postoperative atelectasis. In mild to moderate cases of these disorders, CPAP provides an alternative to intubation and mechanical ventilation. It increases the functional residual capacity by distending collapsed alveoli, which improves PaO_2 and decreases intrapulmonary shunting and oxygen consumption. It also reduces the work of breathing.

Through the nose

Nasal CPAP has proved successful for long-term treatment of obstructive sleep apnea. In this type of CPAP, high-flow compressed air is directed into a mask that covers only the patient's nose. The pressure supplied through the mask serves as a back-pressure splint, preventing the unstable upper airway from collapsing during inspiration.

Not so positive

CPAP may cause gastric distress if the patient swallows air during the treatment (most common when CPAP is delivered without intubation). The patient may feel claustrophobic. Because mask CPAP can also cause nausea and vomiting, it shouldn't be used in patients who are unresponsive or at risk for vomiting and aspiration. In rare cases, CPAP causes barotrauma or lowers cardiac output.

Nursing considerations

• If the patient is intubated or has a tracheostomy, you can accomplish CPAP with a mechanical ventilator by adjusting the settings. Assess vital signs and breath sounds during CPAP.
• If CPAP is to be delivered through a mask, a respiratory therapist usually sets up the system and fits the mask. The mask should be transparent and lightweight, with a soft, pliable seal. A tight seal isn't required as long as pressure can be maintained. Obtain ABG results and bedside pulmonary function studies to establish a baseline.

After the fact

• Check for decreased cardiac output and blood pressure, which may result from increased intrathoracic pressure associated with CPAP.
• Watch closely for changes in respiratory rate and pattern. Uncoordinated breathing patterns may indicate severe respiratory muscle fatigue that can't be helped by CPAP. Report this to the practitioner; the patient may need mechanical ventilation.
• Check the CPAP system for pressure fluctuations.
• Keep in mind that high airway pressures increase the risk of pneumothorax, so monitor for chest pain and decreased breath sounds.
• Use oximetry to monitor oxygen saturation.
• Check closely for air leaks around the mask near the eyes (an area difficult to seal); escaping air can dry the eyes, causing conjunctivitis or other problems.

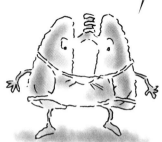

Careful—CPAP masks can leak air around the eyes and cause conjunctivitis. This mask won't do me any harm, though.

ET intubation

ET intubation involves insertion of a tube into the lungs through the mouth or nose to establish a patent airway. It protects patients from aspiration by sealing off the trachea from the digestive tract and permits removal of tracheobronchial secretions in patients who can't cough effectively. ET intubation also provides a route for mechanical ventilation.

Conversation stopper

Drawbacks of ET intubation are that it bypasses normal respiratory defenses against infection, reduces cough effectiveness, may be uncomfortable, and prevents verbal communication.
   Potential complications of ET intubation include:
• aspiration of blood, secretions, or gastric contents
• bronchospasm or laryngospasm
• cardiac arrhythmias
• hypoxemia (if attempts at intubation are prolonged or oxygen delivery interrupted)
• injury to the lips, mouth, pharynx or vocal cords
• tooth damage or loss
• tracheal stenosis, erosion, and necrosis.

Open up

In orotracheal intubation, the oral cavity is used as the route of insertion. It's preferred in emergency situations because it's easier and faster. However, maintaining exact tube placement is more difficult because the tube must be well secured to avoid kinking and prevent bronchial obstruction or accidental extubation. It's

The seven Ps of RSI

Rapid sequence intubation (RSI) is used to rapidly produce optimal conditions for intubation in emergency situations, especially for difficult patients. Seven steps are outlined below.

 Prepare
- Administer I.V.
- Administer oxygen (O_2).
- Institute cardiac and oxygenation saturation monitoring.
- Prepare medications and equipment.

 Pre-oxygenate
- Administer 100% O_2 for 3 minutes using a tight-fitting face mask with reservoir.

 Pretreatment
- Administer a sedating agent, such as etomidate (Amidate), thiopental (Pentothal), propofol (Diprivan), or ketamine (Ketalar).
- Administer additional drugs to minimize the effects of intubation, such as lidocaine (to prevent increased intracranial pressure), atropine (to decrease bradycardia), or succinylcholine (Anectine) (to reduce muscle fasciculations).

 Paralysis
- Administer a short-acting neuromuscular blocking agent, such as succinylcholine or vecuronium (Norcuron).

- Begin or continue to administer mechanical ventilation.

 Placement
- The larynx is compressed against the esophagus (Sellick maneuver) to prevent aspiration.
- The patient is intubated.
- The cuff is inflated.

 Placement and proof
- Endotracheal (ET) tube placement is verified by observation, auscultation, end-tidal carbon dioxide ($ETco_2$) detector, and chest X-ray.

 Postintubation management
- Secure the ET tube using tape or a commercial device.
- Maintain continuous $ETco_2$ monitoring.
- Continue sedation or paralysis as indicated.
- Monitor the patient's response, including vital signs, arterial blood gas values, cardiac monitor, and arterial oxygen saturation.

Reprinted from *Procedures in Emergency Medicine*, 4th ed., Hedges, J.R. and Roberts, J.R., eds., Philadelphia: W.B. Saunders Co., 2003. Used with permission.

also uncomfortable for conscious patients because it stimulates salivation, coughing, and retching.

Be quick about it

Rapid sequence intubation (RSI) is the standard of care for ET intubation. RSI minimizes the complications of endotracheal intubation, such as airway trauma and aspiration, and is more comfortable for the patient. (See *The Seven Ps of RSI*.)

Not for everyone

Orotracheal intubation is contraindicated in patients with orofacial injuries, acute cervical spinal injury, and degenerative spinal disorders.

Through the nose

Oral ET intubation is the preferred method of airway management in patients who are apneic. However, nasal intubation may be an alternative if the oral route is contraindicated. In nasal intubation, a nasal passage is used as the route of insertion. Nasal intubation is preferred for elective insertion when the patient is capable of spontaneous ventilation for a short period.

A conscious choice

Nasal intubation is more comfortable than oral intubation and is typically used in conscious patients who are at risk for imminent respiratory arrest or who have cervical spinal injuries. It's contraindicated in patients with facial or basilar skull fractures.

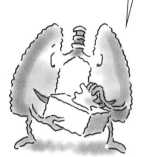

This tissue I can replace. I have less luck with the tissue damaged by nasal intubation.

Difficult and damaging

Although it's more comfortable than oral intubation, nasal intubation is more difficult to perform. Because the tube passes blindly through the nasal cavity, it causes more tissue damage, increases the risk of infection by nasal bacteria introduced into the trachea, and increases the risk of pressure necrosis of the nasal mucosa.

Nursing considerations
• If possible, explain the procedure to the patient and family.
• Obtain the correct size of ET tube. The typical size for an oral ET tube is 7.5 mm (indicates the size of the lumen) for women and 8 mm for men.
• Administer medication, as ordered, to decrease respiratory secretions, induce amnesia or analgesia, and help calm and relax the conscious patient. Remove dentures and bridgework, if present.

Note breath sounds

• After securing the ET tube, reconfirm tube placement by noting bilateral breath sounds and $ETco_2$ readings.
• Auscultate breath sounds and watch for chest movement to ensure correct tube placement and full lung ventilation.
• A chest X-ray may be ordered to confirm tube placement.
• Disposable $ETco_2$ detectors are commonly used to confirm tube placement in EDs, postanesthesia care units, and critical care units (CCUs) that don't use continual $ETco_2$ monitoring. Follow the manufacturer's instructions for proper use of the device. Don't

Understanding manual ventilation

A handheld resuscitation bag is an inflatable device that can be attached to a face mask or directly to a tracheostomy or endotracheal (ET) tube to allow manual delivery of oxygen or room air to the lungs of a patient who can't breathe by himself.

Although usually used in an emergency, manual ventilation can also be performed while the patient is disconnected temporarily from a mechanical ventilator (such as during a tubing change), during transport, or before suctioning. In such instances, use of the handheld resuscitation bag maintains ventilation. Oxygen administration with a resuscitation bag can help improve a compromised cardiorespiratory system.

Ventilation guidelines

To manually ventilate a patient with an ET or tracheostomy tube, follow these guidelines:

• If oxygen is readily available, connect the handheld resuscitation bag to the oxygen. Attach one end of the tubing to the bottom of the bag and the other end to the nipple adapter on the flowmeter of the oxygen source.

• Turn on the oxygen and adjust the flow rate according to the patient's condition.

• Before attaching the handheld resuscitation bag, suction the ET or tracheostomy tube to remove any secretions that may obstruct the airway.

• Remove the mask from the ventilation bag, and attach the handheld resuscitation bag directly to the tube.

• Keeping your nondominant hand on the connection of the bag to the tube, exert downward pressure to seal the mask against his face. For an adult patient, use your dominant hand to compress the bag every 5 seconds to deliver approximately 1 L of air.

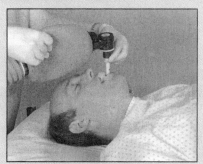

• Deliver breaths with the patient's own inspiratory effort if any is present. Don't attempt to deliver a breath as the patient exhales.

• Observe the patient's chest to ensure that it rises and falls with each compression. If ventilation fails to occur, check the connection and the patency of the patient's airway; if necessary, reposition his head and suction.

• Be alert for possible underventilation, which commonly occurs because the handheld resuscitation bag is difficult to keep positioned while ensuring an open airway. In addition, the volume of air delivered to the patient varies with the type of bag used and the hand size of the person compressing the bag. An adult with a small- or medium-sized hand may not consistently deliver 1 L of air. For these reasons, have someone assist with the procedure, if possible.

• Keep in mind that air is forced into the patient's stomach with manual ventilation, placing the patient at risk for aspiration of vomitus (possibly resulting in pneumonia) and gastric distention.

• Record the date and time of the procedure, reason and length of time the patient was disconnected from mechanical ventilation and received manual ventilation, any complications and the nursing action taken, and the patient's tolerance of the procedure.

use the detector with a heated humidifier or nebulizer because humidity, heat, and moisture can interfere with the device.

• Follow standard precautions, and suction through the ET tube as the patient's condition indicates to clear secretions and prevent mucus plugs from obstructing the tube.

• After suctioning, use a handheld resuscitation bag to hyperoxygenate the patient who's being maintained on a ventilator. (See *Understanding manual ventilation.*)

• If available, use a closed tracheal suctioning system, which permits the ventilated patient to remain on the ventilator during suctioning.

Mechanical ventilation

Mechanical ventilation involves the use of a machine to move air into a patient's lungs. Mechanical ventilators use positive or negative pressure to ventilate patients.

When to ventilate

Indications for mechanical ventilation include:
• acute respiratory failure due to ARDS, pneumonia, acute exacerbations of COPD, pulmonary embolus, heart failure, trauma, tumors, or drug overdose
• respiratory center depression due to stroke, brain injury, or trauma
• neuromuscular disturbances caused by neuromuscular diseases, such as Guillain-Barré syndrome, multiple sclerosis, and myasthenia gravis; trauma, including spinal cord injury; or CNS depression.

Accentuate the positive

Positive pressure ventilators exert positive pressure on the airway, which causes inspiration while increasing tidal volume (V_T). A high-frequency ventilator uses high respiratory rates and low V_T to maintain alveolar ventilation.

The inspiratory cycles of these ventilators may be adjusted for volume, pressure, or time:
• A volume-cycled ventilator (the type used most commonly) delivers a preset volume of air each time, regardless of the amount of lung resistance.
• A pressure-cycled ventilator generates flow until the machine reaches a preset pressure, regardless of the volume delivered or the time required to achieve the pressure.
• A time-cycled ventilator generates flow for a preset amount of time.

Several different modes of ventilatory control are found on the ventilator. The choice of mode depends on the patient's respiratory condition.

Nursing considerations

• Provide emotional support to the patient during all phases of mechanical ventilation to reduce anxiety and promote successful treatment. Even if the patient is unresponsive, continue to explain all procedures and treatments.

Be alarmed

• Make sure the ventilator alarms are on at all times to alert you to potentially hazardous conditions and changes in the patient's status. If an alarm sounds and the problem can't be easily identified, disconnect the patient from the ventilator and use a handheld resuscitation bag to ventilate him.
• Assess cardiopulmonary status frequently—at least every 2 to 4 hours or more often if indicated. Assess vital signs and auscultate breath sounds. Monitor pulse oximetry or $ETCO_2$ levels and hemodynamic parameters as ordered. Monitor intake and output and assess for fluid volume excess or dehydration.
• Administer a sedative or neuromuscular blocking agent, as ordered, to relax the patient or eliminate spontaneous breathing efforts that can interfere with the ventilator's action.

Be extra vigilant

• Remember that the patient receiving a neuromuscular blocking agent requires close observation because he can't breathe or communicate. In addition, if the patient is receiving a neuromuscular blocking agent, make sure he also receives a sedative. Neuromuscular blocking agents cause paralysis without altering the patient's LOC. Reassure the patient and his family that the paralysis is temporary.

Oxygen therapy

In oxygen therapy, oxygen is delivered by mask or nasal prongs to prevent or reverse hypoxemia and reduce the workload of breathing.

Fully equipped

Therapy equipment depends on the patient's condition and the required fraction of inspired oxygen. High-flow systems, such as Venturi masks and ventilators, deliver a precisely controlled air oxygen mixture. Low-flow systems, such as nasal prongs or masks, allow variation in the oxygen percentage delivery based on the patient's respiratory pattern.

Concentrate on concentration

Nasal prongs deliver oxygen at flow rates from 0.5 to 6 L/minute. Masks deliver up to 100% oxygen concentrations but can't be used to deliver controlled oxygen concentrations.

Nursing considerations

• Be sure to humidify oxygen flow exceeding 3 L/minute to help prevent drying of mucous membranes. However, humidity isn't added with Venturi masks because water can block the Venturi jets.

• Assess for signs of hypoxia, including decreased LOC, tachycardia, arrhythmias, diaphoresis, restlessness, altered blood pressure or respiratory rate, clammy skin, and cyanosis. If these occur, notify the practitioner, obtain pulse oximetry readings, and check the oxygen equipment to see if it's malfunctioning.

• Use a low flow rate if your patient has COPD. However, don't use a simple face mask, because low flow rates won't flush carbon dioxide from the mask and the patient will rebreathe carbon dioxide. Watch for alterations in LOC, heart rate, and respiratory rate, which may signal carbon dioxide narcosis or worsening hypoxemia.

Surgery

If drugs or other therapeutic modes fail to maintain the patient's airway patency and protect healthy tissues from disease, surgery may be necessary. Some types of respiratory surgeries are chest tube insertion and tracheotomy.

> Chest-tube insertion gives me the chance to reinflate—maybe a little TOO much this time!

Chest-tube insertion

Chest-tube insertion may be needed when treating patients with pneumothorax, hemothorax, empyema, pleural effusion, or chylothorax. The tube, which is inserted into the pleural space, allows blood, fluid, pus, or air to drain and allows the lung to reinflate. Most chest tubes are placed at the fourth intercostal space in the anterior axillary line. This site allows for drainage of blood and air.

Gotta have some negative pressure

The tube restores negative pressure to the pleural space through an underwater-seal drainage system. The water in the system prevents air from being sucked back into the pleural space during inspiration. If a leak through the bronchi can't be sealed, suction applied to the underwater-seal system removes air from the pleural space faster than it can collect.

Nursing considerations

After chest-tube insertion

• Assess respiratory function and obtain vital signs and oxygen saturation levels immediately after insertion. Routinely assess chest-tube function. Describe and record the amount of drainage. Notify the practitioner immediately if the amount of drainage is greater than 200 ml in 1 hour (indicates bleeding).

• The fluid in the water-seal chamber typically rises on inspiration and decreases on expiration. However, if the patient is receiving positive-pressure ventilation, the opposite is normal.

• Avoid creating dependent loops, kinks, or pressure in the tubing. Don't lift the drainage system above the patient's chest because fluid may flow back into the pleural space. Keep two rubber-tipped clamps at the bedside to clamp the chest tube if the system cracks or to locate an air leak in the system. (See *Checking for chest-tube leaks*.)

• If the drainage collection chamber fills, replace it according to your facility's policy. To do so, double-clamp the chest tube close to the insertion site (using two clamps facing in opposite directions), exchange the system, remove the clamps, and retape the connection.

• To prevent a tension pneumothorax (which can result when clamping stops air and fluid from escaping), never leave the chest tube clamped for more than 1 minute.

• Notify the practitioner immediately if the patient develops cyanosis, rapid or shallow breathing, subcutaneous emphysema, chest pain, or excessive bleeding.

Tracheotomy

A tracheotomy is a surgical procedure that creates an opening into the trachea, called a *tracheostomy*. This opening allows insertion of an indwelling tube to keep the patient's airway open. The tracheostomy tube may be made of plastic, polyvinyl chloride, or metal and comes in various sizes, lengths, and styles, depending on the patient's needs. A patient receiving mechanical ventilation needs a cuffed tube to prevent backflow of air around the tube. A cuffed tracheostomy tube also prevents an unconscious or a paralyzed patient from aspirating food or secretions.

Emergency or planned procedure

In emergency situations, such as foreign body obstruction and laryngeal edema with anaphylactic shock, tracheotomy may be done at the bedside.

Nursing considerations

• Before an emergency tracheotomy, briefly explain the procedure to the patient as time permits and quickly obtain supplies or a tracheotomy tray.

• Ensure that samples for ABG analysis and other diagnostic tests have been collected and that the patient or a responsible family member has signed a consent form.

Checking for chest-tube leaks

When trying to locate a leak in your patient's chest-tube system, try:

• briefly clamping the tube at various points along its length, beginning at the tube's proximal end and working down toward the drainage system

• paying special attention to the seal around the connections

• pushing any loose connections back together and taping them securely.

Bubble may mean trouble

The bubbling of the system stops when a clamp is placed between an air leak and the water seal. If you clamp along the tube's entire length and the bubbling doesn't stop, you probably need to replace the drainage unit because it may be cracked.

Afterward ward

- After the procedure, assess the patient's respiratory status, breath sounds, oxygen saturation levels, vital signs, and heart rhythm. Note any crackles, rhonchi, wheezes, or diminished breath sounds.
- Assess the patient for such complications as hemorrhage, edema into tracheal tissue causing airway obstruction, aspiration of secretions, hypoxemia, and introduction of air into surrounding tissue causing subcutaneous emphysema.
- Document the procedure; the amount, color, and consistency of secretions, stoma, and skin conditions; the patient's respiratory status; the duration of any cuff deflation; and cuff pressure readings with inflation.

Common disorders

Some common respiratory disorders seen in the ED include airway obstruction, inhalation injuries, near drowning, pneumothorax, and status asthmaticus.

Airway obstruction

The body uses coughing as its main mechanism to clear the airway. Yet coughing may not clear the airway during some disease states, or even under normal, healthy conditions if an obstruction is present.

Upper airway obstruction is an interruption in the flow of air through the nose, mouth, pharynx, or larynx. Obstruction of the upper airway is considered a life-threatening situation; if not recognized early, it will progress to respiratory arrest. Respiratory arrest will lead to cardiac arrest, which requires cardiopulmonary resuscitation (CPR).

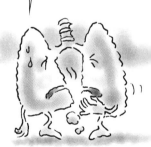

If coughing doesn't clear a patient's airway, he may have an obstruction.

What causes it

A patient's airway can become obstructed or compromised by vomitus, food, edema, or his tongue, teeth, or saliva. Although there are several causes of upper airway obstruction, the most common cause is the tongue. Because muscle tone decreases when a person is unconscious or unresponsive, the potential for the tongue and epiglottis to obstruct the airway increases. Partial airway obstruction is commonly caused by edema or a small foreign object that doesn't completely obstruct the airway.

t's anatomical

The presence of edema—edema of tongue (caused by trauma), laryngeal edema, and smoke inhalation edema—in anatomical structures of the upper airway can lead to an upper airway obstruction. Other potential causes include:

- anaphylaxis
- aspiration of a foreign object
- burns to the head, face, or neck area
- cerebral disorders (stroke)
- croup
- epiglottitis
- laryngospasms
- peritonsilar or pharyngeal abscesses
- tenacious secretions in the airway
- trauma of the face, trachea, or larynx
- tumors of the head or neck.

How it happens

In airway obstructions, the patient is partially able or not able to take in oxygen through inhalation. Hypoxemia results the longer the obstruction remains.

What to look for

Prompt detection and intervention can prevent a partial airway obstruction from progressing to a complete airway obstruction. Signs of a partial airway obstruction include diaphoresis, tachycardia, coughing, and elevated blood pressure. Patients with a partial obstruction may also experience no symptoms. With a complete airway obstruction, the following symptoms may be observed:

- sudden onset of choking or gagging
- stridor
- cyanosis
- wheezing, whistling, or any other unusual breath sound that indicates breathing difficulty
- diminished breath sounds (bilateral or unilateral)
- sense of impending doom.

What tests tell you

Physical examination may indicate decreased breath sounds. Tests aren't usually necessary to diagnose an upper airway obstruction but may include X-rays (particularly a chest X-ray), bronchoscopy, and laryngoscopy. If there are persistent symptoms of an upper airway obstruction, a chest X-ray, neck X-rays, laryn-

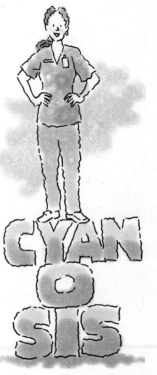

Stay on top of cyanosis by closely examining airway obstruction.

Opening an obstructed airway

To open an obstructed airway, use the head-tilt, chin-lift maneuver or the jaw-thrust maneuver as described here.

Head-tilt, chin-lift maneuver

In many cases of airway obstruction, the muscles controlling the patient's tongue have relaxed, causing the tongue to obstruct the airway. If the patient doesn't appear to have a neck injury, use the head-tilt, chin-lift maneuver to open his airway. Use these four steps to carry out this maneuver:

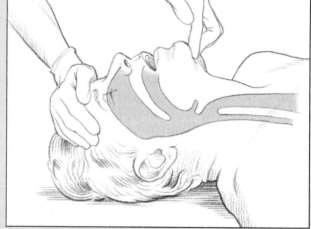

Place your hand that's closest to the patient's head on his forehead.

Apply firm pressure—firm enough to tilt the patient's head back.

Place the fingertips of your other hand under the bony portion of the patient's lower jaw, near the chin.

Lift the patient's chin. Be sure to keep his mouth partially open (as shown at right). Avoid placing your fingertips on the soft tissue under the patient's chin because this may inadvertently obstruct the airway you're trying to open.

Using the jaw-thrust maneuver

If you suspect a neck injury, use the jaw-thrust maneuver to open the patient's airway. Use these four steps to carry out this maneuver:

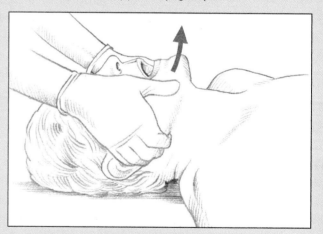

Kneel at the patient's head with your elbows on the ground.

Rest your thumbs on the patient's lower jaw near the corners of his mouth, pointing your thumbs toward his feet.

Place your fingertips around the lower jaw.

To open the airway, lift the lower jaw with your fingertips (as shown at right).

goscopy, or CT scan may be ordered to rule out the presence of a tumor, foreign body, or infection.

How it's treated

• Rapid assessment of airway patency, breathing, and circulation are foremost. (See *Opening an obstructed airway*.)

- Promptly assess the obstruction's cause. When an obstruction relates to the tongue or an accumulation of tenacious secretions, place the head in a slightly extended position and insert an oral airway.
- Promptly remove objects visible in the mouth with suction, fingers, or Magill forceps.
- If the patient can breathe (partial obstruction), encourage him to sit forward and cough to relieve the obstruction. However, be aware that this might worsen the obstruction and may totally occlude the airway.
- ET intubation and removal of the foreign object during insertion of the laryngoscope enables visualization of the obstruction.
- If an oral or ET airway doesn't provide ventilation, emergency cricothyroidotomy is indicated.

What to do

- Assess for the cause of the obstruction.
- Assess the patient's breath sounds bilaterally.
- Monitor oxygen saturation (using pulse oximetry) and cardiac rhythm continuously.
- Continually assess for stridor, cyanosis, and changes in LOC, and notify the practitioner immediately if any of these changes occur.
- Prepare for ET intubation if an airway can't be established.
- Prepare for a cricothyroidotomy if the patient's ventilation isn't established by oral or ET intubation.
- Anticipate cardiac arrest if the obstruction isn't cleared promptly.
- Monitor chest X-ray and ABG results after the obstruction is relieved.

Inhalation injuries

Inhalation injuries result from trauma to the pulmonary system after inhalation of toxic substances or inhalation of gases that are nontoxic but interfere with cellular respiration. Inhaled exposure forms include fog, mist, fume, dust, gas, vapor, or smoke. Inhalation injuries commonly accompany burns.

What causes it

There are many causes of inhalation injuries, including carbon monoxide poisoning and chemical and thermal inhalation.

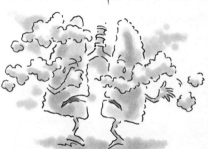

Fog, fumes, dust, gas—you name it! If it floats, it can probably cause inhalation injury.

Carbon monoxide poisoning

Carbon monoxide is a colorless, odorless, tasteless gas produced as a result of combustion and oxidation. Inhaling small amounts of this gas over a long period of time (or inhaling large amounts in a short period of time) can lead to poisoning. Carbon monoxide is considered a chemical asphyxiant. Accidental poisoning can result from exposure to heaters, smoke from a fire, or use of a gas lamp, gas stove, or charcoal grill in a small, poorly ventilated area.

> Accidental carbon monoxide poisoning can make any barbeque blue, so make sure to grill in a well-ventilated area.

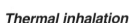

Chemical inhalation

A wide variety of gases may be generated when materials burn. The acids and alkalis produced in the burning process can produce chemical burns when inhaled. The inhaled substances can reach the respiratory tract as insoluble gases and lead to permanent damage. Synthetic materials also produce gases that can be toxic. Plastic material has the ability to produce toxic vapors when heated or burned.

Inhaling unburned chemicals in a powder or liquid form can also cause pulmonary damage. Such substances as ammonia, chlorine, sulfur dioxide, and hydrogen chloride are considered pulmonary irritants.

Thermal inhalation

Pulmonary complications remain the leading cause of death following thermal inhalation trauma. This type of trauma is commonly caused by the inhalation of hot air or steam. The mortality rate exceeds 50% when inhalation injury accompanies burns of the skin. This type of injury should be suspected when the circumstances associated with the patient's injuries involves flames in a confined area, even if burns on the surface of the patient's skin aren't visible.

Other complications

Pulmonary complications can arise from tight eschar formation on the chest from circumferential chest burns. The eschar can restrict chest movement or can impair ventilation from compression of the anatomical structures of the throat and neck. Visual assessment of the chest will reveal the ease of respirations, depth of chest movement, rate of respirations, and respiratory effort.

How it happens

Carbon monoxide poisoning

There are several gases (such as carbon monoxide and hydrogen cyanide) that are nontoxic to the respiratory system directly yet interfere with cellular respiration. Carbon monoxide has a greater attraction to hemoglobin than oxygen. When carbon monoxide enters the blood, it binds with the hemoglobin to form carboxyhemoglobin. Carboxyhemoglobin reduces the oxygen-carrying capacity of hemoglobin. This reduction results in decreased oxygenation to the cells and tissues.

Chemical inhalation

Irritating gases (chlorine, hydrogen chloride, nitrogen dioxide, phosgene, and sulfur dioxide) commonly combine with water in the lungs to form corrosive acids. These acids cause denaturization of proteins, cellular damage, and edema of the pulmonary tissues. Smoke inhalation injuries generally fall into this category. Chemical burns to the airway are similar to burns on the skin, except that they're painless. The tracheobronchial tree is insensitive to pain. The inhalation of small quantities of noxious chemicals can also damage the alveoli and bronchi.

Thermal inhalation

Inhaled hot air or steam is rapidly cooled by the upper airway. Because the hot air or steam is confined to this area, the upper airway suffers the greatest damage. Inhaled hot air or steam can also injure the lower respiratory tract because water holds heat better than dry air. Even so, this injury is rare because reflexive closure of the vocal cords and laryngeal spasm commonly prevent full inhalation of the hot air or steam.

What to look for

Physical findings with an inhalation injury vary depending on the gas or substance inhaled and the duration of the exposure.

Carbon monoxide poisoning

Carboxyhemoglobin reduces the oxygen-carrying capacity of hemoglobin. This reduction commonly causes the patient's face to turn bright red and the lips cherry red. The symptoms of carbon monoxide (CO) poisoning vary with the concentration of carboxyhemoglobin. (See *Oxygen saturation in CO poisoning*.)

When it's a little...

Mild poisoning generally indicates a CO level from 11% to 20%. Symptoms at this concentration commonly include:
- slight shortness of breath
- headache
- decreased visual acuity
- decreased cerebral function.

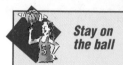

Stay on the ball

Oxygen saturation in CO poisoning

When assessing for carbon monoxide (CO) poisoning, be aware that pulse oximetry devices measure oxygenated and deoxygenated hemoglobin but don't measure dysfunctional hemoglobin such as carboxyhemoglobin. Therefore, the oxygen saturation levels in the presence of carbon monoxide poisoning will be within normal ranges, as the carboxyhemoglobin levels aren't measured.

When it's a lot...

Moderate poisoning indicates a CO level from 21% to 41%. Symptoms at this concentration include:

- altered mental status
- confusion
- headache
- tinnitus
- dizziness
- drowsiness
- irritability
- nausea
- changes in skin color
- electrocardiograph (ECG) changes
- tachycardia
- hypotension
- stupor.

And when it's way too much...

Severe poisoning is defined as a level of CO from 42% to 60%. Symptoms include:

- convulsions
- coma
- generalized instability.

In the final stage (fatal poisoning), the CO level reaches 61% to 80% and results in death.

Chemical inhalation

The most common effects of smoke or chemical inhalation include atelectasis, pulmonary edema, and tissue anoxia. Respiratory distress usually occurs early in the course of smoke inhalation secondary to hypoxia. Patients also exhibiting no respiratory difficulties may suddenly develop respiratory distress. Intubation and mechanical ventilation equipment should be available for immediate use.

Thermal inhalation

The entire respiratory tract has the potential to be damaged by thermal inhalation injury; however, injury rarely progresses to the lungs. Ulcerations, erythema, and edema of the mouth and epiglottis are the initial symptoms of this type of injury. Edema may rapidly progress to upper airway obstruction. You may also note stridor, wheezing, rales, increased secretions, hoarseness, and shortness of breath. Direct thermal injury to the upper

"Hoarse"-ness is a common symptom of thermal inhalation...just like the silence I'm hearing now is a common symptom of bad puns.

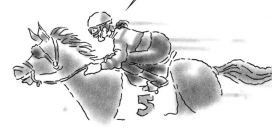

airway yields burns of the face and lips, burned nasal hairs, and laryngeal edema.

What tests tell you

Initial laboratory studies commonly include electrolytes, liver function studies, BUN and creatinine, and a complete blood count (CBC). Obtaining these studies will provide baseline data for analysis. ABG analysis will provide valuable information on the acid-base status, ventilation, and oxygenation status of the patient. In patients with suspected CO poisoning, a carboxyhemoglobin level will be obtained. Cardiac monitoring will monitor ischemic changes, and ECG and chest X-ray will also be evaluated. A depressed ST segment on ECG is a common finding in the moderate stage of CO poisoning.

How it's treated

• Assessment of the patient's airway, breathing, and circulation is the first step.
• Obtain a history of the exposure and attempt to identify the toxic agent of exposure.
• Immediately provide oxygen to the patient. Intubation and mechanical ventilation may be required if the patient demonstrates severe respiratory distress or an altered mental state.
• Upper airway edema requires emergent ET intubation.
• Bronchodilators, antibiotics, and I.V. fluids may be prescribed.
• The preferred treatment for CO poisoning is administering 100% humidified oxygen and continuing until carboxyhemoglobin levels fall to the nontoxic range of 10%.
• Chest physical therapy may assist in the removal of necrotic tissue.
• The use of hyperbaric oxygen for CO poisoning remains controversial, although it's known to lower carboxyhemoglobin levels faster than humidified oxygen.
• Fluid resuscitation is an important component of managing inhalation injury; however, careful monitoring of fluid status is essential because of the risk of pulmonary edema.

What to do

• Remove the patient's clothing, but take care to prevent self-contamination from the toxic substance if the clothing has possibly been exposed to it.
• Establish I.V. access for medication, blood products, and fluid administration.
• Obtain laboratory specimens to evaluate ventilation, oxygenation, and baseline values.
• Obtain chest X-ray, ECG, and pulmonary function studies.

- Implement cardiac monitoring to assess for ischemic changes or arrhythmias.
- Monitor for signs of pulmonary edema that may accompany fluid resuscitation.
- In the event of bronchospasms, provide oxygen, bronchodilators via a nebulizer and, possibly, aminophylline.
- Monitor fluid balance and intake and output closely.
- Administer antibiotics as prescribed.
- Assess lung sounds frequently, and notify the practitioner immediately of changes in those sounds or oxygenation.
- Provide a supportive and educative environment for the patient, his family, and significant others. (See *Inhalation injury in children.*)
- Monitor laboratory studies for changes that may indicate multisystem complications.

Near drowning

Near drowning refers to surviving—at least temporarily—the physiologic effects of hypoxemia and acidosis that result from submersion in fluid. Hypoxemia and acidosis are the primary problems in victims of near drowning. Although we know that drowning claims nearly 8,000 lives annually in the United States, no statistics are available for near-drowning incidents.

What causes it

Near drowning results from an inability to swim or, in swimmers, from panic, a boating accident, a heart attack, a blow to the head while in the water, heavy drinking before swimming, or a suicide attempt.

Near drowning takes three forms:
- *dry*, in which the victim doesn't aspirate fluid but suffers respiratory obstruction or asphyxia (10% to 15% of patients)
- *wet*, in which the victim aspirates fluid and suffers from asphyxia or secondary changes due to fluid aspiration (about 85% of patients)
- *secondary*, in which the victim suffers a recurrence of respiratory distress (usually aspiration pneumonia or pulmonary edema) within minutes or 1 to 2 days after a near-drowning incident.

How it happens

Regardless of the tonicity of the fluid aspirated, hypoxemia is the most serious consequence of near drowning, followed by metabolic acidosis. Other consequences depend on the kind of water aspirated.

Ages and stages

Inhalation injury in children

It's essential that your care of a child with inhalation injury address the emotional and psychological needs of the child and his family. Initially, care will focus on oxygenating and stabilizing the child and managing the physical components of his injury. However, your care must eventually encompass the psychological needs of the frightened child and the emotional needs of his parents.

Parents may feel guilt if the injury could have been prevented or even if it couldn't. Be sure to provide information to the parents about their child's condition, prognosis, treatment plan, and discharge needs. In addition to ongoing communication, psychological intervention may be needed to discuss feelings of guilt, emotional stress, or fears of the parent and child.

Physiologic changes in near drowning

This flowchart shows the primary cellular alterations that occur during near drowning. Separate pathways are shown for saltwater and freshwater incidents. Hypothermia presents a separate pathway that may preserve neurologic function by decreasing the metabolic rate. All pathways lead to diffuse pulmonary edema.

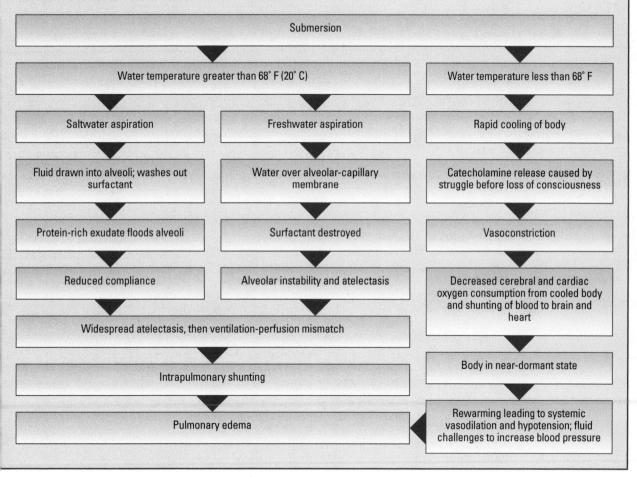

After freshwater aspiration, changes in the character of lung surfactant result in exudation of protein-rich plasma into the alveoli. These changes, plus increased capillary permeability, lead to pulmonary edema and hypoxemia. (See *Physiologic changes in near drowning.*)

After saltwater aspiration, the hypertonicity of seawater exerts an osmotic force that pulls fluid from pulmonary capillaries into the alveoli. The resulting intrapulmonary shunt causes hypoxemia. Also, the pulmonary capillary membrane may be injured and induce pulmonary edema. In both kinds of near drowning, pulmonary edema and hypoxemia take place secondary to aspiration.

What to look for

Near-drowning victims can display a host of clinical problems, including:
- fever
- confusion
- unconsciousness
- irritability
- lethargy
- restlessness
- substernal chest pain
- shallow or gasping respirations
- cough that produces a pink, frothy fluid
- vomiting
- abdominal distention
- apnea
- asystole
- bradycardia
- tachycardia.

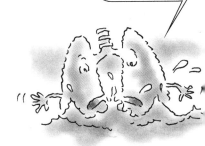

I like some aspirations: a good job, a happy home life. But freshwater and saltwater are aspirations I could do without.

What tests tell you

Diagnosis requires a history of near drowning, including the type of water aspirated, along with characteristic features and auscultation of crackles and rhonchi.

ABG analysis shows decreased oxygen content, low bicarbonate levels, and low pH. Electrolyte levels may be elevated or decreased, depending on the type of water aspirated. Leukocytosis may occur. ECG shows arrhythmias and waveform changes.

How it's treated

- Emergency treatment begins with CPR and administration of 100% oxygen.
- If hypothermia is an issue, measures must be taken to warm the patient.
- Ongoing support and monitoring of circulation and oxygenation should be maintained, and hemodynamic monitoring should be instituted.

What to do

- Stabilize the patient's neck in case he has a cervical injury.
- Assess for a patent airway, and be prepared to administer high-flow oxygen and assist with ET intubation.

• Assess the patient's core body temperature, and be prepared to institute rewarming as necessary.
• Continue CPR, intubate the patient, and provide respiratory assistance, such as mechanical ventilation with positive end-expiratory pressure (PEEP), if needed.
• Assess ABG and pulse oximetry values.
• If the patient's abdomen is distended, insert a nasogastric tube. (Intubate the patient first if he's unconscious.)
• Start I.V. lines and insert an indwelling urinary catheter.
• Give medications as ordered; drug treatment for near-drowning victims is controversial. Such treatment may include sodium bicarbonate for acidosis, corticosteroids and osmotic diuretics for cerebral edema, antibiotics to prevent infections, and broncho-dilators to ease bronchospasms.
• Observe for pulmonary complications and signs of delayed drowning (confusion, substernal pain, adventitious breath sounds). Suction often. Pulmonary artery catheters may be useful in assessing cardiopulmonary status.
• Monitor vital signs, intake and output, and peripheral pulses.
• Check for skin perfusion and watch for signs of infection.
• To facilitate breathing, raise the head of the bed slightly.
• Prepare to administer prophylactic antibiotics as needed.
• Correct acid-base imbalances.
• Prepare the patient for transfer to a CCU or, if patient is a child, to a pediatric unit or facility.

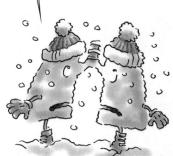

Make sure to check the near drowning patient's core body temperature to assess for hypothermia.

Pneumothorax

Pneumothorax is an accumulation of air in the pleural cavity that leads to partial or complete lung collapse. The amount of air trapped in the intrapleural space determines the degree of lung collapse. In some cases, venous return to the heart is impeded, causing a life-threatening condition called *tension pneumothorax*.

Pneumothorax can be classified as *traumatic* or *spontaneous*. Traumatic pneumothorax may be further classified as *open* or *closed*. (Note that an open, or penetrating, *wound* may cause *closed* pneumothorax.) Spontaneous pneumothorax, which is also considered *closed*, is most common in older patients with COPD but can appear in young, healthy patients as well.

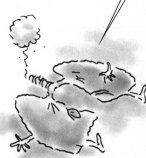

Air plus pleural cavity equals partial or complete lung collapse.

What causes it

The causes of pneumothorax vary according to classification.

Traumatic pneumothorax

Traumatic pneumothorax may be open or closed.

Open book

Causes of open pneumothorax include:
- penetrating chest injury (stab or gunshot wound)
- insertion of a central venous catheter
- thoracentesis or closed pleural biopsy
- transbronchial biopsy
- chest surgery.

Closed call

Causes of closed pneumothorax include:
- blunt chest trauma
- interstitial lung disease such as eosinophilic granuloma
- tubercular or cancerous lesions that erode into the pleural space
- air leakage from ruptured blebs
- rupture resulting from barotrauma caused by high intrathoracic pressures during mechanical ventilation.

Spontaneous pneumothorax

Spontaneous pneumothorax is usually caused by the rupture of a subpleural bleb (a small cystic space) at the surface of a lung.

Tension pneumothorax

Causes of tension pneumothorax include:
- penetrating chest wound treated with an airtight dressing
- fractured ribs
- mechanical ventilation
- chest tube occlusion or malfunction
- high-level PEEP that causes alveolar blebs to rupture.

How it happens

Traumatic pneumothorax

Open pneumothorax results from atmospheric air flowing directly into the pleural cavity (under negative pressure). As the air pressure in the pleural cavity becomes positive, the lung on the affected side collapses, causing decreased total lung capacity. As a result, the patient develops a $\dot{V}/\dot{Q}$ imbalance that leads to hypoxia.

Closed pneumothorax results when an opening is created between the intrapleural space and the parenchyma of the lung. Air enters the pleural space from within the lung, causing increased pleural pressure and preventing lung expansion during inspiration.

Understanding tension pneumothorax

In tension pneumothorax, air accumulates intrapleurally and can't escape. As intrapleural pressure increases, the lung on the affected side collapses.

On inspiration, the mediastinum shifts toward the unaffected lung, impairing ventilation.

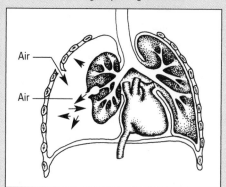

On expiration, the mediastinal shift distorts the vena cava and reduces venous return.

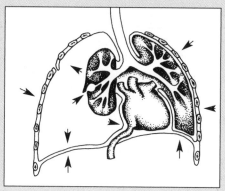

Spontaneous pneumothorax

In spontaneous pneumothorax, the rupture of a subpleural bleb causes air leakage into the pleural spaces, which causes the lung to collapse. Hypoxia results from decreased total lung capacity, vital capacity, and lung compliance.

Tension pneumothorax

Tension pneumothorax results when air in the pleural space is under higher pressure than air in the adjacent lung. (See *Understanding tension pneumothorax.*) Here's what happens:

• Air enters the pleural space from the site of pleural rupture, which acts as a one-way valve. Thus, air enters the pleural space on inspiration but can't escape as the rupture site closes on expiration.

• More air enters with each inspiration, and air pressure begins to exceed barometric pressure.

• The air pushes against the recoiled lung, causing compression atelectasis, and pushes against the mediastinum, compressing and displacing the heart and great vessels.

• The mediastinum eventually shifts away from the affected side, affecting venous return and putting ever greater pressure on the heart, great vessels, trachea, and contralateral lung. Without immediate treatment, this emergency can rapidly become fatal.

I try my best to hang loose—tension just isn't my thing, and neither is tension pneumothorax.

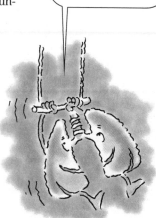

What to look for

Assessment findings depend on the severity of the pneumothorax. Spontaneous pneumothorax that releases a small amount of air into the pleural space may cause no signs or symptoms. Generally, tension pneumothorax causes the most severe respiratory signs and symptoms.

Every breath hurts

Your patient's history reveals sudden, sharp, pleuritic chest pain. The patient may report that chest movement, breathing, and coughing exacerbate the pain. He may also report shortness of breath.

Further findings

Inspection reveals asymmetric chest wall movement with overexpansion and rigidity on the affected side. The skin may be cool, clammy, and cyanotic. Palpation of the chest wall may reveal crackling beneath the skin (subcutaneous emphysema) and decreased vocal fremitus.

In addition, percussion may reveal hyperresonance on the affected side. Auscultation may disclose decreased or absent breath sounds on the affected side. Vital signs may follow the pattern of respiratory distress seen with respiratory failure.

Did we mention the tension?

Tension pneumothorax also causes:
• distended jugular veins as a result of high intrapleural pressure, mediastinal shift, and increased cardiovascular pressure
• hypotension and tachycardia due to decreased cardiac output
• tracheal deviation to the opposite side (a late sign).

What tests tell you

• Chest X-rays reveal air in the pleural space and a mediastinal shift, which confirm pneumothorax.
• ABG analysis reveals hypoxemia, usually with elevated $Paco_2$ and normal bicarbonate ion levels in the early stages.
• ECG may reveal decreased QRS amplitude, precordial T-wave inversion and rightward shift of the frontal QRS axis.

How it's treated

Treatment of pneumothorax depends on the cause and severity.

With trauma

Open or closed pneumothorax may necessitate surgical repair of affected tissues, followed by chest-tube placement with an underwater seal.

With less lung collapse

Spontaneous pneumothorax with less than 30% lung collapse, no signs of increased pleural pressure, and no dyspnea or indications of physiologic compromise may be corrected with:
• aspiration of air from the intrapleural space with a large-bore needle attached to a syringe to restore negative pressure within the pleural space
• oxygen administration to improve hypoxia
• vital signs monitoring to detect physiologic compromise.

With more lung collapse

Lung collapse greater than 30% may necessitate other measures, such as:
• placing a chest tube in the second or third intercostal space in the midclavicular line to reexpand the lung by restoring negative intrapleural pressure
• connecting the chest tube to an underwater seal or a low-pressure suction to reexpand the lung.

With tension

Treatment for tension pneumothorax typically involves:
• analgesics to promote comfort and encourage deep breathing and coughing
• immediate large-bore needle insertion into the pleural space through the second intercostal space to reexpand the lung, followed by insertion of a chest tube if large amounts of air escape through the needle after insertion.

What to do

• Assess the patient's respiratory status, including auscultation of bilateral breath sounds.
• Monitor oxygen saturation levels closely for changes; obtain ABG analysis as ordered.
• Monitor hemodynamic parameters frequently, as appropriate and indicated. Anticipate the need for cardiac monitoring because hypoxemia can predispose the patient to arrhythmias.
• Initiate and maintain vascular access.
• Watch for complications, signaled by pallor, gasping respirations, and sudden chest pain. Carefully monitor vital signs at least every hour for indications of shock, increasing respiratory distress, or mediastinal shift. If your patient's respiratory status dete-

riorates, anticipate the need for ET intubation and mechanical ventilation and assist as necessary.
• Assist with chest-tube insertion and connect to suction as ordered. Monitor your patient for possible complications associated with chest-tube insertion.
• Maintain bed rest in high Fowler's position.

Status asthmaticus

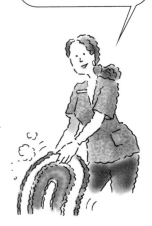

Look at it this way—you aren't spring cleaning, you're reducing the risk of extrinsic asthma.

Status asthmaticus is a life-threatening situation resulting from an acute asthma attack. It begins with impaired gas exchange and—without rapid intervention—may lead to respiratory failure and, eventually, death.

Asthma overview

Asthma is a chronic inflammatory airway disorder that causes episodic airway obstruction and hyperresponsiveness of the airway to multiple stimuli. It results from bronchospasms, increased mucus secretion, and mucosal edema. If left untreated or if the patient doesn't respond to drug therapy after 24 hours, status asthmaticus is diagnosed.

Making things worse

Asthma exacerbations are acute or subacute episodes of worsening shortness of breath, coughing, and wheezing, with measurable decreases in expiratory airflow.

What causes it

Many asthmatics, especially children, have intrinsic and extrinsic asthma.

Outside factors

Extrinsic (or *atopic*) asthma begins in childhood. Patients are typically sensitive to specific external allergens. Extrinsic allergens that can trigger an asthma attack include pollen, animal dander, house dust or mold, kapok or feather pillows, food additives containing sulfites, and other sensitizing substances.

Extrinsic asthma in childhood is commonly accompanied by other hereditary allergies, such as eczema and allergic rhinitis.

Factors within

Patients with intrinsic (or *nonatopic*) asthma react to internal, nonallergenic factors. Intrinsic factors that can trigger an asthma attack include irritants, emotional stress, fatigue, endocrine changes, temperature variations, humidity variations, exposure to noxious fumes, anxiety, coughing or laughing, and genetic factors.

Most episodes take place after a severe respiratory tract infection, especially in adults.

Irritants in the workplace

Many adults acquire an allergic form of asthma or exacerbation of existing asthma from exposure to agents in the workplace. Irritants include chemicals in flour, acid anhydrides, and excreta of dust mites in carpet.

Genetic messes

Asthma is associated with two genetic influences:

☝ ability to develop asthma because of an abnormal gene (atopy)

✌ tendency to develop hyperresponsive airways (without atopy).

A potent mix

Environmental factors interact with inherited factors to cause asthmatic reactions with associated bronchospasms.

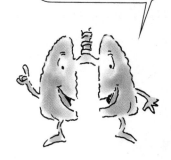

Irritants in the workplace—and no, the guy who hogs the copier doesn't count—can exacerbate existing asthma.

How it happens

Status asthmaticus begins with an asthma attack. In asthma, bronchial linings overreact to various stimuli, causing episodic smooth-muscle spasms that severely constrict the airways. Here's how asthma develops into status asthmaticus:

• Immunoglobulin (Ig) E antibodies attached to histamine-containing mast cells and receptors on cell membranes initiate intrinsic asthma attacks.

• When exposed to an antigen, such as pollen, the IgE antibody combines with it.

• On subsequent exposure to the antigen, mast cells degranulate and release mediators.

• Mast cells in the lung are stimulated to release histamine and the slow-reacting substance of anaphylaxis.

Attachment disorder

• Histamine attaches to receptor sites in the larger bronchi, where it causes swelling in smooth muscles.

• Mucous membranes become inflamed, irritated, and swollen. The patient may experience dyspnea, prolonged expiration, and an increased respiratory rate.

• Leukotrienes attach to receptor sites in the smaller bronchi and cause local swelling of the smooth muscle.

• Leukotrienes also cause prostaglandins to travel by way of the bloodstream to the lungs, where they enhance the effect of hista-

mine. A wheeze may be audible during coughing—the higher the pitch, the narrower the bronchial lumen.
• Histamine stimulates the mucous membranes to secrete excessive mucus, further narrowing the bronchial lumen.

A not-so-good goblet

• Goblet cells secrete viscous mucus that's difficult to cough up, resulting in coughing, rhonchi, higher-pitched wheezing, and increased respiratory distress. Mucosal edema and thickened secretions further block the airways.
• On inhalation, the narrowed bronchial lumen can still expand slightly, allowing air to reach the alveoli. On exhalation, increased intrathoracic pressure closes the bronchial lumen completely. Air enters but can't escape.
• When status asthmaticus occurs, hypoxemia worsens and the expiratory rate and volume decrease even further.
• Obstructed airways impede gas exchange and increase airway resistance. The patient labors to breathe.
• As breathing and hypoxemia tire the patient, the respiratory rate drops to normal, $Paco_2$ levels rise, and the patient hypoventilates from exhaustion.
• Respiratory acidosis develops as $Paco_2$ increases.
• The situation becomes life-threatening when no air is audible on auscultation (a silent chest) and $Paco_2$ rises to over 70 mm Hg.
• Without treatment, the patient experiences acute respiratory failure.

What to look for

A patient who comes to the ED during a suspected asthma attack will demonstrate:
• absent or minimal wheezing
• inability to speak more than a few words before pausing for breath
• fatigue
• decreasing LOC
• inability to lay flat
• pulsus paradoxus greater than 20 mm Hg
• long expiratory phase
• Spo_2 less than 90%
• hypoxemia
• hypercarbia (elevated $Paco_2$)
• metabolic acidosis
• increased respiratory rate
• use of accessory muscles
• cyanosis (a late sign and usually unreliable).

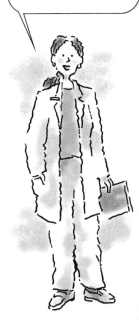

One instance where silence isn't golden: when it's in your patient's chest and means his asthma attack has become life-threatening.

What tests tell you

• Pulmonary function tests reveal decreased vital capacity and increased total lung and residual capacities during an acute attack. Peak and expiratory flow rate measurements are less than 60% of baseline.
• Pulse oximetry commonly shows that oxygen saturation is less than 90%.
• Chest X-ray may show hyperinflation with areas of atelectasis and flat diaphragm due to increased intrathoracic volume.
• ABG analysis reveals decreasing Pa_{O_2} and increasing Pa_{CO_2}.
• ECG shows sinus tachycardia during an attack.
• Sputum analysis may indicate increased viscosity, mucus plugs, presence of Curschmann's spirals (casts of airways), Charcot-Leyden crystals, and eosinophils. Culture may disclose causative organisms if infection is the trigger.
• CBC with differential shows an increased eosinophil count secondary to inflammation and an elevated white blood cell count and granulocyte count if an acute infection is present.

How it's treated

In acute status asthmaticus, the patient is monitored closely for respiratory failure. Oxygen, bronchodilators, epinephrine, corticosteroids, and nebulizer therapies may be ordered. The patient may be intubated and placed on mechanical ventilation if Pa_{CO_2} increases or if he experiences respiratory arrest.
     Treatment may include the use of:
• humidified oxygen to correct dyspnea, cyanosis, and hypoxemia and to maintain an oxygen saturation greater than 90%
• mechanical ventilation, which is necessary if the patient doesn't respond to initial ventilatory support and drugs or develops respiratory failure

Bucking bronchos

• bronchodilators, such as epinephrine and albuterol (Ventolin), to decrease bronchoconstriction, reduce bronchial airway edema, and increase pulmonary ventilation
• subcutaneous epinephrine to counteract the effects of mediators of an asthma attack
• anticholinergics to increase the effects of bronchodilators
• corticosteroids, such as methylprednisolone (Medrol), to decrease bronchoconstriction, reduce bronchial airway edema, and increase pulmonary ventilation
• mast cell stabilizers, such as cromolyn (Intal) and nedocromil (Tilade), in patients with atopic asthma who have seasonal disease because, when given prophylactically, they block the acute obstructive effects of antigen exposure by inhibiting the degranu-

lation of mast cells, thereby preventing the release of chemical mediators responsible for anaphylaxis
• relaxation exercises to increase circulation and aid recovery from an asthma attack.

What to do

• Monitor SpO_2.
• Monitor ABGs as indicated.
• Provide supplemental oxygen.
• Administer bronchodilators.
• Establish and maintain vascular access.
• Prepare for possible ET intubation.
• Assess the patient's respiratory status, especially if he isn't intubated.
• Check the respiratory rate.
• Auscultate for breath sounds.
• Monitor oxygen saturation.
• Assess the patient's mental status for confusion, agitation, or lethargy.
• Assess the patient's heart rate and rhythm.
• Initiate cardiac monitoring, and be alert for cardiac arrhythmias related to bronchodilator therapy or hypoxemia.
• Obtain ordered tests and report results promptly.
• When the acute phase is over, position the patient for maximum comfort, usually in semi-Fowler's position. Encourage coughing to clear secretions.
• Offer emotional support and reassurance.

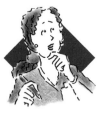

Quick quiz

1.   When auscultating for breath sounds in a patient's lungs, you hear crackles, which are caused by:
    A.   secretions blocking the bronchial airways.
    B.   collapsed or fluid-filled alveoli snapping open.
    C.   foreign body obstructing the trachea.
    D.   consolidation.

Answer: B. Crackles are caused by alveoli opening and are usually associated with fluid in the alveolar space.

2. Which ABG analysis results would you expect to find in a patient with acute respiratory failure?

- A. pH 7.25, Pao_2 48, $Paco_2$ 55
- B. pH 7.40, Pao_2 82, $Paco_2$ 45
- C. pH 7.50, Pao_2 60, $Paco_2$ 30
- D. pH 7.30, Pao_2 85, $Paco_2$ 48

Answer: A. The patient with a Pao_2 less than 50, a decreased pH, and an elevated $Paco_2$ is hypoxemic and in respiratory acidosis.

3. ET tubes have inflatable cuffs to:

- A. measure pressure on tracheal tissues.
- B. drain gastric contents.
- C. prevent backflow of oxygen.
- D. treat laryngeal edema.

Answer: C. ET tube cuffs prevent backflow of oxygen so that it's delivered fully to the lungs.

4. Which condition is a cause of spontaneous pneumothorax?

- A. Fractured ribs
- B. Rupture of a small cystic area on the lung's surface
- C. Interstitial lung disease
- D. Mechanical ventilation

Answer: B. In spontaneous pneumothorax, the rupture of a subpleural bleb results in air leakage into the pleural spaces, causing lung collapse. Hypoxia results from decreased total lung capacity, vital capacity, and lung compliance.

5. Why are chemical burns to the airway from inhalation injury usually painless?

- A. The chemical alters the patient's sense of perception.
- B. The patient immediately becomes unconscious after the injury.
- C. The tracheobronchial tree is insensitive to pain.
- D. The burn damages the nerves, and the patient can't sense the pain.

Answer: C. Chemical burns to the airway are similar to burns on the skin, except that they're painless. The tracheobronchial tree is insensitive to pain. The inhalation of small quantities of noxious chemicals can also damage the alveoli and bronchi.

6. The preferred treatment for CO poisoning is:
   A. administration of 100% humidified oxygen.
   B. sedation.
   C. hyperbaric oxygen therapy.
   D. corticosteroid therapy.

Answer: A. The preferred treatment for CO poisoning is administering 100% humidified oxygen until carboxyhemoglobin levels fall to the nontoxic range of 10%.

Scoring

☆☆☆ If you answered all six questions correctly, breathe a big sigh of relief. You're a respiratory mastermind!

☆☆ If you answered four or five questions correctly, don't wait to exhale. You're an inspiration!

☆ If you answered fewer than four questions correctly, you're on the verge of expiration. Take a deep breath and dive back into the chapter!

6

Gastrointestinal emergencies

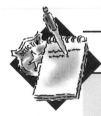

Just the facts

In this chapter, you'll learn:

♦ emergency assessment of the GI system

♦ diagnostic tests and procedures for GI emergencies

♦ GI disorders in the emergency department and their treatments.

Understanding GI emergencies

Being able to identify subtle changes in a patient's GI system can mean the difference between effective and ineffective emergency care. GI signs and symptoms can have many baffling causes. When your patient comes to the emergency department (ED) with a GI emergency, your assessment can be used to determine whether the patient's signs and symptoms are related to his current medical problem or indicate a new problem.

When faced with an emergency involving the GI system, you must assess the patient thoroughly and stay alert for subtle changes that may indicate a potential deterioration in his condition. A thorough assessment forms the basis for your interventions, which then must be instituted quickly to minimize what can be life-threatening risks to the patient.

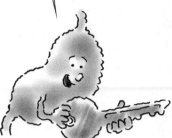

The keys to many GI emergency mysteries are careful assessment and quick action.

Assessment

Unless the patient requires immediate stabilizing treatment, begin by taking a thorough health history. Then probe further by conducting a thorough physical examination using inspection, auscultation, palpation, and percussion.

If you can't interview the patient because of his condition, you may gather history information from the patient's medical record.

In some cases, you may need to ask his family or the emergency medical response team that transported him to the ED.

Health history

Begin by introducing yourself and explaining what happens during the health history and physical examination. Then obtain information about the patient's chief complaint, medications used, family history, and lifestyle patterns. Conduct this part of the assessment as privately as possible because the patient may feel embarrassed when talking about GI function.

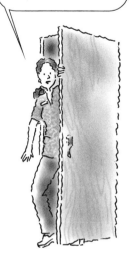

A patient may be embarrassed to talk about GI function, so make your health history assessment as private as possible.

Chief complaint

A patient with a GI problem usually complains of:
- altered bowel habits
- heartburn
- nausea
- pain
- vomiting.

To investigate these and other signs and symptoms, ask about the onset, duration, and severity of each. Inquire about the location of the pain, precipitating factors, alleviating factors, and associated symptoms. (See *Asking the right questions.*)

Previous health status

To determine if the patient's problem is new or recurring, ask about GI illnesses, such as an ulcer, gallbladder disease, inflammatory bowel disease, and GI bleeding. Also ask if he has had abdominal surgery or trauma.

Further questions

Ask the patient additional questions, such as:
- Are you allergic to any foods or medications?
- Have you noticed a change in the color, amount, and appearance of your stool? Have you ever seen blood in your stool?
- Have you recently traveled abroad? (This question applies if the patient seeks care for diarrhea, because diarrhea, hepatitis, and parasitic infections can result from ingesting contaminated food or water.)
- Ask him about his dental history. Poor dentition may impair his ability to chew and swallow food.

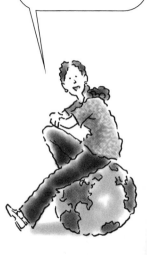

Ask about travel—sometimes a patient returns from abroad with diarrhea, hepatitis, or parasites as souvenirs!

Medications used

Ask the patient if he's taking medication. Several drugs, including aspirin, sulfonamides, nonsteroidal anti-inflammatory drugs

Asking the right questions

When assessing a patient with gastrointestinal-related signs and symptoms, be sure to ask the right questions. To establish a baseline for comparison, ask about the patient's current state of health, including questions about the onset, duration, quality, severity, and location of problems as well as precipitating factors, alleviating factors, and associated symptoms.

Onset

How did the problem start? Was it gradual or sudden? With or without previous symptoms? What was the patient doing when he noticed it? If he has diarrhea, has he been traveling? If so, when and where?

Duration

When did the problem start? Has the patient had the problem before? Has he had abdominal surgery? If yes, when? If he's in pain, find out when the problem began. Is the pain continuous, intermittent, or colicky (cramplike)?

Quality

Ask the patient to describe the problem. Has he ever had it before? Was it diagnosed? If he's in pain, find out whether the pain feels sharp, dull, aching, or burning.

Severity

Ask the patient to describe how badly the problem bothers him—for example, have him rate it on a pain scale of 0 to 10. Does it keep him from his normal activities? Has it improved or worsened since he first noticed it? Does it wake him at night? If he's in pain, does he double over from it?

Location

Where does the patient feel the problem? Does it spread, radiate, or shift? Ask him to point to where he feels it the most.

Precipitating factors

Does anything seem to bring on the problem? What makes it worse? Does it occur at the same time each day or with certain positions? Does the patient notice it after eating or drinking certain foods or after certain activities?

Alleviating factors

Does anything relieve the problem? Does the patient take any prescribed or over-the-counter medications for relief? Has he tried anything else for relief?

Associated symptoms

What else bothers the patient when he has the problem? Has he had nausea, vomiting, dry heaves, diarrhea, constipation, bloating, or flatulence? Has he lost his appetite or lost or gained any weight? If so, how much? When was the patient's last bowel movement? Was it unusual? Has he seen blood in his vomitus or stool? Has his stool changed in size or color or included mucus? Ask the patient whether he can eat normally and hold down foods and liquids. Also ask about alcohol consumption.

(NSAIDs), analgesics, and some antihypertensives, can cause nausea, vomiting, diarrhea, constipation, and other GI problems. Be sure to ask about laxative use because habitual laxative intake can cause constipation.

Family history

Because some GI disorders are hereditary, ask the patient whether anyone in his family has had a GI disorder, including:
• alcoholism
• colon cancer
• Crohn's disease
• diabetes
• stomach ulcer
• ulcerative colitis.

Lifestyle patterns

Psychological and sociologic factors can profoundly affect health. To determine factors that may have contributed to your patient's problem, ask about his occupation, home life, financial situation, stress level, and recent life changes.

Be sure to ask about alcohol, illegal drug, caffeine, and tobacco use as well as food consumption, exercise habits, and oral hygiene. Also ask about sleep patterns, such as hours of sleep and whether sleep is restful.

Cultural factors may affect a patient's dietary habits, so ask about any dietary restrictions the patient has, such as following a vegetarian diet.

Physical examination

Physical examination of the GI system usually includes evaluation of the mouth, abdomen, liver, rectum, and spleen. Before beginning your examination, explain the techniques you'll be using and warn the patient that some procedures might be uncomfortable. Perform the examination in a private, quiet, warm, and well-lighted room.

Assessing the mouth

Use inspection and palpation to assess the oral cavity:
• First, inspect the patient's mouth and jaw for asymmetry and swelling. Check his bite, noting malocclusion from an overbite or underbite. If the patient has dentures, do they fit? Are they intact or broken?
• Inspect the inner and outer lips, teeth, and gums with a penlight. Note bleeding, gum ulcerations, and missing, displaced, or broken teeth. Palpate the gums for tenderness and the inner lips and cheeks for lesions.
• Assess the tongue, checking for coating, tremors, swelling, and ulcerations. Note unusual breath odors.
• Lastly, examine the pharynx, looking for uvular deviation, tonsillar abnormalities, lesions, plaques, and exudate.

Assessing the abdomen

To ensure an accurate assessment be sure to:
• drape the patient appropriately
• keep the room warm because chilling can cause abdominal muscles to tense

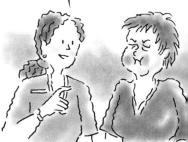

There's no need to hold back; unusual breath odors are common in patients with GI emergencies.

• warm your hands and the stethoscope
• speak softly and encourage the patient to perform breathing exercises or use imagery during uncomfortable procedures
• assess painful areas last to avoid making the patient tense.

In order, please

The GI system requires abdominal auscultation before percussion and palpation because the latter can alter intestinal activity and bowel sounds. So, when assessing the abdomen, perform the four basic steps in the following sequence:

inspection

auscultation

percussion

palpation.

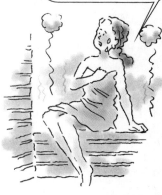

Keeping the room, your hands, and your stethoscope warm (but not this warm) can ease patient discomfort during abdominal examination.

Abdominal inspection

Before inspecting the abdomen, mentally divide it into four quadrants. (See *Identifying abdominal landmarks*, page 270.)

General inspection

Begin by performing a general inspection of the patient:
• Observe the skin, oral mucosa, nail beds, and sclera for jaundice or signs of anemia.
• Observe the abdomen for symmetry, checking for bumps, bulges, or masses. A bulge may indicate bladder distention or hernia.
• Note the patient's abdominal shape and contour. The abdomen should be flat to rounded in people of average weight. A protruding abdomen may be caused by obesity, pregnancy, ascites, or abdominal distention. A slender person may have a slightly concave abdomen.

The cause of abdominal bulge is pretty obvious here, but in other patients it may be due to distention or hernia.

To striae or not to striae

• Next, inspect the abdominal skin, which normally appears smooth and intact. Striae, or stretch marks, can be caused by pregnancy, excessive weight gain, or ascites. New striae are pink or blue; old striae are silvery white. In patients with darker skin, striae may be dark brown. Note dilated veins. Record the length of any surgical scars on the abdomen.
• Note abdominal movements and pulsations. Usually, waves of peristalsis aren't visible unless the patient is very thin, in which case they may be visible as slight wavelike motions. Marked visible rippling may indicate bowel obstruction; re-

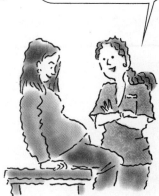

Identifying abdominal landmarks

To aid accurate abdominal assessment and documentation of findings, you can mentally divide the patient's abdomen into regions. Use the quadrant method—the easiest and most commonly used method—to divide the abdomen into four equal regions using two imaginary perpendicular lines crossing above the umbilicus.

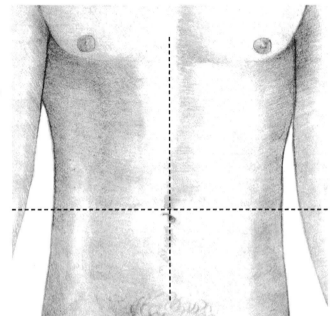

Right upper quadrant
- Liver and gallbladder
- Pylorus
- Duodenum
- Head of pancreas
- Hepatic flexure of colon
- Portions of ascending and transverse colon

Left upper quadrant
- Left liver lobe
- Stomach
- Body of pancreas
- Splenic flexure of colon
- Portions of transverse and descending colon

Right lower quadrant
- Cecum and appendix
- Portion of ascending colon
- Lower portion of right kidney
- Bladder (if distended)

Left lower quadrant
- Sigmoid colon
- Portion of descending colon
- Lower portion of left kidney
- Bladder (if distended)

port it immediately. In a thin patient, pulsation of the aorta is visible in the epigastric area. Marked pulsations may occur with hypertension, aortic insufficiency, and other conditions causing widening pulse pressure.

Abdominal auscultation

Auscultation provides information about bowel motility and the underlying vessels and organs.

Follow the clock

Use a stethoscope to auscultate for bowel and vascular sounds. Lightly place the stethoscope diaphragm in the right lower quadrant, slightly below and to the right of the umbilicus.

Do you hear what I hear?

Auscultate in a clockwise fashion in each of the four quadrants, spending at least 2 minutes in each area. Note the character and quality of bowel sounds in each quadrant. In some cases, you may need to auscultate for 5 minutes before you hear sounds. Be sure to allow enough time to listen in each quadrant before you decide that bowel sounds are absent.

> The gurgling, the splashing—nothing makes me happier than a normal bowel sound!

Tube tip

Before auscultating the abdomen of a patient with a nasogastric (NG) tube or other abdominal tube connected to suction, briefly clamp the tube or turn off the suction. Suction noises can obscure or mimic actual bowel sounds.

Sound class

Bowel sounds are classified as normal, hypoactive, or hyperactive:
• *Normal* bowel sounds are high-pitched, gurgling noises caused by air mixing with fluid during peristalsis. The noises vary in frequency, pitch, and intensity and occur irregularly from 5 to 34 times per minute. They're loudest before mealtimes. Borborygmus, or stomach growling, is the loud, gurgling, splashing sound heard over the large intestine as gas passes through it.
• *Hypoactive* bowel sounds are heard infrequently. They're associated with ileus, bowel obstruction, or peritonitis and indicate diminished peristalsis. Paralytic ileus, torsion of the bowel, or use of opioids and other medications can decrease peristalsis.
• *Hyperactive* bowel sounds are loud, high-pitched, tinkling sounds that occur frequently and may be caused by diarrhea, constipation, or laxative use.

Sound off

Next, use the bell of the stethoscope to auscultate for vascular sounds. Normally, you should detect no vascular sounds. Note a bruit, venous hum, or friction rub. (See *Interpreting abnormal abdominal sounds*, page 272.)

Abdominal percussion

Use abdominal percussion to determine the size and location of abdominal organs and detect excessive accumulation of fluid and air. Begin percussion in the right lower quadrant and proceed clockwise, covering all four quadrants. Keep the approximate locations of the patient's organs in mind as you progress. Use direct or indirect percussion:
• In *direct* percussion, strike your hand or finger directly over the patient's abdomen.

Interpreting abnormal abdominal sounds

This chart lists abnormal abdominal sounds along with the location and possible cause of each.

Sound and description	Location	Possible cause
Abnormal bowel sounds		
Hyperactive sounds (unrelated to hunger)	Any quadrant	Diarrhea, laxative use, or early intestinal obstruction
Hypoactive, then absent sounds	Any quadrant	Paralytic ileus or peritonitis
High-pitched tinkling sounds	Any quadrant	Intestinal fluid and air under tension in a dilated bowel
High-pitched rushing sounds coinciding with abdominal cramps	Any quadrant	Intestinal obstruction
Systolic bruits		
Vascular blowing sounds resembling cardiac murmurs	Over abdominal aorta	Partial arterial obstruction or turbulent blood flow
	Over renal artery	Renal artery stenosis
	Over iliac artery	Iliac artery obstruction
Venous hum		
Continuous, medium-pitched tone created by blood flow in a large engorged vascular organ such as the liver	Epigastric and umbilical regions	Increased collateral circulation between portal and systemic venous systems, such as in cirrhosis
Friction rub		
Harsh, grating sound like two pieces of sandpaper rubbing together	Over liver and spleen	Inflammation of the peritoneal surface of the liver, such as from a tumor

- With *indirect* percussion, use the middle finger of your dominant hand or a percussion hammer to strike a finger resting on the patient's abdomen.

Percussion precaution

Don't percuss the abdomen of a patient with an abdominal aortic aneurysm or a transplanted abdominal organ. Doing so can precipitate a rupture or organ rejection.

Tympany and dullness

Normally, you should hear two sounds during percussion of the abdomen: tympany and dullness. When you percuss over hollow organs, such as an empty stomach or bowel, you should hear a clear, hollow sound like a drum beating. This sound, *tympany*, predominates because air is normally present in the stomach and bowel. The degree of tympany depends on the amount of air and gastric dilation.

When you percuss over solid organs, such as the liver, kidney, or feces-filled intestines, the sound changes to dullness. Note where percussed sounds change from tympany to dullness, which may indicate a solid mass or enlarged organ.

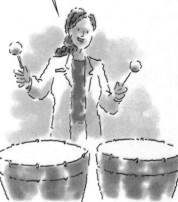

Tympany should be the predominant sound you hear when percussing the abdomen. And now for my drum roll…

Abdominal palpation

Abdominal palpation includes light and deep touch to determine the size, shape, position, and tenderness of major abdominal organs and detect masses and fluid accumulation. Palpate all four quadrants, leaving painful and tender areas for last.

Light palpation

Use light palpation to identify muscle resistance and tenderness as well as the location of some superficial organs. To do so, gently press your fingertips ½″ to ¾″ (1.5 to 2 cm) into the abdominal wall. Use the lightest touch possible because too much pressure blunts your sensitivity.

Deep palpation

Use deep palpation by pressing the fingertips of both hands about 1½″ (3.5 cm) into the abdominal wall. Move your hands in a slightly circular fashion so that the abdominal wall moves over the underlying structures.

Deep palpation may evoke rebound tenderness when you suddenly withdraw your fingertips, a possible sign of peritoneal inflammation. (See *Eliciting abdominal pain*, page 274.)

Assessing the liver

You can estimate the size and position of the liver through percussion and palpation.

Percussion discussion

Percussing the liver allows you to estimate its size. Hepatomegaly is commonly associated with hepatitis and other liver disease. Liver borders may be obscured and difficult to assess. (See *Percussing the liver*, page 275.)

Eliciting abdominal pain

Rebound tenderness and the iliopsoas and obturator signs can indicate such conditions as appendicitis and peritonitis. You can elicit these signs of abdominal pain, as illustrated here.

Rebound tenderness

To test for rebound tenderness, help the patient into a supine position with his knees flexed to relax the abdominal muscles. Place your hands gently on the right lower quadrant at McBurney's point (located about midway between the umbilicus and the anterior superior iliac spine). Slowly and deeply dip your fingers into the area; then release the pressure in a quick, smooth motion. Pain on release—rebound tenderness—is a positive sign. The pain may radiate to the umbilicus.

Caution: To minimize the risk of rupturing an inflamed appendix, don't repeat this maneuver.

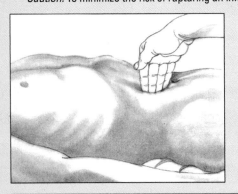 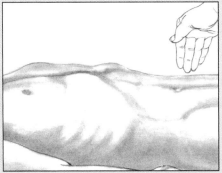

Iliopsoas sign

To elicit the iliopsoas sign, help the patient into a supine position with his legs straight. Instruct him to raise his right leg upward as you exert slight pressure with your hand. Repeat the maneuver with the left leg. When testing either leg, increased abdominal pain is a positive result, indicating irritation of the psoas muscle.

Obturator sign

To elicit the obturator sign, help the patient into a supine position with his right leg flexed 90 degrees at the hip and knee. Hold the leg just above the knee and at the ankle; then rotate the leg laterally and medially. Pain in the hypogastric region is a positive sign, indicating irritation of the obturator muscle.

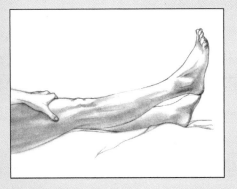 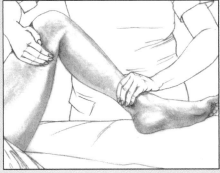

Percussing the liver

Begin percussing the abdomen along the right midclavicular line, starting below the level of the umbilicus. Move upward until the percussion notes change from tympany to dullness, usually at or slightly below the costal margin. Mark the point of change with a felt-tip pen.

Then percuss downward along the right midclavicular line, starting above the nipple. Move downward until percussion notes change from normal lung resonance to dullness, usually at the 5th to 7th intercostal space. Again, mark the point of change with a felt-tip pen. Estimate liver size by measuring the distance between the two marks.

Anatomic landmarks for liver percussion

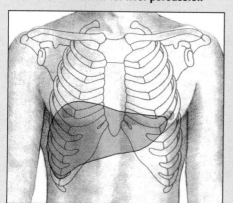

Hand position for liver percussion

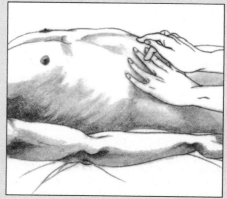

Palpation problem

It's usually impossible to palpate the liver in an adult patient. If palpable, the liver border feels smooth and firm, with a rounded, regular edge. A palpable liver may indicate hepatomegaly. To palpate for hepatomegaly:

Start at the lower left quadrant.

Have the patient take a deep breath and hold it while you palpate using the tips of your fingers.

Slowly move your hand up toward the costal margin and palpate while the patient exhales.

Assessing the rectum

If your patient is age 40 or older, a rectal examination may be part of your GI assessment. Explain the procedure to reassure the patient.

Perianal is primary

To perform a rectal examination, first inspect the perianal area following these steps:
• Put on gloves and spread the buttocks to expose the anus and surrounding tissue, checking for fissures, lesions, scars, inflammation, discharge, rectal prolapse, and external hemorrhoids.
• Ask the patient to strain as if he's having a bowel movement; this may reveal internal hemorrhoids, polyps, or fissures.

Rectum is next

After examining the perianal area, palpate the rectum:
• Apply a water-soluble lubricant to your gloved index finger. Tell the patient to relax and explain to him that he'll feel some pressure.
• Insert your finger into the rectum toward the umbilicus. To palpate, rotate your finger. The walls should feel soft and smooth without masses, fecal impaction, or tenderness.
• Remove your finger from the rectum and inspect the glove for stool, blood, or mucus. Test fecal material adhering to the glove for occult blood using a guaiac test.

Assessing the spleen

Unless the spleen is enlarged, it isn't palpable. To attempt to palpate the spleen, stand on the patient's right side. Use your left hand to support his posterior left lower rib cage, and ask him to take a deep breath. Then with your right hand on his abdomen, press up and in toward the spleen.

Stop in the name of spleen

If you do feel the spleen, stop palpating immediately because compression can cause rupture.

Diagnostic tests

Many tests provide information to guide your care of a patient with a GI emergency. Even if you don't participate in testing, you should know why the test was ordered, what the results mean, and what your responsibilities are before, during, and after the test. Diagnostic tests commonly ordered include abdominal X-ray, colonoscopy, computed tomography (CT) scan, esophagogastroduodenoscopy (EGD), fecal studies, liver spleen scan, magnetic resonance imaging (MRI), and peritoneal fluid analysis.

Abdominal X-ray

An abdominal X-ray, also called *flat plate of the abdomen* or *kidney-ureter-bladder radiography*, is used to detect and evaluate tumors, kidney stones, abnormal gas collection, and other abdominal disorders. The test consists of two plates: one taken with the patient supine and the other taken while he stands.

Reading the rays

On X-ray, air appears black, fat appears gray, and bone appears white. Although a routine X-ray doesn't reveal most abdominal organs, it does show the contrast between air and fluid. For example, intestinal blockage traps large amounts of detectable fluids and air inside organs. When an intestinal wall tears, air leaks into the abdomen and becomes visible on X-ray.

Practice pointers

• Explain the procedure to the patient.
• Radiography requires no special pretest or posttest care. It's usually done at the bedside using portable X-ray equipment.

Colonoscopy

Colonoscopy, also referred to as *lower GI endoscopy*, is used to:
• diagnose inflammatory and ulcerative bowel disease
• pinpoint lower GI bleeding
• detect lower GI abnormalities, such as tumors, polyps, hemorrhoids, and abscesses.

Practice pointers

• Explain the procedure and its purpose, and tell the patient he'll receive I.V. premedication and conscious sedation for the procedure.
• Make sure that an informed consent form has been signed.
• Check the time that the patient last ate; if possible, withhold all fluids and food for at least 6 to 8 hours before the test.
• Assist with bowel preparation as indicated.
• To decrease the risk of aspiration in a patient receiving electrolyte lavage solution through an NG tube, ensure proper tube placement and elevate the head of the bed or position the patient on his side. Have suction equipment available. (See *Lavage: Increased risk in elderly patients*, page 278.)
• Warn the patient that he may feel the urge to defecate when the scope is inserted; encourage slow, deep breathing through the mouth, as appropriate.

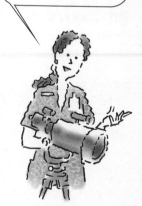

Colonoscopy provides a direct view of visceral linings using fiber optics. Good thing the instruments used are a lot smaller than this!

• Initiate an I.V. line if one isn't already in place for a patient who will be receiving conscious sedation.
• Obtain the patient's baseline vital signs and oxygen saturation levels. Monitor cardiac rhythm.
• Administer medications as ordered, such as midazolam for sedation. Provide supplemental oxygen as ordered.
• During the procedure, monitor the patient's vital signs, airway patency, oxygen saturation, cardiac rhythm, skin color, abdominal distention, level of consciousness (LOC), and pain tolerance.

Postprocedure

• After the procedure, assess your patient's vital signs and cardiopulmonary status, breath sounds, oxygen saturation, and LOC every 15 minutes for the first hour, every 30 minutes for the next hour, and then hourly until the patient stabilizes.
• Administer supplemental oxygen as ordered and as indicated by oxygen saturation levels.
• Watch for adverse effects of sedation, such as respiratory depression, apnea, hypotension, excessive diaphoresis, bradycardia, and laryngospasm. Notify the practitioner if any occur.
• Assess the patient's stool for evidence of frank or occult bleeding.
• Monitor the patient for signs and symptoms of perforation, such as vomiting, severe abdominal pain, abdominal distention or rigidity, and fever. Notify the practitioner if any occur.
• Document the procedure, interventions, and assessment findings.

Ages and stages

Lavage: Increased risk in elderly patients

Elderly patients are at increased risk for experiencing adverse effects from lavage solution, including nausea, vomiting, abdominal cramps, abdominal fullness, dizziness, and fluid and electrolyte imbalances. What's more, elderly patients may have difficulty ingesting the required amount of solution because of these adverse effects.

CT scan

In a CT scan, a computer translates multiple X-ray beams into three-dimensional oscilloscope images of the patient's biliary tract, liver, and pancreas. The test can be done with or without a contrast medium, but contrast is preferred unless the patient is allergic to contrast media.

Scads of scans

CT scan is used to:
• distinguish between obstructive and nonobstructive jaundice
• identify abscesses, cysts, hematomas, tumors, and pseudocysts
• evaluate the cause of weight loss and look for occult malignancy
• diagnose and evaluate pancreatitis.

CT scans evaluate everything from A to P—abscesses to pancreatitis—and more.

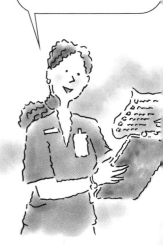

Practice pointers

• Explain the procedure to the patient and tell him that he should lie still, relax, and breathe normally during the test. Explain that, if the practitioner orders an I.V. contrast medium, he may experience discomfort from the needle puncture and a localized feeling of warmth on injection.
• Ascertain when the patient last ate or drank; restrict food and fluids as soon as possible, but continue any drug regimen as ordered.
• Confirm if the patient has an allergy to iodine or shellfish. If he has a seafood or dye allergy, give him a pretest preparation kit containing prednisone and diphenhydramine as ordered to reduce the risk of a reaction to the dye. Report immediately any adverse reactions, such as nausea, vomiting, dizziness, headache, and urticaria.
• If the patient is on nothing-by-mouth status, increase the I.V. fluid rate as ordered after the procedure to flush the contrast medium from his system. Monitor serum creatinine and blood urea nitrogen levels for signs of acute renal failure, which may be caused by the contrast medium.

EGD

EGD, also called *upper GI endoscopy*, is used to identify abnormalities of the esophagus, stomach, and small intestine, such as esophagitis, inflammatory bowel disease, Mallory-Weiss syndrome, lesions, tumors, gastritis, and polyps.

Bypass surgery

EGD eliminates the need for extensive exploratory surgery and can be used to detect small or surface lesions missed by radiography. It can also be used for sclerotherapy or to remove foreign bodies by suction (for small, soft objects) or electrocautery, snare, or forceps (for large, hard objects).

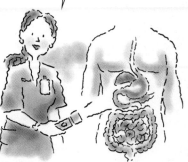

EGD focuses on the esophagus, stomach, and small intestine.

Practice pointers

Before the procedure

• Explain the procedure and its purpose to the patient.
• Tell him the that he'll receive I.V. premedication and conscious sedation during the procedure as well as a local anesthetic spray in his mouth and nose.
• Make sure that an informed consent form has been signed.
• Insert an NG tube to aspirate contents and minimize the risk of aspiration.

• Make sure that the patient's dentures and eyeglasses are removed before the test.
• If the procedure is to be performed at the bedside, have the necessary equipment available for the procedure and initiate an I.V. line if one isn't already in place.
• Monitor the patient before and throughout the procedure, including airway patency, vital signs, oxygen saturation, cardiac rhythm, abdominal distention, LOC, and pain tolerance.

After the procedure

• Monitor your patient's vital signs, oxygen saturation, cardiac rhythm, and LOC.
• Administer oxygen therapy as ordered.
• Place the patient in a side-lying position with the head of the bed flat until sedation wears off.
• Withhold all food and fluids until your patient's gag reflex returns. After it does, offer ice chips and sips of water, gradually increasing the patient's intake as tolerated and allowed.
• Observe for adverse effects of sedation, such as respiratory depression, apnea, hypotension, excessive diaphoresis, bradycardia, and laryngospasm. Notify the practitioner if any occur.
• Monitor the patient for signs and symptoms of perforation, such as difficulty swallowing, pain, fever, and bleeding indicated by black stools or bloody vomitus.
• Document the procedure, interventions, and assessment findings.

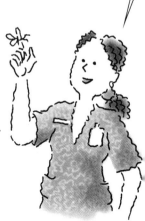

Remember to keep an eye out for adverse effects of sedation.

Fecal studies

Normal stool appears brown and formed but soft. These abnormal findings may indicate a problem:
• Narrow, ribbonlike stool signals spastic or irritable bowel, partial bowel obstruction, or rectal obstruction.
• Constipation may be caused by diet or medications.
• Diarrhea may indicate spastic bowel or viral infection.
• Mixed with blood and mucus, soft stool can signal bacterial infection; mixed with blood or pus, colitis.
• Yellow or green stool suggests severe, prolonged diarrhea; black stool suggests GI bleeding or intake of iron supplements or raw-to-rare meat. Tan or white stool shows hepatic duct or gallbladder-duct blockage, hepatitis, or cancer. Red stool may signal colon or rectal bleeding; however, drugs and foods can also cause this coloration.
• Most stool contains 10% to 20% fat. A higher fat content can turn stool pasty or greasy, a possible sign of intestinal malabsorption or pancreatic disease.

Practice pointers

• Collect the stool specimen in a clean, dry container, and immediately send it to the laboratory.
• Don't use stool that has been in contact with toilet-bowl water or urine.
• Use commercial fecal occult blood slides as a simple method of testing for blood in stool. Follow package directions because certain medications and foods can interfere with test results.

Liver-spleen scan

In a liver-spleen scan, a scanner or gamma camera records the distribution of radioactivity within the liver and spleen after I.V. injection of a radioactive colloid. Kupffer's cells in the liver take up most of this colloid, while smaller amounts lodge in the spleen and bone marrow.

Detective device

By registering the extent of this absorption, the imaging device detects such abnormalities as tumors, cysts, and abscesses. Because the test demonstrates disease nonspecifically (as a cold spot, which is an area that fails to take up the colloid), test results usually require confirmation by ultrasonography, CT or gallium scan, or biopsy.

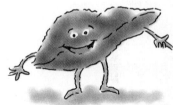

There's going to be a gamma camera recording me next week. The question is, what should I wear?

Practice pointers

• Describe the test to the patient and explain that it's used to examine the liver and spleen through pictures taken with a special scanner or camera.
• Tell the patient he'll receive an injection of a radioactive substance (technetium-99m sulfide) through an I.V. line in his hand or arm to allow better visualization of the liver and spleen.
• Immediately report any adverse reactions, such as flushing, fever, light-headedness, or difficulty breathing.

MRI

MRI is used to examine the liver and abdominal organs. It's useful in evaluating liver disease by characterizing tumors, masses, or cysts found on previous studies. An image is generated by energizing protons in a strong magnetic field. Radio waves emitted as protons return to their former equilibrium and are recorded. No ionizing radiation transmits during the scan.

MRI mire

Disadvantages of MRI include the closed, tubelike space required for the scan. Newer MRI centers offer a less confining "open-MRI" scan. In addition, the test can't be performed on patients with implanted metal prostheses or devices.

Practice pointers

• Explain the procedure to the patient and stress the need to remove metal objects such as jewelry before the procedure.
• Explain to the patient that he must lie still for 1 to 1½ hours for the procedure.
• Generally, you'll accompany the patient to the MRI suite. If he becomes claustrophobic during the test, administer mild sedation as ordered.

Peritoneal fluid analysis

Peritoneal fluid analysis includes examination of gross appearance, erythrocyte and leukocyte counts, cytologic studies, microbiological studies for bacteria and fungi, and determinations of protein, glucose, amylase, ammonia, and alkaline phosphatase levels.

Peritoneal through paracentesis

Abdominal paracentesis is a bedside procedure involving aspiration of fluid from the peritoneal space through a needle, trocar, or cannula inserted in the abdominal wall.
    Paracentesis is used to:
• diagnose and treat massive ascites resistant to other therapy
• detect intra-abdominal bleeding after traumatic injury
• obtain a peritoneal fluid sample for laboratory analysis
• decrease intra-abdominal pressure and alleviate dyspnea.

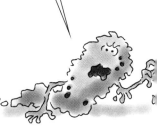

Bacteria like me can find a home in peritoneal fluid, but after peritoneal fluid analysis I might get evicted.

Practice pointers

• Explain the procedure to the patient.
• Make sure that an informed consent form has been signed.
• Instruct the patient to empty his bladder. Usually, an indwelling urinary catheter is inserted.
• Record the patient's baseline vital signs, weight, and abdominal girth. Indicate the abdominal area measured with a felt-tipped marking pen.

Positioning for abdominal paracentesis

When positioning a patient for abdominal paracentesis, help him sit up in bed or allow him to sit on the edge of the bed with additional support for his back and arms.

In this position, gravity causes fluid to accumulate in the lower abdominal cavity. The internal organs provide counter-resistance and pressure to aid fluid flow.

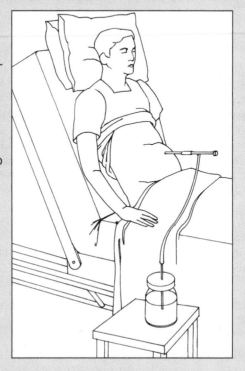

During...

• The trocar is inserted with the patient supine. After insertion, assist the patient to sit up in bed. (See *Positioning for abdominal paracentesis.*)
• Remind the patient to remain as still as possible during the procedure.
• Throughout the procedure, monitor the patient's vital signs, oxygen saturation, and cardiac rhythm every 15 minutes and observe for tachycardia, hypotension, dizziness, pallor, diaphoresis, and increased anxiety, especially if the practitioner aspirates more than 1,500 ml of peritoneal fluid at one time.
• If the patient shows signs of hypovolemic shock, slow the drainage rate by raising the collection container vertically so it's closer to the height of the needle, trocar, or cannula. Stop the drainage if necessary. Limit aspirated fluid to between 1,500 and 2,000 ml.

• After the practitioner removes the needle, trocar, or cannula and, if necessary, sutures the incision, apply a dry sterile pressure dressing.

...and after

After the procedure

• Monitor the patient's vital signs, oxygen saturation, and cardiac rhythm, and check the dressing for drainage every 15 minutes for the first hour, every 30 minutes for the next 2 hours, every hour for 4 hours, and then every 4 hours for 24 hours.
• Observe the patient for signs of hemorrhage or shock, such as hypotension, tachycardia, pallor, and excessive diaphoresis. These signs may indicate puncture of the inferior epigastric artery, hematoma of the anterior cecal wall, or rupture of the iliac vein or bladder. Observe for hematuria.
• Observe the patient for signs of a perforated intestine, such as increasing pain or abdominal tenderness.
• Document the procedure, and record the patient's weight and abdominal girth to detect recurrent ascites.

Treatments

GI emergencies present many treatment challenges because they stem from various mechanisms occurring separately or simultaneously, including tumors, hyperactivity and hypoactivity, malabsorption, infection and inflammation, vascular disorders, intestinal obstruction, and degenerative disease. Treatment options include drug therapy and GI intubation.

Drug therapy

Drug therapy may be used for such disorders as acute GI bleeding, peptic ulcer disease, and hepatic failure. Some of the most commonly used drugs in critical care include ammonia detoxicants, antacids, antidiuretic hormone, antiemetics, histamine-2 (H_2) receptor antagonists, and proton pump inhibitors.

How fast?

Some of these drugs, such as antacids and antiemetics, provide relief immediately. Other drugs, such as ammonia detoxicants and H_2-receptor antagonists, may take several days or longer to alleviate the problem. (See *Watch out for sedatives* and *Common GI drugs.*)

Stay on the ball

Watch out for sedatives

Administer sedatives cautiously in a patient with underlying liver disease. Be sure to establish a baseline for the patient's level of consciousness (LOC) before administering the medication to ensure valid assessments of the patients LOC after the medication has been given.

Common GI drugs

This chart lists common GI drugs along with their indications and adverse reactions.

Drugs	Indications	Adverse reactions
Ammonia detoxicant		
lactulose (Chronulac)	• To prevent and treat portosystemic encephalopathy in patients with severe hepatic disease (increasing clearance of nitrogenous products and decreasing serum ammonia levels through laxative effects) • Laxative to treat constipation	Abdominal cramps, diarrhea, flatulence
Antacids		
aluminum hydroxide (Alu-Cap)	• Antacid used for heartburn, acid indigestion, and adjunct therapy with peptic ulcer disease	Constipation, intestinal obstruction, encephalopathy
aluminum hydroxide and magnesium hydroxide (Maalox)	• Antacid used for heartburn, acid indigestion, and adjunct therapy with peptic ulcer disease	Diarrhea, hypermagnesemia in patients with severe renal impairment
calcium carbonate (Caltrate)	• Antacid used for heartburn, acid indigestion, and adjunct therapy with peptic ulcer disease • Calcium supplement	Nausea, vomiting, possibly hypercalcemia (with excessive use)
Antidiuretic hormone		
vasopressin (Pitressin)	• Injection administered I.V. or intra-arterially into the superior mesenteric artery used as treatment in acute, massive GI hemorrhage (such as peptic ulcer disease, ruptured esophageal varices, and Mallory-Weiss syndrome)	Angina, cardiac arrhythmias (bradycardia, heart block), cardiac arrest, water intoxication, seizures, bronchospasms, coronary thrombosis, possibly mesenteric and small bowel infarction with mesenteric artery intra-arterial infusion
Antiemetics		
dolasetron (Anzemet), ondansetron (Zofran)	• Prevention and treatment of postoperative nausea and vomiting and in conjunction with cancer chemotherapy	Diarrhea, arrhythmias, electrocardiogram changes (prolonged PR and QT intervals and widened QRS complex), liver test abnormalities, pruritus
metoclopramide (Reglan)	• Prevention and treatment of postoperative nausea and vomiting and in conjunction with cancer chemotherapy • Delayed gastric emptying secondary to diabetic gastroparesis	Restlessness, anxiety, depression, suicidal ideation, seizures, bradycardia, bronchospasm, transient hypertension

(continued)

Common GI drugs *(continued)*

Drugs	Indications	Adverse reactions
Histamine-2 receptor antagonists		
famotidine (Pepcid)	• Treatment of duodenal and gastric ulcers, gastroesophageal reflux disease (GERD), and Zollinger-Ellison syndrome • Prevention of gastric stress ulcers	Headache, palpitations, diarrhea, constipation
ranitidine (Zantac)	• Treatment of duodenal and gastric ulcers, GERD, and Zollinger-Ellison syndrome • Prevention of gastric stress ulcers	Malaise, reversible confusion, depression or hallucinations, blurred vision, jaundice, leukopenia, angioedema
Proton pump inhibitors		
lansoprazole (Prevacid), omeprazole (Prilosec), pantoprazole (Protonix)	• Treatment of duodenal and gastric ulcers, erosive esophagitis, GERD, Zollinger-Ellison syndrome, and *Helicobacter pylori* eradication • Prophylaxis for gastric stress ulcer (in critically ill patients)	Diarrhea, abdominal pain, nausea, constipation, chest pain, dizziness, hyperglycemia

GI intubation

NG and other specialized tubes may be used in treating the patient with acute intestinal obstruction, bleeding, esophageal varices, or another GI dysfunction.

Gastric lavage

Gastric lavage is an emergency treatment for the patient with GI hemorrhage caused by peptic ulcer disease or ruptured esophageal or gastric varices and as emergency treatment for some drug overdoses. It involves intubation with a large-bore, single- or double-lumen tube; instillation of irrigating fluid; and aspiration of gastric contents. In some cases, a vasoconstrictor, such as norepinephrine (Levophed), may be added to the irrigating fluid to enhance this action.

Rarely seen

Complications are rare and include:
• bradycardia
• electrolyte imbalance or metabolic acidosis

Measuring NG tube length

To determine how long the nasogastric (NG) tube must be to reach the stomach, hold the end of the tube at the tip of the patient's nose. Extend the tube to the patient's earlobe and then down to the xiphoid process.

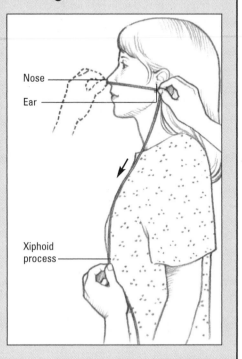

• fluid overload
• vomiting and aspiration.

Nursing considerations

• Explain the procedure to the patient.
• Determine the length of the tube for insertion. (See *Measuring NG tube length.*)
• Lubricate the end of the tube with a water-soluble lubricant and insert it into the patient's mouth or nostril as ordered. Advance the tube through the pharynx and esophagus and into the stomach.
• Check the tube for placement by attaching a piston or bulb syringe and aspirating stomach contents. Examine the aspirate and place a small amount on the pH test strip. Probability of gastric placement is increased if the aspirate has a typical gastric fluid appearance (grassy-green, clear and colorless with mucus shreds, or brown) and has a pH of less than or equal to 5.

• When the tube is in place, lower the head of the bed to 15 degrees and reposition the patient on his left side, if possible.
• Fill the syringe with 30 to 50 ml of irrigating solution and begin instillation. Instill about 250 ml of fluid, wait 30 seconds, and then begin to withdraw the fluid into the syringe. If you can't withdraw any fluid, allow the tube to drain into an emesis basin.
• If the practitioner orders a vasoconstrictor to be added to the irrigating fluid, wait for the prescribed period before withdrawing fluid to allow absorption of the drug into the gastric mucosa.

Fluid watch

• Carefully measure and record fluid return. If the volume of fluid return doesn't at least equal the amount of fluid instilled, abdominal distention and vomiting result.
• Continue lavage until return fluid is clear or as ordered. Remove the tube or secure it as ordered. If appropriate, send lavage specimens to the laboratory for toxicology studies and send gastric contents for pH and guaiac studies.
• Never leave the patient alone during gastric lavage.
• Monitor the patient's cardiac rhythm and observe for possible complications, such as bradycardia, hypovolemia, vomiting, and aspiration.
• Monitor the patient's vital signs and oxygen saturation every 30 minutes until his condition stabilizes.
• Document the procedure and any appropriate interventions.

> *Don't worry; I'll be back. I know it means trouble when the fluid return doesn't at least equal the fluid instilled during lavage.*

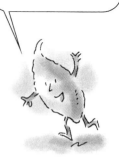

Multilumen esophageal tube placement

In esophagogastric tamponade, an emergency treatment, a multilumen esophageal tube is inserted to control esophageal or gastric hemorrhage resulting from ruptured varices. It's usually a tentative measure until sclerotherapy can be done. (See *Comparing esophageal tubes.*)

The tube is inserted through a nostril, or sometimes the mouth, and then passed into the stomach. The tube's esophageal and gastric balloons are inflated to exert pressure on the varices to stop bleeding, while a lumen allows esophageal and gastric contents to be aspirated.

Balloon inflation for longer than 48 hours may cause pressure necrosis, which can lead to further hemorrhage. Follow your facility's policy and procedure for balloon inflation and deflation.

Nursing considerations
Before the procedure
• Describe the procedure to the patient. Explain that a helmet may be used to apply traction to keep balloon pressure at the gastroesophageal junction. Place the patient in semi-Fowler's posi-

Comparing esophageal tubes

There are three common types of esophageal tubes: the Linton tube, the Minnesota esophagogastric tamponade tube, and the Sengstaken-Blakemore tube.

Linton tube

The Linton tube, a three-lumen, single-balloon device, has ports for esophageal and gastric aspiration. Because the tube doesn't have an esophageal balloon, it isn't used to control bleeding for esophageal varices.

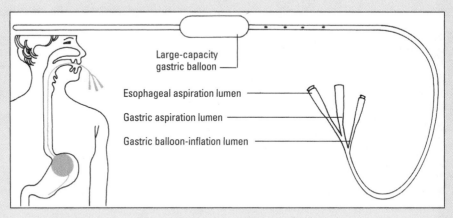

Large-capacity gastric balloon

Esophageal aspiration lumen

Gastric aspiration lumen

Gastric balloon-inflation lumen

Minnesota esophagogastric tamponade tube

The Minnesota esophagogastric tamponade tube has four lumens and two balloons. It has pressure-monitoring ports for both balloons.

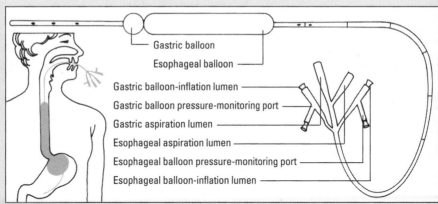

Gastric balloon

Esophageal balloon

Gastric balloon-inflation lumen

Gastric balloon pressure-monitoring port

Gastric aspiration lumen

Esophageal aspiration lumen

Esophageal balloon pressure-monitoring port

Esophageal balloon-inflation lumen

Sengstaken-Blakemore tube

The Sengstaken-Blakemore tube, a three-lumen device with esophageal and gastric balloons, has a gastric aspiration port that allows drainage from below the gastric balloon and is also used to instill medication.

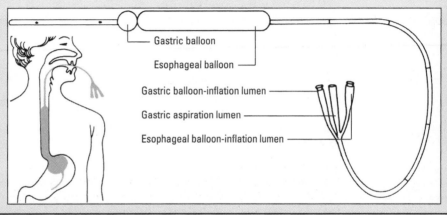

Gastric balloon

Esophageal balloon

Gastric balloon-inflation lumen

Gastric aspiration lumen

Esophageal balloon-inflation lumen

tion. (If unconscious, place the patient on his left side, with the head of the bed elevated to 15 degrees.) An unresponsive patient may also require endotracheal intubation.
• Tape a pair of scissors to the head of the bed in case of acute respiratory distress.
• Check tube balloons for air leaks and patency before insertion.
• Never leave the patient alone during tamponade.

When it's done

After the procedure
• Closely monitor the patient's condition and lumen pressure. If the pressure changes or decreases, check for bleeding and notify the practitioner immediately.
• Monitor the patient's cardiac rhythm, vital signs, and oxygen saturation every 30 to 60 minutes. A change may indicate new bleeding.
• Monitor the patient's respiratory status and observe for respiratory distress. If respiratory distress develops, have someone notify the practitioner. If the airway is obstructed, cut both balloon ports and remove the tube. Notify the practitioner immediately.
• Maintain suction on the ports. Irrigate the gastric aspiration port to prevent clogging.
• Deflate the esophageal balloon for about 30 minutes every 12 hours or according to your facility's policy and procedure.
• Observe the patient for signs of esophageal rupture, such as shock, increased respiratory difficulty, and increased bleeding. Notify the practitioner if such signs are present.
• Keep the patient warm, comfortable, and as still as possible.

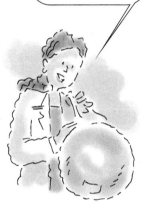

Check your facility's policy for how often you should deflate the patient's esophageal balloon.

Nasoenteric decompression tube
The nasoenteric decompression tube is used to aspirate intestinal contents for analysis and to correct intestinal obstruction. It's inserted nasally and advanced beyond the stomach into the intestinal tract. The tube may also prevent nausea, vomiting, and abdominal distention after GI surgery.
   A balloon or rubber bag at one end of the tube holds mercury (or air or water) to stimulate peristalsis and aid the tube's passage through the pylorus and into the intestinal tract. (See *Common nasoenteric decompression tubes.*)

Nursing considerations
The patient with a nasoenteric decompression tube needs special care and continuous monitoring to:
• ensure tube patency
• maintain suction and bowel decompression

Common nasoenteric decompression tubes

The type of nasoenteric decompression tube chosen for your patient will depend on the size of the patient and his nostrils, the estimated duration of intubation, and the reason for the procedure.

Most tubes are impregnated with a radiopaque mark so that placement can easily be confirmed by X-ray or another imaging technique. Among the most commonly used types of nasoenteric decompression tubes are the Cantor tube, Miller-Abbott tube, Harris tube, and Dennis tube.

Cantor tube
The Cantor tube is a 10' (3-m) long, single-lumen tube and has a balloon that can hold mercury at its distal tip. It may be used to relieve bowel obstructions and to aspirate intestinal contents.

Miller-Abbott tube
The Miller-Abbott tube is 10' long and has two lumens: one for inflating the distal balloon with air and one for instilling mercury or water. It's also used in case of bowel obstruction. This type of tube allows aspiration of intestinal contents.

Harris tube
The single-lumen Harris tube is only 6' (1.8 m) long, also ending with a balloon that holds mercury. Used primarily for treating a bowel obstruction, the Harris tube—usually with a Y tube attached—allows lavage of the intestinal tract.

Dennis tube
The 10' long, three-lumen Dennis sump tube is used to decompress the intestinal tract before or after GI surgery. Each lumen is marked to denote its use: irrigation, drainage, and balloon inflation.

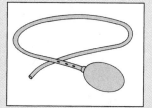 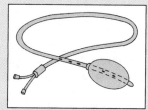 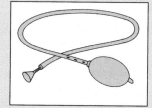 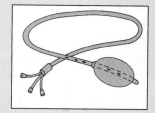

• detect such complications as fluid and electrolyte imbalance.

Dealing with obstruction

If your patient's tube appears to be obstructed, follow your facility's policy and procedure and notify the practitioner if you're unable to restore patency. He may order such measures as those described here, to restore patency quickly and efficiently:
• First, disconnect the tube from suction and irrigate with normal saline solution. Use gravity flow to help clear the obstruction unless otherwise ordered.
• If irrigation doesn't reestablish patency, the tube may be obstructed by its position against the gastric mucosa. Tug slightly on the tube to move it away from the mucosa.
• If gently tugging doesn't work, the tube may be kinked and need additional manipulation. However, don't reposition or irrigate a tube in a patient who had GI surgery, in one who had the tube inserted during surgery (because this may disturb new sutures), or in a patient who was difficult to intubate.

Common disorders

GI disorders commonly encountered in the ED include abdominal trauma, acute GI bleeding, appendicitis, cholecystitis, and diverticulitis.

Abdominal trauma

Abdominal trauma accounts for approximately one-fourth of all trauma events and is associated with a high rate of morbidity and mortality. It can occur as a single event or be associated with multiple injuries, further compounding their seriousness.

What causes it

Abdominal trauma is commonly classified as *penetrating* or *blunt*, depending on the type of injury.

An explosive situation

Penetrating abdominal trauma involves an injury by a foreign object, such as a knife (the most common cause of stabbing injury), bullet (the most common cause of missile injury), pitchfork, or other pointed object that penetrates the abdomen.

Typically, penetrating abdominal trauma is fairly limited, usually involving isolated organs and lacerated tissues. In some cases, however, extensive tissue damage can occur if a bullet explodes in the abdominal cavity.

To put it bluntly

Blunt abdominal trauma results from sudden compression or positive pressure inflicted by a direct blow to the organ and surrounding tissue. Blunt abdominal trauma commonly occurs in motor vehicle collisions, assaults, and falls. Of these, blunt abdominal trauma from motor vehicle collisions is the most common.

Blunt abdominal trauma can cause extensive injury to the peritoneum and abdominal organs. The liver and spleen are the two organs most commonly injured from blunt abdominal trauma. The other organs, such as the stomach, intestines, and pancreas, as well as the diaphragm and vascular structures, can also be injured, although these injuries are less common.

How it happens

Injuries to the abdomen usually involve one or more of these conditions:

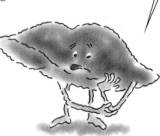

Blunt abdominal trauma is commonly caused by car collisions, and commonly affects the liver. Now I'm uncommonly scared to drive.

• hypovolemia resulting from massive fluid or blood loss, especially if the spleen is injured
• hypoxemia resulting from damage to the diaphragm or associated chest trauma
• respiratory or cardiac failure resulting from associated chest injury.

Tissue damage caused by penetrating trauma, such as an impaled object or foreign body, is related to the object size as well as the depth and velocity of penetration. For example, penetrating abdominal trauma from a bullet has many variables; the extent of injury depends on the distance at which the weapon was fired, the type of ammunition, the velocity of the ammunition, and the entrance and (if present) exit wounds.

Other considerations

Additional factors to consider when assessing the extent of abdominal trauma from a bullet include type of weapon; caliber, barrel, and length of the gun; and powder composition. An intact bullet causes less damage than a bullet that explodes on impact. A bullet that explodes within the abdomen may break up and scatter fragments, burn tissue, fracture bone, disrupt vascular structures, or cause a bullet embolism.

Trauma physics

Injury resulting from blunt abdominal trauma is related to the amount of force, compression, and cavitation. Blunt force that strikes the abdomen at high velocity transfers that force to underlying organs and tissue. The direct impact of force is transmitted internally and the energy dissipates to internal structures.

Buckle up

Recently, seat belts have been associated with a blunt abdominal trauma. Referred to as "seat belt syndrome," abdominal injury in a motor vehicle collision in which the patient was wearing a seat belt can involve injuries to the large and small intestines, liver, spleen, abdominal vessels and, possibly, the lumbar spine.

What to look for

Assessment findings may vary based on the type and extent of abdominal trauma. In some cases, the patient may be asymptomatic, especially if the trauma occurred days or weeks before the patient arrives at the ED. In other situations, the patient may have multiple injuries and a severely compromised status that require immediate intervention.

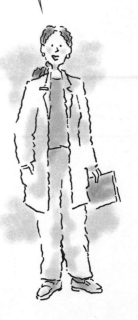

Think of "the FCC"—Force, Compression, and Cavitation—as you evaluate blunt trauma's impact.

Stay on the ball

Identifying injuries to the liver and spleen

The liver and spleen are the two organs most commonly injured from abdominal trauma.

Spleen signs

When performing your assessment, suspect injury to the spleen if your patient:
- has a history of blunt trauma to the left upper quadrant
- complains of pain or exhibits bruising in the left upper quadrant
- demonstrates a positive Kehr's sign (evidence of left shoulder pain due to irritation of the diaphragm with blood from the peritoneum).

Liver look-fors

Suspect a liver injury if your patient:
- has a history of direct trauma to the right upper quadrant (between the eighth rib and central abdominal area)
- has pain or bruising over the right upper quadrant
- complains of referred pain to the right shoulder
- demonstrates hemodynamic instability.

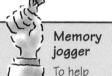

Memory jogger

To help remember what information to obtain during assessment of the patient with abdominal trauma, use the acronym **SAMPLE:**

Signs and symptoms

Allergies

Medications

Past medical history

Last meal

Events leading to injury.

Have a look-see

When assessing the patient with abdominal trauma, be alert for:
- bruising, abrasions, and lacerations of the abdomen (see *Identifying injuries to the liver and spleen*)
- bruising along the area of the seat belt line
- positive Grey-Turner's sign (purplish discoloration along the flank) or Cullen's sign (purplish discoloration around the umbilicus)
- obvious wounds, such as gunshot wounds or stab wounds
- change in bowel sounds (The presence of bowel sounds in the chest suggests diaphragmatic rupture and should be reported immediately.)
- pain, rigidity, tenderness, or guarding on palpation.

What tests tell you

Diagnostic testing depends on the patient's condition and extent of injuries. In addition, diagnostic tests performed are based on the area affected by the trauma. Some possible diagnostic tests include:
- peritoneal lavage to detect blood in the peritoneal cavity

• CT scan, which may reveal hemorrhage, hematomas, or skeletal injuries
• ultrasonography, which may show free fluid in the abdominal cavity
• abdominal and chest X-rays to detect fluid, free air, ileus, or rupture of the diaphragm
• pelvic X-rays, which may demonstrate bony abnormalities.
    Other tests that may be performed include:
• arterial blood gas (ABG) analysis to evaluate respiratory and acid-base status
• complete blood count (CBC) to evaluate degree of blood loss
• coagulation studies to determine the patient's clotting ability
• serum electrolyte levels to determine possible imbalances.

How it's treated

Treatment of abdominal trauma focuses on immediately stabilizing the patient; assessing and maintaining his airway, breathing, and circulation (ABC); assessing LOC; and preparing him for transport and possible surgery.
    If the patient has a wound, treatment may include controlling bleeding, usually by applying firm, direct pressure, and cleaning the wound. Pain medication and antibiotic therapy are instituted as indicated. In addition, I.V. therapy is started to ensure fluid balance and maintain the patient's hemodynamic status.

What to do

• Assess the patient's ABCs and initiate emergency measures if necessary; administer supplemental oxygen as ordered.
• Monitor vital signs and note significant changes.
• Assess oxygen saturation and cardiac rhythm for arrhythmias. Assess neurologic status, including LOC and pupillary and motor response.
• Obtain blood studies, including type and crossmatch.
• Insert two large-bore I.V. catheters and infuse normal saline or lactated Ringer's solution as ordered.
• Quickly and carefully assess the patient for other areas of trauma.
• Assess wounds and provide wound care as appropriate. Cover open wounds and control bleeding by applying pressure.
• Assess for increased abdominal distention.
• Administer blood products as appropriate.
• Monitor for signs of hypovolemic shock.
• Provide pain medication, as appropriate.
• Prepare the patient and family for diagnostic testing and possible surgery.
• Provide reassurance to the patient and his family.

Acute GI bleeding

GI bleeding can occur anywhere along the GI tract. Although GI bleeding stops spontaneously in most patients, acute bleeding accounts for significant morbidity and mortality.

Maybe multiple morbidities

Many patients who require emergency care experience upper GI bleeding. Additionally, they may have underlying comorbidities that contribute to the risk of upper GI bleeding, such as:
- coronary artery disease
- history of myocardial infarction
- renal failure
- history of chronic liver damage secondary to alcohol abuse or hepatitis
- history of radiation therapy
- chronic pain condition, such as arthritis, requiring treatment with NSAIDs.

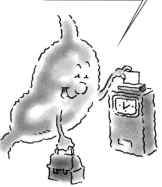

Most GI bleeding clocks out on its own, but the kind that sticks around carries a risk of morbidity and mortality.

What causes it

Upper GI bleeding includes bleeding in the esophagus, stomach, and duodenum. Bleeding below the Treitz ligament is considered lower GI bleeding; the most common site is in the colon.

Upper causes

Causes of upper GI bleeding include:
- angiodysplasias
- arteriovenous malformations (AVMs)
- erosive gastritis
- esophagitis
- Mallory-Weiss tear
- peptic ulcer disease
- rupture of esophageal varices.

Lower causes

The most common causes of lower GI bleeding include:
- AVMs
- diverticulitis
- hemorrhoids
- inflammatory bowel disease
- neoplasm
- polyps.

How it happens

In GI bleeding, the patient experiences a loss of circulating blood volume, regardless of the cause of bleeding. Because the arterial

blood supply near the stomach and esophagus is extensive, bleeding can lead to a rapid loss of large amounts of blood, subsequent hypovolemia, and shock. Here's what else happens:
• Loss of circulating blood volume leads to a decreased venous return.
• Cardiac output and blood pressure decrease, causing poor tissue perfusion. In response, the body compensates by shifting interstitial fluid to the intravascular space.
• The sympathetic nervous system is stimulated, resulting in vasoconstriction and increased heart rate.
• The renin-angiotensin-aldosterone system is activated, leading to fluid retention and increasing blood pressure.
• If blood loss continues, cardiac output decreases, leading to cellular hypoxia. Eventually, all organs fail due to hypoperfusion.

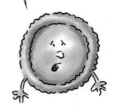

No matter what the cause, too much GI blood loss can lead to hypovolemia and shock.

What to look for

Because GI bleeding can occur anywhere along the GI tract, assessment is crucial to determine the level and possible location of bleeding.

Source signs

The appearance of blood in tube drainage, vomitus, and stool indicates the source of GI bleeding:
• *Hematemesis* (bright red blood in NG tube drainage or vomitus) typically indicates an upper GI source. However, if the blood has spent time in the stomach where it was exposed to gastric acid, the drainage or vomitus resembles coffee grounds.
• *Hematochezia* (bright red blood from the rectum) typically indicates a lower GI source of bleeding. It may also suggest an upper GI source if the transit time through the bowel was rapid.
• *Melena* (black, tarry, sticky stool) usually indicates an upper GI bleeding source. However, it can result from bleeding in the small bowel or proximal colon.

Thirty percent of total blood volume is GI bleeding's critical calculation. A patient losing more than that may go into hypovolemic shock.

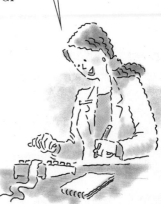

Signs and symptoms

Typically, the patient exhibits signs and symptoms based on the amount and rate of bleeding. With acute GI bleeding and blood loss greater than 30% of the patient's blood volume, he exhibits signs and symptoms of hypovolemic shock, including:
• apprehension
• cool, clammy skin
• diaphoresis
• hypotension
• pallor
• restlessness

• syncope
• tachycardia.

What tests tell you

These findings aid in diagnosing acute GI bleeding:
• Upper GI endoscopy reveals the source of esophageal or gastric bleeding.
• CBC reveals the amount of blood loss.
• ABG analysis can indicate metabolic acidosis from hemorrhage and possible hypoxemia.
• 12-lead electrocardiogram (ECG) may reveal evidence of cardiac ischemia secondary to hypoperfusion.
• Abdominal X-ray may indicate air under the diaphragm, suggesting ulcer perforation.
• Angiography may aid in visualizing the bleeding site.

How it's treated

Treatment goals include stopping the bleeding and providing fluid replacement while maintaining the patient's function. Treatment may include:
• fluid volume replacement with crystalloid solutions initially, followed by colloids and blood component therapy
• respiratory support
• gastric intubation with gastric lavage (unless the patient has esophageal varices) and gastric pH monitoring
• drug therapy, such as antacids, H_2-receptor antagonists, and proton pump inhibitors
• endoscopic or surgical repair of bleeding sites.

What to do

• Type and crossmatch at least 2 units of blood.
• Start at least two large-bore I.V. lines (16G or 18G preferred). Assess the patient for blood loss and begin fluid replacement therapy as ordered, initially delivering crystalloid solutions such as normal saline or lactated Ringer's solution, followed by blood component products.
• Ensure your patient's patent airway. Monitor cardiac and respiratory status and assess LOC at least every 15 minutes until he stabilizes and then as indicated by his status. Assist with insertion of hemodynamic monitoring devices and assess hemodynamic parameters.

Don't forget oxygen

• Administer supplemental oxygen as ordered. Monitor oxygen saturation levels.

- Monitor the patient's skin color and capillary refill for signs of hypovolemic shock.
- Obtain serial hemoglobin and hematocrit levels. Administer albumin or blood as ordered.
- Monitor the patient's intake and output closely, including all losses from the GI tract. Check all stools and gastric drainage for occult blood.
- Assist with or insert an NG tube and perform lavage using room temperature saline to clear blood and clots from the stomach.
- Assess the patient's abdomen for bowel sounds and gastric pH as ordered. Expect to resume enteral or oral feedings after bowel function returns and when there's no evidence of further bleeding.
- Provide appropriate emotional support to the patient.
- Prepare the patient for endoscopic repair or surgery, if indicated. Anticipate transfer of the patient to the critical care unit.

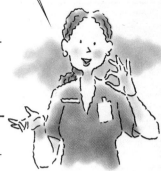

Just a little bit of emotional support can go a long way for a patient who has suffered dramatic blood loss.

Appendicitis

Appendicitis is the most common major surgical emergency. It occurs when the appendix becomes inflamed. More precisely, this disorder is an inflammation of the vermiform appendix, a small, fingerlike projection attached to the cecum just below the ileocecal valve. Although the appendix has no known function, it does regularly fill and empty itself of food.

What causes it

Appendicitis may be due to:
- barium ingestion
- fecal mass (fecalith)
- mucosal ulceration
- stricture
- viral infection.

How it happens

Mucosal ulceration triggers inflammation, which temporarily obstructs the appendix. The obstruction blocks mucus outflow. Pressure in the now-distended appendix increases, and the appendix contracts. Bacteria multiply, and inflammation and pressure continue to increase, restricting blood flow to the organ and causing severe abdominal pain.

Inflammation can lead to infection, clotting, tissue decay, and perforation of the appendix. If the appendix ruptures or perforates, the infected contents spill into the abdominal cavity, causing peritonitis, the most common and most dangerous complication.

What to look for

Initially, look for these signs or symptoms:
• abdominal pain, generalized or localized in the right upper abdomen and eventually localizing in the right lower abdomen (McBurney's point)
• anorexia
• boardlike abdominal rigidity
• nausea and vomiting
• retractive respirations
• increasingly severe abdominal spasms and rebound spasms (rebound tenderness on the opposite side of the abdomen suggests peritoneal inflammation).

...and then later

Later, look for these signs or symptoms:
• constipation (although diarrhea is also possible)
• fever of 99° to 102° F (37.2° to 38.9° C)
• tachycardia
• sudden cessation of abdominal pain (indicates perforation or infarction of the appendix).

What tests tell you

These tests help diagnose appendicitis:
• White blood cell (WBC) count is moderately elevated, with increased immature cells.
• Ultrasound of the abdomen and pelvis can be helpful in diagnosing a nonperforated appendix. A CT scan can help identify an abscess.

How it's treated

An appendectomy is the only effective treatment for appendicitis. If peritonitis develops, treatment involves GI intubation, parenteral replacement of fluids and electrolytes, and administration of antibiotics.

What to do

If appendicitis is suspected or you're preparing for an appendectomy, follow these steps:
• Administer I.V. fluids to prevent dehydration. Never administer cathartics or enemas because they may rupture the appendix.
• Maintain the patient on nothing-by-mouth (NPO) status, and administer analgesics judiciously because they may mask symptoms of rupture.

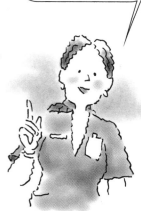

Sometimes there's only one way to go with treatment. In the case of appendicitis, it's surgical removal.

Education edge

Teaching the patient with appendicitis

• Explain what happens in appendicitis.
• Help the patient understand the required surgery and its possible complications.
• If time allows, provide preoperative teaching, including coughing and deep breathing exercises and incentive spirometry.
• Discuss postoperative care and activity limitations. Tell the patient to follow the doctor's orders for driving, returning to work, and resuming physical activity.

• Place the patient in Fowler's position to reduce pain. (This position is also helpful postoperatively.)
• Never apply heat to the lower right abdomen or perform palpation; these actions may cause the appendix to rupture.
• Provide support to the patient and family; prepare them for surgery as indicated.
• Begin educating the patient about his condition and care. (See *Teaching the patient with appendicitis.*)

Cholecystitis

Cholecystitis refers to an acute or chronic inflammation of the gallbladder, usually associated with a gallstone impacted in the cystic duct, causing painful gallbladder distention. The acute form is most common during middle age, whereas the chronic form is more common in the elderly. Prognosis is good with treatment.

What causes it

The exact cause of cholecystitis is unknown. However, certain risk factors have been identified, including:
• high-calorie, high-cholesterol diet associated with obesity
• elevated estrogen levels from hormonal contraceptives, post-menopausal therapy, pregnancy, or multiparity
• diabetes mellitus, ileal disease, hemolytic disorders, liver disease, or pancreatitis
• genetic factors
• weight-reduction diets with severe calorie restriction and rapid weight loss.

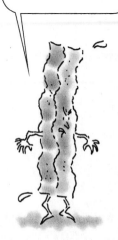

Okay, so I'm part of a high-calorie, high-cholesterol diet. There are other risk factors for cholecystitis, you know!

How it happens

Certain conditions (such as age, obesity, and estrogen imbalance) cause the liver to secrete bile that's abnormally high in cholesterol or that lacks the proper concentration of bile salts. Excessive water and bile salts are reabsorbed, making the bile less soluble. Cholesterol, calcium, and bilirubin then precipitate into gallstones.

What to look for

In acute cholecystitis, look for:
• classic attack signs and symptoms with severe midepigastric or right upper quadrant pain radiating to the back or referred to the right scapula, commonly after meals rich in fats
• recurring fat intolerance
• belching that leaves a sour taste in the mouth
• flatulence
• indigestion
• diaphoresis
• nausea
• chills and low-grade fever
• possible jaundice and clay-colored stools with common duct obstruction
• local and rebound tenderness.

What tests tell you

These tests help diagnose cholecystitis:
• Ultrasonography reveals calculi in the gallbladder with 96% accuracy. Percutaneous transhepatic cholangiography distinguishes between gallbladder disease and cancer of the pancreatic head in patients with jaundice.
• CT scan may identify ductal stones.
• Endoscopic retrograde cholangiopancreatography (ERCP) visualizes the biliary tree after endoscopic examination of the duodenum, cannulation of the common bile and pancreatic ducts, and injection of a contrast medium.
• Cholescintigraphy detects obstruction of the cystic duct.

Bad to the stone

• If stones are identified in the common bile duct by radiologic examination, a therapeutic ERCP may be performed before cholecystectomy to remove the stones.
• Oral cholecystography shows calculi in the gallbladder and biliary duct obstruction.

- Laboratory tests showing an elevated icteric index and elevated total bilirubin, urine bilirubin, and alkaline phosphatase levels support the diagnosis.
- WBC count is slightly elevated during a cholecystitis attack.
- Serum amylase levels distinguish gallbladder disease from pancreatitis.
- Serial enzyme tests and an ECG should precede other diagnostic tests if heart disease is suspected.

How it's treated

- During an acute attack, treatment may include insertion of an NG tube and I.V. line as well as antibiotic administration.
- Surgery is the treatment of choice for cholecystitis. Cholecystectomy (removal of the gallbladder) restores biliary flow. The surgery may be performed conventionally via a large incision, or laparoscopically using a laser. The laparoscopic procedure aids in speeding recovery and reducing the risk of infection and herniation.
- In patients who are poor surgical candidates for cholecystectomy, a cholecystostomy (incision into the fundus of the gallbladder to remove and drain retained stones or inflammatory debris) or choledochotomy (incision into the common bile duct to remove gallstones or other obstructions) may be performed.
- A low-fat diet is prescribed to prevent attacks. Vitamin K is also prescribed for itching, jaundice, and bleeding tendencies caused by vitamin K deficiency.
- Ursodiol, a drug that dissolves the solid cholesterol in gallstones, provides an alternative for patients who are poor surgical risks or who refuse surgery. However, use of ursodiol is limited by the need for prolonged treatment (2 years), the incidence of adverse reactions, and the frequency of calculi reformation after treatment.
- Lithotripsy, the ultrasonic breakup of gallstones, is usually unsuccessful and the rate of recurrence after this treatment is significant. The relative ease, short length of stay, and cost-effectiveness of laparoscopic cholecystectomy have made dissolution and lithotripsy less viable options.

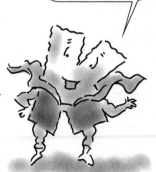

Lack of vitamin K isn't okay; it can lead to itching, jaundice, and bleeding tendencies.

What to do

- Monitor the patient's vital signs and intake and output.
- Insert an NG tube as ordered and attach it to low, intermittent suction.
- Administer medications to control complaints of nausea and vomiting.
- Give opioid analgesics for pain.

• Assist in stabilizing the patient's nutritional and fluid balance before surgery.
• Withhold food and fluids by mouth; determine the time when the patient last ate.
• Provide preoperative care including teaching and administration of preoperative medications.
• Ensure that an informed consent form has been signed and is on the patient's chart.

Diverticulitis

Diverticulitis is a form of diverticular disease. In diverticular disease, bulging, pouchlike herniations (diverticula) in the GI wall push the mucosal lining through the surrounding muscle. Diverticula occur most commonly in the sigmoid colon, but they may develop anywhere from the proximal end of the pharynx to the anus. Other typical sites are the duodenum, near the pancreatic border or the ampulla of Vater, and the jejunum.

Diverticula in the stomach are rare and are usually a precursor to peptic or neoplastic disease. Diverticular disease of the ileum (Meckel's diverticulum) is the most common congenital anomaly of the GI tract. Diverticular disease has two clinical forms:

diverticulosis—diverticula that are present but produce no symptoms

diverticulitis—inflamed diverticula that may cause potentially fatal obstruction, infection, and hemorrhage.

What causes it

The exact cause of diverticular disease is unknown, but it may result from:
• diminished colonic motility and increased intraluminal pressure
• defects in colon wall strength.

How it happens

Diverticula probably result from high intraluminal pressure on an area of weakness in the GI wall where blood vessels enter. Diet may be a contributing factor because insufficient fiber reduces fecal residue, narrows the bowel lumen, and leads to high intra-abdominal pressure during defecation.

Packed in the sac

In diverticulitis, undigested food and bacteria accumulate in the diverticular sac. This accumulation causes the formation of a hard

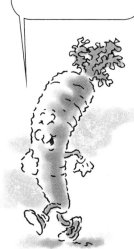

A lack of fiber may contribute to the formation of diverticula, so at the risk of my own safety, I say eat those veggies!

mass that cuts off the blood supply to the thin walls of the sac, making them more susceptible to attack by colonic bacteria. Inflammation follows and may lead to perforation, abscess, peritonitis, obstruction, or hemorrhage. Occasionally, the inflamed colon segment adheres to the bladder or other organs and causes a fistula.

What to look for
• Meckel's diverticulum usually produces no symptoms.
• In diverticulosis, recurrent left lower abdominal quadrant pain is relieved by defecation or passage of flatus. Constipation and diarrhea alternate.
• In diverticulitis, the patient may have moderate left lower abdominal quadrant pain, mild nausea, gas, irregular bowel habits, low-grade fever, leukocytosis, rupture of the diverticula (in severe diverticulitis), and fibrosis and adhesions (in chronic diverticulitis).

What tests tell you
These tests aid diagnosis of diverticular disease:
• An upper GI series confirms or rules out diverticulosis of the esophagus and upper bowel.
• Barium enema confirms or rules out diverticulosis of the lower bowel.
• Biopsy rules out cancer; however, a colonoscopic biopsy isn't recommended during acute diverticular disease because of the strenuous bowel preparation it requires.
• Blood studies may show an elevated erythrocyte sedimentation rate in diverticulitis, especially if the diverticula are infected.

How it's treated
Treatment of mild diverticulitis without signs of perforation must prevent constipation and combat infection. It may include bed rest, a liquid diet, stool softeners, a broad-spectrum antibiotic, opioids to control pain and relax smooth muscle, and an antispasmodic, such as dicyclomine (Antispas) or hyoscyamine (Levsin), to control muscle spasms.

What to do
If the patient with a history of diverticulosis comes to the ED, observe his stool carefully for frequency, color, and consistency; monitor pulse and temperature for changes which may signal developing inflammation or complications. Care of the patient with diverticulitis depends on the severity of symptoms:

• In mild disease, administer medications, as ordered. Explain diagnostic tests and preparations for such tests; observe stool carefully; and maintain accurate records of temperature, pulse rate, respiratory rate, and intake and output. Begin patient teaching for discharge. (See *Teaching the patient with diverticulitis.*)

Severe steps

If the patient's condition is more severe:
• Insert an I.V. line to administer fluids for rehydration.
• Maintain the patient on NPO status and anticipate insertion of an NG tube to low intermittent suction if the patient experiences persistent vomiting.
• Administer antispasmodic agents to reduce colon spasms; give analgesics to manage pain and antibiotics for infection as ordered.
• Assess the patient for signs and symptoms of peritonitis, such as tachycardia, hypotension, abdominal rigidity, rebound tenderness, and fever.
• Monitor the patient carefully if he requires angiography and catheter placement for vasopressin infusion. Inspect the insertion site frequently for bleeding, check pedal pulses frequently, and keep the patient from flexing his legs at the groin.
• Watch for signs and symptoms of vasopressin-induced fluid retention (apprehension, abdominal cramps, seizures, oliguria, and anuria) and severe hyponatremia (hypotension; rapid, thready pulse; cold, clammy skin; and cyanosis).
• Prepare the patient for surgery as indicated; provide preoperative teaching and support to the patient and his family.

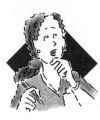

Quick quiz

1. A patient with abdominal trauma exhibits a bluish discoloration around his umbilicus. You should document this as:
- A. Grey-Turner's sign.
- B. iliopsoas sign.
- C. obturator sign.
- D. Cullen's sign.

Answer: D. Cullen's sign refers to a bluish discoloration that appears around the umbilicus.

2. Auscultation of a patient's abdomen reveals hypoactive bowel sounds. You should interpret this sign as indicating:
- A. turbulent blood flow in the arteries.
- B. inflammation of the peritoneal surface.
- C. diminished peristaltic activity.
- D. obstruction in the intestine.

Answer: C. Hypoactive bowel sounds indicate that peristalsis is slowed or diminished, and are associated with ileus, bowel obstruction, peritonitis, or use of such medications as opioids.

3. Which sign or symptom would you be least likely to observe in a patient with acute cholecystitis?
- A. Fever greater than 101.4° F (38.6° C)
- B. Right upper quadrant pain radiating to right shoulder
- C. Belching that leaves a sour taste in the mouth
- D. Recurrent fat intolerance

Answer: A. In cholecystitis, the patient usually has right upper quadrant pain that radiates to the back or shoulder, a history of fat intolerance, and belching that leaves a sour taste in the mouth. The patient may have a fever, but it's usually low-grade.

4. Which intervention would be appropriate for a patient diagnosed with appendicitis?
- A. Maintaining the patient on NPO status
- B. Applying a heating pad to the abdomen
- C. Administering an enema before surgery
- D. Giving frequent doses of opioid analgesics

Answer: A. For the patient with appendicitis, you should maintain the patient on NPO status and administer I.V. fluids. In addition, analgesics are given cautiously because they may mask the signs and symptoms of rupture. Heat and enemas are never used because they could lead to rupture.

Scoring

☆☆☆   If you answered all four questions correctly, you deserve a gourmet meal! You're a GI genius!

☆☆   If you answered three questions correctly, read up and try again! Your hunger for GI information makes it easy to swallow.

☆   If you answered fewer than three questions correctly, you may be fact-starved. Chew over the chapter and then take the test again.

7

Musculoskeletal emergencies and wound management

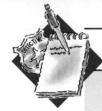

Just the facts

In this chapter, you'll learn:

♦ musculoskeletal assessment techniques

♦ tests to diagnose musculoskeletal emergencies

♦ common musculoskeletal emergencies, their causes, and treatments.

Understanding musculoskeletal emergencies

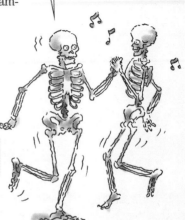

They may not be life-threatening, but musculoskeletal emergencies can sure mess up a patient's groove!

Musculoskeletal injuries are common in hospital emergency departments (EDs). They aren't life-threatening, but they do result in significant pain, long-term disability, and possible disfigurement. These emergencies can involve the entire musculoskeletal system and include strains, sprains, contusions, fractures, or tramatic amputation along with injuries to the muscles, tendons, and ligaments.

Be prepared to call on your full range of nursing skills when providing orthopedic care. While some musculoskeletal problems are subtle and difficult to assess, others are obvious or even traumatic, and affect the patient physically and emotionally.

Assessment

Your sharp assessment skills will help you uncover orthopedic abnormalities and evaluate the patient's ability to perform activities of daily living (ADLs). However, because many musculoskeletal injuries are emergencies, you may have to rely on the patient's family for information about his history. With any musculoskeletal injury or complaint, you must carefully evaluate neurologic and vascular status.

Health history

If possible, question the patient about his current and past illnesses and injuries, including allergies, medications, and social history.

Current illness or injury

Ask the patient about his chief complaint. Questions about the patient's pain level, factors and events that came before the illness or injury, and his capabilities after the illness or injury will help you decide how to initiate intervention.

Any ouchies?

For example, when a patient comes to the ED with hip pain, ask him: When did the pain start? Did he sustain an injury before the pain? If so, what type of injury—blunt trauma (a fall, a motor vehicle collision) or penetrating trauma (stabbing, puncture wound)?

How did it happen? For example, did he suffer hip injury after being hit by a car, or did he fall from a ladder and land on his coccyx? This information will help guide your assessment and predict hidden trauma.

Out-of-joint, fractured, or all muscle

Patients with joint injuries usually complain of pain, swelling, or stiffness in the affected area. They may experience decreased range of motion (ROM) or be unable to bear weight. Patients with bone fractures have sharp pain when they move the affected area and will attempt to guard the affected area. Some swelling may be present. Patients with muscular injury commonly describe their pain as a burning sensation. Muscular injuries are commonly associated with swelling, bruising, and weakness.

Ask the patient if his ability to carry out ADLs is affected. Has he noticed abnormal sounds (grating, crunching, clicking) when he moves certain parts of his body? Has he used ice, heat, or other remedies to treat the problem?

Past illness or injury

Inquire whether the patient has ever had gout, arthritis, tuberculosis, or cancer, which may cause bony metastases. Has he been diagnosed with osteoporosis or degenerative joint disease? Also ask the patient whether he uses an assistive device, such as a cane, walker, or brace. If so, watch him use the device to assess how he moves.

Medications

Question the patient about the medications he takes regularly because many drugs can affect the musculoskeletal system. Corticosteroids, for example, can cause muscle weakness, myopathy, osteoporosis, pathologic fractures, and avascular necrosis of the heads of the femur and humerus. Also ask whether he's using over-the-counter or herbal medicines or cultural remedies.

Family history

Ask the patient if his family suffers from joint disease. Disorders with a hereditary component include:
• gout
• osteoarthritis of the interphalangeal joints
• rheumatoid arthritis
• spondyloarthropathies (such as ankylosing spondylitis, Reiter's syndrome, psoriatic arthritis, and enteropathic arthritis).

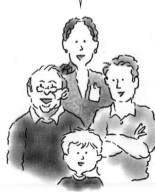

Without a doubt, gout is a hereditary disorder.

Social history

Ask the patient about his job, hobbies, and personal habits. Knitting, playing football or tennis, working at a computer, or doing construction work can all cause repetitive stress injuries or injure the musculoskeletal system in other ways. Even carrying a heavy knapsack or purse can cause injury or increase muscle size.

What goes in

Inquire about his social habits; smoking, drug or alcohol use, and amount of caffeine consumed. (Caffeine can cause demineralization of bones, causing bones to be more brittle.) Perform an abuse screen based on facility policy. Most facilities have general questions to ask all patients. These questions screen for potential abuse situations, especially intimate partner violence.

Physical assessment

Because the central nervous system and musculoskeletal system are interrelated, you should assess them together. To assess the musculoskeletal system, use inspection and palpation to test all the major bones, joints, and muscles. Perform a complete examination if the patient has generalized symptoms, such as aching in several joints. Perform an abbreviated examination if he has pain in only one body area, such as his ankle.

The five P's of musculoskeletal injury

To swiftly assess a musculoskeletal injury, remember the five P's: pain, paresthesia, paralysis, pallor, and pulse.

Pain

Ask the patient whether he feels pain. If he does, assess its location, severity, and quality.

Paresthesia

Assess the patient for loss of sensation by touching the injured area with the tip of an open safety pin. Abnormal sensation or loss of sensation indicates neurovascular involvement.

Paralysis

Assess whether the patient can move the affected area. If he can't, he might have nerve or tendon damage.

Pallor

Paleness, discoloration, and coolness on the injured side may indicate neurovascular compromise.

Pulse

Check all pulses distal to the injury site. A decreased or absent pulse means reduced blood supply to the area.

First thing's first

Always perform a primary assessment of the patient's airway, breathing, circulation, and disability, and base your initial treatment on that assessment. Then evaluate the neurovascular status of each injured limb. Because any patient experiencing trauma to an extremity risks neurovascular injuries and tissue ischemia, use the "Five P's" to evaluate limb circulation, sensation, and motor function. (See *The five P's of musculoskeletal injury.*)

After you've established the patient's airway, breathing, and circulation (ABCs), begin your physical assessment. As you do, ask questions that relate to the patient's history and the events leading to his injury.

With feeling

As you palpate, note:
- skin temperature
- pain and the point of tenderness
- bony crepitus
- joint instability
- peripheral nerve function (sensory and motor).

A watchful eye

During inspection, be mindful of:
- color
- disruption of skin integrity
- position of the extremity
- edema, swelling, or ecchymosis
- ROM or lack of ROM
- symmetry, alignment, deformity.

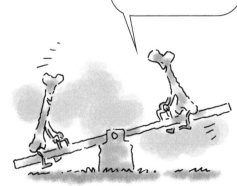

Checking alignment isn't child's play, it's a vital part of musculoskeletal assessment.

Assessing the bones and joints

After you finish your head-to-toe evaluation using inspection and palpation, you can perform ROM exercises to determine whether the joints are healthy. Never force movement; ask the patient to tell you when he experiences pain. Also, watch his facial expressions for signs of pain or discomfort.

Head, jaw, and neck

First, inspect the patient's face for swelling, symmetry, and evidence of trauma. The mandible should be in the midline, not shifted to the right or left.

Is the TMJ A-OK?

Next, evaluate ROM in the temporomandibular joint (TMJ). Place the tips of your first two or three fingers in front of the middle of the patient's ear and ask him to open and close his mouth. Then place your fingers into the depressed area over the joint, noting the motion of the mandible. The patient should be able to open and close his jaw and protract and retract his mandible easily, without pain or tenderness. If you hear or palpate a click as the patient's mouth opens, suspect an improperly aligned jaw. TMJ dysfunction may also lead to swelling of the area, crepitus, or pain.

Check the neck

Before performing an examination of the neck, radiological studies of the cervical spine may be indicated to rule out injury. Spinal cord injury should be suspected whenever there is a history of significant trauma, such as a high-speed motor vehicle collision; fall from higher than 3′ (1 m); significant trauma with loss of consciousness; loss or decrease of movement or sensation in the extremities; significant swelling, pain, or tenderness to the neck; or penetrating trauma to the neck. (See chapter 3, Neurologic emergencies, for more information on spinal cord injury.)

Before cervical spine clearance, the neck should be examined by removing the cervical collar and manually immobilizing the neck. Inspect the front, back, and sides of the patient's neck. Observe for obvious signs of injury to the cervical spine. Also assess the patient's ability to move his extremities and feel pain. Palpate the cervical area for pain, tenderness, deformity, and crepitus. *Crepitus* is an abnormal grating sound, not the occasional crack we hear from our joints, and indicates fracture. Be sure to replace the collar when the neck examination is complete.

Memory jogger

Here's an easy way to keep adduction and abduction straight.

Adduction is moving a limb toward the body's midline; think of it as adding two things together.

Abduction is moving a limb away from the body's midline; think of it as taking something away, like abducting, or kidnapping.

Head circles and chin-ups

When the doctor states that the cervical spine has been cleared of injury, you can remove the cervical collar. Now check ROM in the neck. Ask the patient to try touching his right ear to his right shoulder, and his left ear to his left shoulder. The usual ROM is 40 degrees on each side. Next, ask him to touch his chin to his chest and then point his chin toward the ceiling. The neck should flex forward 45 degrees and extend backward 55 degrees.

To assess rotation, ask the patient to turn his head to each side without moving his trunk. His chin should be parallel to his shoulders. Lastly, ask him to move his head in a circle; normal rotation is 70 degrees.

Spine

Before performing an examination of the spine, radiologic studies may be indicated to rule out injury. As with cervical spine injury, injury to the spinal vertebrae should be suspected when there's significant trauma or clinical signs of injury.

The patient should be immobilized (as indicated in chapter 3) and log-rolled with the assistance of three people. The remainder of the spine should be examined just as the cervical spine was. When the spine has been cleared of injury and the doctor states so, immobilization can be discontinued. Observe the spine; it should be in midline position without deviation to either side. Lateral deviation suggests scoliosis.

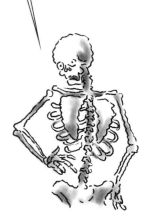

Pay no mind to the deviation of my head here; what you need to heed is any lateral deviation of the spine, which suggests scoliosis.

Spine-tingling procedure

Palpate the spinal processes and the areas lateral to the spine. Have the patient bend at the waist and let his arms hang loosely at his sides; palpate the spine with your fingertips. Repeat the palpation using the side of your hand, lightly striking the lateral areas. Note tenderness, swelling, or spasm.

Shoulders and elbows

Start by observing the patient's shoulders, noting asymmetry, muscle atrophy, or deformity. Swelling or loss of normal, rounded shape could mean that one or more bones is dislocated or out of alignment. Remember, even if the patient seeks care for shoulder pain, the problem may not have started in the shoulder. Shoulder pain may come from other sources, including a heart attack or ruptured ectopic pregnancy.

Palpate the shoulders with the palmar surfaces of your fingers to locate bony landmarks; note crepitus or tenderness. Using your entire hand, palpate the shoulder muscles for firmness and symmetry. Also palpate the elbow and the ulna for subcutaneous nodules that signal rheumatoid arthritis.

Lift and rotate

If the patient's shoulders don't seem dislocated, assess rotation. Start with the patient's arm straight at his side—the neutral position. Ask him to lift his arm straight up to shoulder level and then to bend his elbow horizontally until his forearm is at a 90-degree angle to his upper arm. His arm should be parallel to the floor, and his fingers should be extended with palms down.

To assess external rotation, have him bring his forearm up until his fingers point toward the ceiling. To assess internal rotation, have him lower his forearm until his fingers point toward the floor. Normal ROM is 90 degrees in each direction.

Flex and extend

To assess flexion and extension, start with the patient's arm in the neutral position. To assess flexion, ask him to move his arm anteriorly over his head, as if reaching for the sky. Full flexion is 180 degrees. To assess extension, have him move his arm from the neutral position posteriorly as far as possible. Normal extension ranges from 30 to 50 degrees.

Swing into position

To assess abduction, ask the patient to move his arm from the neutral position laterally as far as possible. Normal ROM is 180 degrees. To assess adduction, have the patient move his arm from the neutral position across the front of his body as far as possible. Normal ROM is 50 degrees.

He's up to his elbows

Next, assess the elbows for flexion and extension. Have the patient rest his arm at neutral position. Ask him to flex his elbow from this position and then extend it. Normal ROM is 90 degrees for flexion and extension.

To assess supination and pronation of the elbow, have the patient place the side of his hand on a flat surface with the thumb on top. Ask him to rotate his palm down toward the table for pronation and upward for supination. The normal angle of elbow rotation is 90 degrees in each direction.

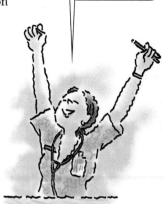

Reach for the sky—a good motto, and an even better way to check arm flexion!

Wrists and hands

Inspect the wrists and hands for contour, and compare them for symmetry. Also check for nodules, redness, swelling, deformities, and webbing between fingers. Use your thumb and index finger to palpate both wrists and each finger joint. Note tenderness, nodules, or bogginess. To avoid causing pain, be especially gentle with elderly patients and those with arthritis.

Rotate and flap

Assess ROM in the wrist. Ask the patient to rotate his wrist by moving his entire hand—first to the left and then to the right—as if he's waxing a car. Normal ROM is 55 degrees laterally and 20 degrees medially. Observe the wrist while the patient extends his fingers up toward the ceiling and down toward the floor, as if he's flapping his hand. He should be able to extend his wrist 70 degrees and flex it 90 degrees.

Lift a finger; make a fist

To assess extension and flexion of the metacarpophalangeal joints, ask the patient to keep his wrist still and move only his fingers—first up toward the ceiling and then down toward the floor. Normal extension is 30 degrees; normal flexion, 90 degrees.

Next, ask the patient to touch his thumb to the little finger of the same hand. He should be able to fold or flex his thumb across his palm so that it touches or points toward the base of his little finger.

To assess flexion of all of the fingers, ask the patient to form a fist. Then have him spread his fingers apart to demonstrate abduction and draw them back together to demonstrate adduction.

At arm's length

If you think one arm is longer than the other, take measurements. Extend a measuring tape from the acromial process of the shoulder to the tip of the middle finger. Drape the tape over the outer elbow. The difference between the left and right extremities should be no more than ⅜" (1 cm).

Hips and knees

Inspect the hip area for contour and symmetry. Next inspect knee position, noting whether the patient is bowlegged (having knees that point out), or knock-kneed (having knees that turn in). Then watch the patient walk.

Palpate each hip over the iliac crest and trochanteric area for tenderness or instability. Palpate both knees—they should feel smooth, and the tissues should feel solid. (See *Assessing bulge sign.*)

Hip, hip, hooray!

Assess ROM in the hip; these exercises are typically performed with the patient in a supine position. To assess hip flexion, place your hand under the patient's lower back and have him pull one

Assessing bulge sign

The bulge sign indicates excess fluid in the joint. To assess the patient for this sign, ask him to lie down so that you can palpate his knee. Then give the medial side of his knee two to four firm strokes, as shown top right, to displace excess fluid.

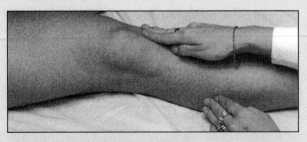

Lateral check

Next, tap the lateral aspect of his knee while checking for a fluid wave on the medial aspect, as shown bottom right.

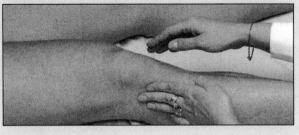

knee as far as he can toward his abdomen and chest. You'll feel the patient's back touch your hand as the normal lumbar lordosis of the spine flattens. As the patient flexes his knee, the opposite hip and thigh should remain flat on the bed. Repeat on the opposite side.

To assess hip abduction, stand alongside the patient and press down on the superior iliac spine of the opposite hip with one hand to stabilize the pelvis. With your other hand, hold the patient's leg by the ankle and gently abduct the hip until you feel the iliac spine move. That movement indicates the limit of hip abduction. Then, while still stabilizing the pelvis, move the ankle medially across the patient's body to assess hip adduction. Repeat on the other side. Normal ROM is about 45 degrees for abduction and 30 degrees for adduction.

To assess hip extension, have the patient lie prone (facedown), and gently extend the thigh upward. Repeat on the other thigh.

As the hip turns

To assess internal and external rotation of the hip, ask the patient to lift one leg up and, keeping his knee straight, turn his leg and foot medially and laterally. Normal ROM for internal rotation is 40 degrees; for external rotation, 45 degrees.

On bended knees

Assess ROM in the knee. If the patient is standing, ask him to bend his knee as if he's trying to touch his heel to his buttocks. Normal ROM for flexion is 120 to 130 degrees. If the patient is lying down, have him draw his knee up to his chest; his calf should touch his thigh.

Knee extension returns the knee to a neutral position of 0 degrees; however, some knees may normally be hyperextended 15 degrees. If the patient can't extend his leg fully or if his knee pops audibly and painfully, consider the response abnormal.

Other abnormalities include pronounced crepitus, which may signal a degenerative disease of the knee, and sudden buckling, which may indicate a ligament injury.

Ankles and feet

Inspect the ankles and feet for swelling, redness, nodules, and other deformities. Check the arch of the foot and look for toe deformities. Also note edema, calluses, bunions, corns, ingrown toenails, plantar warts, trophic ulcers, hair loss, or unusual pigmentation.

Use your fingertips to palpate the bony and muscular structures of the ankles and feet. Palpate each toe joint by compressing it with your thumb and fingers.

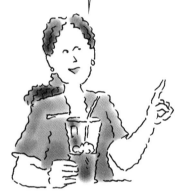

Pop in a glass? Absolutely! But pop in a knee? Abnormal!

The ankle angle

To examine the ankle, have the patient sit in a chair or on the side of a bed. To test plantar flexion, ask him to point his toes toward the floor. Test dorsiflexion by asking him to point his toes toward the ceiling. Normal ROM for plantar flexion is about 45 degrees; for dorsiflexion, 20 degrees.

Next, assess ROM in the ankle. Ask the patient to demonstrate inversion by turning his feet inward, and eversion by turning his feet outward. Normal ROM for inversion is 45 degrees; for eversion, 30 degrees.

To assess the metatarsophalangeal joints, ask the patient to flex his toes and then straighten them.

The long and short of it

Take measurements if you think that one leg is longer than the other. Put one end of the tape at the medial malleolus at the ankle and the other end at the anterior iliac spine. Cross the tape over the medial side of the knee. A difference of more than ⅜" (1 cm) is abnormal.

Assessing the muscles

When assessing the muscles, start by inspecting all major muscle groups for tone, strength, and symmetry. If a muscle appears atrophied or hypertrophied, measure it by wrapping a tape measure around the largest circumference of the muscle on each side of the body and comparing the two numbers.

Other abnormalities of muscle appearance include contracture and abnormal movements, such as spasms, tics, tremors, and fasciculation (fine movements of a small area of muscle).

Tuning in to muscle tone

Muscle tone describes muscular resistance to passive stretching. To test the patient's arm muscle tone, move his shoulder through passive ROM exercises. You should feel a slight resistance. Then let his arm drop. It should fall easily to his side.

Test leg muscle tone by putting the patient's hip through passive ROM exercises and then letting the leg fall to the examination table or bed. Like the arm, the leg should fall easily.

Abnormal findings include muscle rigidity and flaccidity. Rigidity indicates increased muscle tone, possibly caused by an upper motor neuron lesion after a stroke. Flaccidity may result from a lower motor neuron lesion.

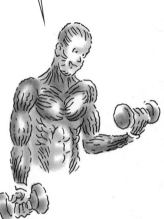

Nurses can't resist me, but I have to resist them pretty often. I tell them it's for the sake of muscle tone.

Wrestling with muscle strength

Observe the patient's gait and movement to gauge his general muscle strength. Grade muscle strength on a scale of 0 to 5, with 0 representing no strength and 5 representing maximum strength. Document the results as a fraction, with the score as the numerator and maximum strength as the denominator. (See *Grading muscle strength*.)

Grading muscle strength

Grade muscle strength on a scale of 0 to 5:
• 5/5 = Normal—Patient moves joint through full range of motion (ROM) and against gravity with full resistance.
• 4/5 = Good—Patient completes ROM against gravity with moderate resistance.
• 3/5 = Fair—Patient completes ROM against gravity only.
• 2/5 = Poor—Patient completes full ROM with gravity eliminated (passive motion).
• 1/5 = Trace—Patient's attempt at muscle contraction is palpable but without joint movement.
• 0/5 = Zero—There is no evidence of muscle contraction.

Testing muscle strength

To test the muscle strength of your patient's arm and ankle muscles, use the techniques shown here.

Biceps strength

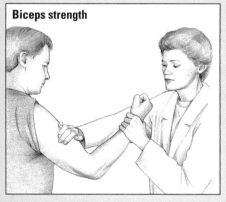

Ankle strength: Plantar flexion

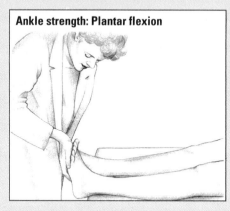

Triceps strength

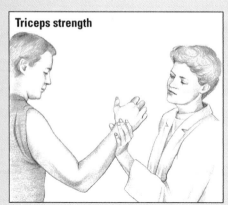

Ankle strength: Dorsiflexion

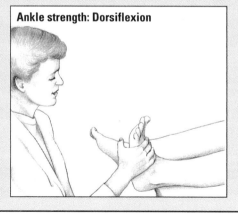

To test specific muscle groups, ask the patient to move the muscles while you apply resistance; then compare the contralateral muscle groups. (*See Testing muscle strength.*)

Shoulder, arm, wrist, and hand strength

Test the strength of the patient's shoulder girdle by asking him to extend his arms with the palms up and hold this position for 30 seconds. If he can't lift both arms equally and keep his palms up, or if one arm drifts down, he probably has shoulder girdle weakness on that side. If he passes the first part of the test, gauge his strength by placing your hands on his arms and applying downward pressure as he resists you.

Testing the bi's and tri's

Next, have the patient hold his arm in front of him with the elbow bent. To test bicep strength, pull down on the flexor surface of his forearm as he resists. To test triceps strength, have him try to straighten his arm as you push upward against the extensor surface of his forearm.

Forcing his hand

Assess the strength of the patient's flexed wrist by pushing against it. Test the strength of the extended wrist by pushing down on it. Test the strength of finger abduction, thumb opposition, and handgrip the same way. (See *Testing handgrip strength*.)

Leg strength

Ask the patient to lie in a supine position on the examining table or bed and lift both legs at the same time. Note whether he lifts both legs at the same time and to the same distance. To test quadricep strength, have him lower his legs and raise them again while you press down on his anterior thighs.

Then ask the patient to flex his knees and put his feet flat on the bed. Assess lower-leg strength by pulling his lower leg forward as he resists and then pushing it backward as he extends his knee.

Lastly, assess ankle strength by having the patient push his foot down against your resistance and then pull his foot up as you try to hold it down.

Testing handgrip strength
When testing handgrip strength, face the patient, extend the first and second fingers of each hand, and ask him to grasp your fingers and squeeze. Don't extend fingers with rings on them; a strong handgrip on those fingers can be painful.

Diagnostic tests

Diagnostic tests help confirm the diagnosis and identify the underlying cause of musculoskeletal emergencies. Common procedures include arthrocentesis, computed tomography (CT) scan, magnetic resonance imaging (MRI), and X-ray.

Arthrocentesis

Arthrocentesis is a joint puncture that's used to collect synovial fluid for analysis to identify the cause of pain and swelling, to assess for infection, and to distinguish forms of arthritis, such as pseudogout and infectious arthritis. The practitioner will probably choose the knee for this procedure, but he may tap synovial fluid from the wrist, ankle, elbow, or first metatarsophalangeal joint.

Telltale findings

In joint infection, synovial fluid looks cloudy and contains more white blood cells (WBCs) and less glucose than normal. When trauma causes bleeding into a joint, synovial fluid contains red blood cells. In specific types of arthritis, crystals can confirm the diagnosis, such as urate crystals indicating gout.

Doing double duty

Arthrocentesis also has therapeutic value. For example, in symptomatic joint effusion, removing excess synovial fluid relieves pain.

Practice pointers

• Describe the procedure to the patient. Explain that he'll be asked to assume a certain position, depending on the joint being aspirated, and that he'll need to remain still.
• After the test, the practitioner may ask you to apply ice or cold packs to the joint to reduce pain and swelling.
• If the practitioner removed a large amount of fluid, tell the patient that he may need to wear an elastic bandage.

CT scan

A CT scan aids diagnosis of bone tumors and other abnormalities. It helps assess questionable fractures, fracture fragments, bone lesions, and intra-articular loose bodies.

Beam me up

A computerized body scanner directs multiple X-ray beams at the body from different angles. The beams pass through the body and strike radiation detectors, producing electrical impulses. A computer then converts these impulses into digital information, which is displayed as a three-dimensional image on a video monitor.

Practice pointers

• Verify patient allergies and hypersensitivities.
• The patient should be in a hospital gown and instructed to remove all jewelry and hairpins.
• Inform the patient he won't be in an enclosed space, that the machine isn't enclosed, and that it's shaped like a doughnut. Let him know that he'll hear a low-pitched spinning sound.
• Tell him there will be no pain involved.

• Instruct him to remain still during the test. Although he'll be alone in the room, assure him that he can communicate with the technician through an intercom system.

MRI

MRI can show irregularities of soft tissue (such as brain tissue), bone, and muscle.

Must be your animal magnetism

The MRI scanner uses a powerful magnetic field and radiofrequency energy to produce images based on the hydrogen content of body tissues. The computer processes signals and displays the resulting high-resolution image on a video monitor. The patient can't feel the magnetic fields, and no harmful effects have been observed.

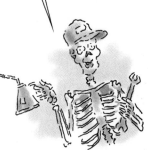

Metal and magnets don't mix! Make sure patients remove all metal objects before entering the MRI.

Practice pointers

• Make sure the patient is in a hospital gown and has removed all metal objects, including bobby pins, jewelry, piercings, watches, eyeglasses, hearing aids, and dental appliances. He should also secure his belongings—including credit, bank, and parking cards—because the scan could erase their magnetic codes.
• Explain to the patient that he'll be positioned on a narrow bed that slides into a large cylinder housing the MRI magnets. Ask if claustrophobia has ever been a problem for him. If so, sedation may help him tolerate the scan.
• Tell the patient he'll hear soft thumping noises during the test.
• Instruct him to remain still during the test. Although he'll be alone in the room, assure him that he can communicate with the technician through an intercom system.

X-rays

Anteroposterior, posteroanterior, and lateral X-rays allow three-dimensional visualization. They help diagnose:
• fractures and dislocations
• bone disease, including solitary lesions, multiple focal lesions in one bone, or generalized lesions involving all bones
• joint disease (such as arthritis), infection, degenerative changes, synoviosarcoma, osteochondromatosis, avascular necrosis, slipped femoral epiphysis, and inflamed tendons and bursae around a joint
• masses and calcifications.

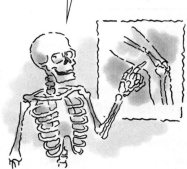

Sure, X-rays help diagnose fractures, but did you know they can also point out joint disease, bone disease, and masses?

If the practitioner needs further clarification of standard X-rays, he may order a CT scan or an MRI.

Practice pointers

- Explain the procedure to the patient.
- Make sure the patient removes all jewelry from the area to be X-rayed.
- Verify that the X-ray order includes pertinent recent history such as trauma, and identifies the point tenderness site. It should also include past fractures, dislocations, or surgery involving the affected area.
- Medicate patients for pain before radiography. Radiography can involve movement of the affected area, increasing the patient's level of discomfort, which can lead to an uncooperative patient, poor radiography quality, and an inaccurate diagnosis.

Treatments

Pain and impaired mobility are good motivators for obtaining medical care. Consequently, most patients with musculoskeletal problems eagerly seek treatment.

Get up and go again

To restore a patient's mobility, several treatments are used alone or in combination:
- drug therapy to control pain, inflammation, or muscle spasticity
- nonsurgical treatments, including closed reduction or immobilization
- surgery with subsequent immobilization in a cast, brace, or other device.

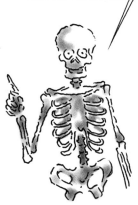

Musculoskeletal emergency patients are usually eager for treatment. Luckily, there's an a-BONE-dance to choose from!

Drug therapy

Salicylates are the first line of defense against arthropathies. Other drug therapy includes analgesics, nonsteroidal anti-inflammatory drugs, corticosteroids, and skeletal muscle relaxants.

Nonsurgical treatments

Some patients with musculoskeletal emergencies require nonsurgical treatment. Treatment options include closed reduction of a fracture or immobilization.

Closed reduction

Closed reduction involves external manipulation of fracture fragments or dislocated joints to restore their normal position and alignment. It may be done under conscious sedation or local, regional, or general anesthesia.

Immobilization

Immobilization devices are commonly used to maintain proper alignmen, limit movement, and help relieve pain and pressure.

Don't move a muscle!

Immobilization devices include:
• plaster and synthetic casts applied after closed or open reduction of fractures, or after other severe injuries
• splints to immobilize fractures, dislocations, or subluxations
• slings to support and immobilize an injured arm, wrist, or hand, or to support the weight of a splint or hold dressings in place
• skin or skeletal traction, using a system of weights and pulleys to reduce fractures, treat dislocations, correct deformities, or decrease muscle spasms
• braces to support weakened or deformed joints
• cervical collars to immobilize the cervical spine, decrease muscle spasms and, possibly, relieve pain
• long spine boards with cervical immobilization devices to fully immobilize the entire spine. (See *Teaching about immobilization devices*.)

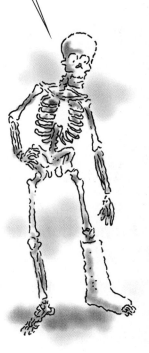

> Casts can be applied after severe injuries or closed or open fracture reductions.

Education edge

Teaching about immobilization devices

When discharging a patient with a musculoskeletal injury who has been prescribed an immobilization device, be sure to include these points:
• Tell him to promptly report signs of complications, including increased pain, drainage, or swelling in the involved area.
• Stress the need for strict compliance with activity restrictions while the immobilization device is in place.
• If the patient was given a walker, cane, or crutches to use with a leg or ankle cast, splint, or knee immobilizer, make sure he's able to demonstrate correct ambulation using the device.
• If the patient has a removable device, such as a knee immobilizer, make sure he knows how to apply it correctly.
• Advise the patient to keep scheduled medical appointments to evaluate healing.

Surgery

Surgical procedures include open reduction and internal fixation. During open reduction, the surgeon restores the normal position and alignment of fracture fragments or dislocated joints. He then inserts internal fixation devices—such as pins, screws, wires, nails, rods, or plates—to maintain alignment until healing begins.

Common disorders

In any musculoskeletal emergency, neurologic and vascular status must be evaluated carefully because a patient with a musculoskeletal illness or injury is at risk for potential neurovascular injuries and tissue ischemia. Musculoskeletal emergencies may include amputations (traumatic), compartment syndrome, contusions, dislocations and fractures, puncture wounds, and strains and sprains.

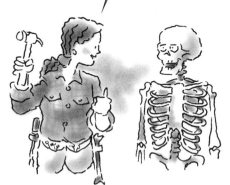

Can you pick up more screws and nails at the store? I need them for home repair, and you need them for bone repair.

Amputations (traumatic)

Amputation is the removal of a part of the body by traumatic means. Two common types of amputations are the complete (guillotine) or incomplete (crush or tear). A *complete amputation* occurs when the appendage has been completely severed from the body. An *incomplete amputation* occurs when an attachment of the appendage to the body is still present, even if minute in size.

What causes it

Amputation is accidental and traumatic, and it can originate from human or mechanical error. Potential for traumatic amputations exists anywhere there are humans working around machinery or hand tools.

How it happens

Complete and incomplete amputations occur with equal frequency. Incomplete amputations acquire greater tissue damage because of the distortion and destruction of the involved and surrounding structures, especially the vasculature. Tissue damage in complete amputations is minor because there's a precise cut between the body and affected part.

What to look for

• Observe the extent and location of the injury. Some amputations will require the patient to go immediately to the operating room.
• Assess what's missing and how much, if any, of the appendage is left intact.
• Determine the amount and color of the blood. Dark blood indicates a venous injury, while bright red blood indicates an arterial injury.
• Palpate pulses distal to the injury. If the pulses aren't palpable, immediate intervention is warranted.
• Capillary refill should be less than 2 seconds to indicate adequate perfusion.
• Pain may be present depending on the extent of nerve involvement and damage.
• Determine the underlying physiological or psychological pathology prompting the injury. For example, did the patient get dizzy and fall into machinery? Or, was his leg amputated by a train as he was trying to kill himself?

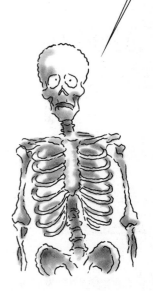

Traumatic is right! One minute my arm is attached, the next minute I'm learning to write left-handed!

What tests tell you

• X-rays will evaluate the extent to which underlying bony structures are involved or damaged, and also determine the level of injury and suitability for replantation.
• Vascular studies, such as arteriograms, determine the extent of vascular compromise caused by the injury.
• Laboratory tests ordered for initial management and preoperative screening may include complete blood count (CBC) with differential, chemistry, type, and screen; prothrombin time; partial thromboplastin time; International Normalized Ratio level; urine drug screen; and urinalysis. These studies reveal infections and evaluate blood loss, electrolyte balance, and kidney function. Bleeding times and clotting times are important factors for patient management.
• An electrocardiogram evaluates cardiac activity and can identify disease processes that cause complications from fluid resuscitation or anesthesia. These studies can also give clues about the injury's cause—for example, whether the patient had a syncopal episode while using the circular saw, which in turn caused the amputation of his finger.

How it's treated

Treatment for amputation may include surgical replantation. Antibiotics are administered before surgery and postoperatively.

What to do

• Assess the patient's ABCs and manage his life-threatening concerns. The patient's ABCs and cervical spine should be cleared before addressing secondary findings.
• Insert two large-bore (18G or larger) I.V. lines; depending on the site of amputation, you may need a central access device.
• Administer oxygen.
• Control bleeding.
• Clean the site using normal saline solution irrigation only; don't scrub or use cleaning solution on the stump.
• Administer tetanus prophylaxis.
• Administer analgesics and antibiotics.
• Apply sterile dressings.
• Prepare the patient for transfer to an appropriate facility or the operating room.
• Provide a psychosocial report for the patient and his family.
• Don't apply a tourniquet to the affected limb.
• Immobilize the limb in its correct anatomical position.
• Take care to preserve the amputated part for possible reimplantation by wrapping it in saline-moistened gauze and placing it in a sealed plastic bag. The bag should then be placed in a bath of ice water. Make sure that the part doesn't freeze. Don't allow the part to be submerged directly in the ice.

Compartment syndrome

Compartment syndrome is a condition in which increased pressure within a closed-tissue space compromises circulation to the capillaries, muscles, and nerves within that space. It's considered one of the few true orthopedic emergencies that occur in the ED. The key to a positive patient outcome is early recognition, diagnosis, and intervention. If left untreated, it can be one of the most devastating and debilitating injuries a patient can experience.

What causes it

Compartment syndrome can result from external or internal causes.

External

• Casts
• Tight dressing
• Splints
• Skeletal traction

Internal

- Frostbite
- Snakebite
- Fractures or contusions
- Bleeding into a muscle
- I.V. infiltration or extravasation

How it happens

Compartments are composed of arteries, veins, nerves, muscles, and bones. The compartments most clinically relevant to the ED practitioner are the upper and lower extremities. Compartment syndrome occurs when there's an increase of pressure within the compartment, causing ischemia to its contents. This ischemia causes severe pain but, because the cause isn't readily observed, it will seem out of proportion to the injury. Compartment syndrome can occur immediately or as long as 4 days after the injury.

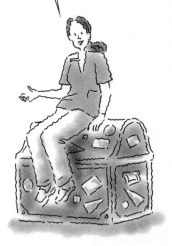

Increased pressure within a small space? Compartment syndrome sounds a lot like my packing strategy!

What to look for

Signs and symptoms of compartment syndrome include:
- swelling
- paresthesia
- pain out of proportion to injury (especially on passive movement)
- diminished pulse (a late sign).

What tests tell you

These tests are used to diagnose compartment syndrome:
- X-rays will help rule out other diagnoses.
- Obtaining a compartment pressure can be accomplished quickly and easily using a commercially available battery-powered monitor.
- Normal pressure is approximately zero but always less than 10 mm Hg.
- Compromise of capillary blood flow occurs at a pressure greater than 20 mm Hg and pressure above 30 to 40 mm Hg indicates an immediate risk because muscle and nerve tissue necrosis will occur if pressure isn't alleviated.
- Laboratory studies should include CBC to evaluate hemoglobin level, hematocrit, WBC, and platelet count; and chemistry for analysis of metabolic stability and renal function. Myoglobinuria is a common adverse effect of compartment syndrome, so close observation of renal function is imperative for a positive patient outcome.

How it's treated

• Mild cases are treated with immediate application of ice and elevation of the affected area to help decrease swelling. When the compartment pressures are over 40 mm Hg, surgical decompression by fasciotomy is required.
• Constant observation, assessment, and re-assessment in conjunction with frequent monitoring of compartment pressures is key to management of compartment syndrome.
• Cases that aren't diagnosed expeditiously require a surgical procedure known as a fasciotomy. This procedure involves surgically opening the fascia through the entire length of both compartments of the affected limb. Opening both compartments prevents swelling and ischemia in a lateral area. The surgical site is left open until all the swelling has resolved (approximately 3 to 5 days), and is then closed by skin grafting.

What to do

• Assess the patient's ABCs and manage his life-threatening concerns. The patient's ABCs and cervical spine should be cleared before addressing secondary findings.
• Obtain a thorough history of the present illness.
• Immediately apply ice and elevation to any traumatic injury to stop the pressure of swelling.
• Remove any constrictive or restrictive clothing, dressings, or devices (especially jewelry).
• Request and administer analgesia.
• Obtain I.V. access.
• Administer tetanus toxoid.

Contusions

A *contusion* is an injury resulting from a direct blow to the affected area.

What causes it

The causes of contusion vary but can include motor vehicle collisions, falls, being struck by a blunt object, or striking an immovable object with a part of the body.

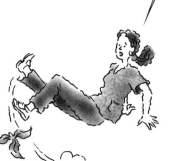

Whoops! I sense a contusion—and a lot of laughter—coming on.

How it happens

A contusion results from minor hemorrhaging underneath unbroken skin. Following the injury, blood extravasates into the surrounding tissue, causing swelling or ecchymosis. This "black-and-blue" mark will change to a yellowish-green color after approximately 2 days as the healing process progresses. The patient may experience minor discomfort from the initial injury but it will subside as swelling decreases and the blood is reabsorbed by the body.

What to look for

• Report of recent trauma to the area causing discomfort
• Bruising or swelling to the injured area (If the patient reports pain that seems out of proportion to the observed injury, you must consider the possibility of compartment syndrome.)

What tests tell you

The diagnosis of a contusion is based on clinical findings. Diagnostic tests are performed based on the mechanism of injury only to rule out underlying pathologic conditions such as a fracture.

How it's treated

Treatment is supportive and is based on symptoms:
• Ice helps decrease swelling and prevent further complications.
• A mild analgesia may be prescribed if appropriate.
• Observation may be necessary depending on the location and severity of the contusion. If symptoms progress or new ones develop, further evaluation and consultation may be warranted.

What to do

• Assess the patient's ABCs and manage his life-threatening concerns. The patient's ABCs and cervical spine should be cleared before addressing secondary findings.
• Obtain a thorough patient history, including mechanism of injury, time, and treatment performed before the patient's arrival.

History of violence

• Be alert when obtaining the patient's history for any red flags indicating abuse. (See *Abuse alerts*, page 332.)
• Provide physical care, including ice application and, if appropriate, immobilization to decrease pain.
• Mild analgesia, such as acetaminophen (Tylenol) or ibuprofen (Motrin), should be effective; if these drugs provide no decrease in pain, you should attempt to rule out compartment syndrome.
• Patient education should include trauma prevention and early signs and symptoms of compartment syndrome. The patient should follow up with his primary care doctor or return to the ED if he experiences worsening symptoms or his condition doesn't improve.

Stay on the ball

Abuse alerts

Red flags indicating abuse might include:
- multiple bruises in various stages of healing
- impatience with treatment times
- desire to leave by a specific time
- lack of direct eye contact when describing what happened
- conflicting stories from patient and caregiver.

If the patient arrives with a significant other, observe their interaction. The patient should be interviewed privately and specifically asked about abuse. If he reports being an abuse victim, take appropriate measures to ensure both his and the medical staff's safety. Contact a social services representative as soon as possible after patient presentation. This representative will provide emotional support during hospitalization and assist the patient with legal processes and aftercare.

Dislocations and fractures

A *dislocation* is an injury that occurs at the articulation of two or more bones, causing these bones to move out of their anatomically correct position. Dislocations may also include associative soft tissue and vascular or nerve injury. (See *Types of dislocations.*)

A *fracture* is an interruption in the continuity and stability of the bone. Fractures themselves, while painful and temporarily debilitating, don't cause fatalities. However, complications of fracture can lead to permanent disability and even death if not recognized and treated. Fractures are classified by five general divisions:

- anatomic location
- direction of fracture lines
- relationship of fragments to each other
- stability
- associated soft tissue injury.

Trauma and force

Direct trauma describes an injury caused by a force that directly impacted or caused the damage, while *indirect trauma* refers to

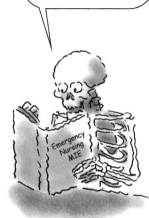

Interruption of stability, relationship of fragments—this fracture stuff sounds awfully emotional.

Types of dislocations

This chart lists the common sites of dislocations, causes, common signs and symptoms, and treatments for each type.

Location	Causes	Signs and symptoms	Treatments
Acromioclavicular separation	• Common athletic injury • Fall or direct blow to the point of the shoulder	• Severe pain in the joint area • Inability to raise the arm or adduct the arm across the chest • Deformity • Point tenderness	• Depends on the degree of dislocation • Reduction, which should take place as soon as possible to avoid complications • Postreduction treatment of minor injuries, including splinting in position of comfort with sling and swath, which the patient should maintain for approximately 7 to 10 days • Open reduction or having the patient wear the splint for a longer period for more severe injuries
Shoulder	*Anterior* • Usually an athletic injury resulting from a fall on an extended arm which is externally rotated and abducted *Posterior* • Rare but may be seen when the arm has been forcefully abducted and internally rotated	• Decreased or limited range of motion (ROM) • Decreased function • Deformity	• Closed reduction after associative fracture is ruled out • Reduction, which should occur immediately if neurovascular compromise is present • Operative interventions when indicated, as when there's soft-tissue interposition, displaced greater tuberosity fracture, and Glenoid rim fracture measuring greater than 5 mm • Surgery, possibly the treatment of choice for athletes
Elbow	• Fall on an extended arm	• Pain that increases with movement • Decreased or limited ROM • Decreased function • Deformity	• Varied, based on direction of dislocation, but usually closed reduction followed by splint application • Surgical repair for a dislocation that's irreducible or one that has associative neurovascular compromise
Wrist	• Fall on an outstretched hand	• Pain, especially with movement • Deformity	• Support in position of comfort • Closed reduction • Surgical intervention

(continued)

Types of dislocations (continued)

Location	Causes	Signs and symptoms	Treatments
Hand or finger	• Fall on an outstretched hand • Direct blow to the fingertip or a jamming force to the fingertip	• Pain • Swelling • Deformity • Inability to move the joint	• Support in position of comfort • Reduction
Hip	• Major trauma such as frontal motor vehicle collision (foot on brake pedal or knee hits dashboard)	• Hip pain • Knee pain • Pain that may radiate to groin • Hip flexed, adducted, and internally rotated (posterior dislocation) • Hip slightly flexed, abducted, and externally rotated (anterior dislocation [rare]) • Patient complaints of joint feeling locked • Inability to move the leg	• Support in position of comfort • Surgical reduction • For postsurgical dislocation, closed reduction under moderate sedation or, if unsuccessful, completed under general anesthesia
Knee	• Major trauma • High-speed motor vehicle collision • Sports injury	• Severe pain • Deformity • Gross swelling • Inability to move the joint	• Splint in position of comfort • Immediate reduction (within 24 hours) • Admission or transfer to the operating room
Patella	• History of spontaneous dislocation • Direct trauma • Rotation of a planted foot	• Knee in flexed position • Pain • Loss of function • Swelling • Tenderness	• Possible spontaneous reduction into place • Splint or cast • Crutches
Ankle	• Commonly associated with a motor vehicle collision (foot on pedal) • Commonly associated with a fracture	• Swelling • Deformity • Pain • Inability to move the joint	• Possible surgical reduction • Splint or cast • Crutches

an injury caused by the transmission of force from one area to another.

Location and direction

Anatomic location describes exactly where in the bone the fracture is located. A long bone is divided into sections:

Classifying fractures

One of the best-known systems for classifying fractures uses a combination of terms—such as *simple, nondisplaced,* and *oblique*—to describe them.

General classification of fractures
- *Simple (closed)*—Bone fragments don't penetrate the skin.
- *Compound (open)*—Bone fragments penetrate the skin.
- *Incomplete (partial)*—Bone continuity isn't completely interrupted.
- *Complete*—Bone continuity is completely interrupted.

Classification by fragment position
- *Comminuted*—The bone breaks into small pieces.
- *Impacted*—One bone fragment is forced into another.
- *Angulated*—Fragments lie at an angle to each other.
- *Displaced*—Fracture fragments separate and are deformed.
- *Nondisplaced*—The two sections of bone maintain essentially normal alignment.
- *Overriding*—Fragments overlap, shortening the total bone length.
- *Segmental*—Fractures occur in two adjacent areas with an isolated central segment.
- *Avulsed*—Fragments are pulled from normal position by muscle contractions or ligament resistance.

Classification by fracture line
- *Linear*—The fracture line runs parallel to the bone's axis.
- *Longitudinal*—The fracture line extends in a longitudinal (but not parallel) direction along the bone's axis.
- *Oblique*—The fracture line crosses the bone at roughly a 45-degree angle to the bone's axis.
- *Spiral*—The fracture line crosses the bone at an oblique angle, creating a spiral pattern.
- *Transverse*—The fracture line forms a right angle with the bone's axis.

- proximal
- middle or distal
- head, shaft, or base.
  The *direction* of the fracture line is categorized as:
- *transverse*—when the fracture is perpendicular to the bone
- *oblique*—when the line runs across the bone at a 45- to 60-degree angle
- *spiral*—when the direction of the fracture line looks twisted
- *comminuted*—when the bone is broken into more than two fragments
- *impacted*—when the ends of the fracture are compressed together. (See *Classifying fractures.*)
  Transverse, oblique, or comminuted fractures generally occur as a result of direct force. Avulsion, spiral, and stress fractures are typically caused by indirect force.

Relationship and stability

The relationship of the fracture fragments to each other is described by *alignment* and *apposition*. *Alignment* describes how the bones are positioned or placed. *Apposition* describes the contact between the fracture surfaces.

Stability describes the tendency of a fracture to displace after reduction. A *stable* fracture doesn't displace; an *unstable* fracture does.

Don't go soft on us now

Associated soft tissue injury is divided into:
- *simple*—when there's no break in the skin
- *compound*—when overlying skin is broken, but there's no direct communication between open skin and the fracture
- *complicated*—when there's associative neurovascular, visceral, ligament, or muscular damage. (Intra-articular fractures are also categorized as complicated.)

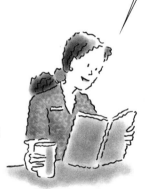

Soft tissue injuries are like good stories; some are simple, and some are complicated.

What causes it

Most dislocations and fractures are caused by direct or indirect trauma, although some have different causes. Stress fractures result from repetitive use or motion. Pathologic fractures occur in a bone weakened by a pre-existing disease. They can be preceded by injury or occur during normal activity. Regardless of underlying disease, the mechanism of injury plays an important role. (See *Understanding fractures*, pages 338 to 345.)

How it happens

The extent and severity of dislocations or fractures depends on extrinsic factors; amount, direction, and duration of force; and the frequency of the injury-causing act.

Dislocation

A dislocation occurs when there's a disruption in the relationship of the bones at their articulation. Reduction of dislocations should be completed as soon as possible to prevent the injury from progressing to adjacent vasculature and nerves.

Fracture

A fracture occurs when the stress applied to the bone exceeds its malleability. The bone's strength is directly related to its density. Factors affecting the osseous structure, such as an underlying disease process, specific medication regimens, and some congenital anomalies, affect its density. Immediately after a fracture occurs, the bone body initiates its own healing process. This process occurs in three phases:

 inflammatory phase

 reparative phase

remodeling phase.

It's a hematoma!

Because the periosteum is torn, a hematoma forms between the two separated areas of bone. In the *inflammatory phase*, the hematoma begins to clot and deprives the osteocytes at the bones' ends of oxygen and nutrients, which causes them to die. A significant inflammatory response ensues, including vasodilation, causing release of inflammatory cells, leukocytes, and macrophages.

Organization is key

Next, in the *reparative phase*, cells within the hematoma (mesenchymal cells) organize, localize, and begin to form bone. Osteoblasts move from inside the bone toward the damaged ends and assist in the healing process.

I'm brand new!

New bone is formed from trabeculae organization—causing the reconnection of the previously separated bone edges—in the *remodeling phase* of healing.

What to look for

The most common signs and symptoms of dislocations and fractures include:
- pain
- swelling
- ecchymosis
- point tenderness.

What's more...

Deformity may also be present, and can be associated with a loss of normal function ranging from minimal to complete, depending on the injury. Associative blood loss shouldn't be overlooked during patient care; blood loss volumes can be minimal to shock-inducing. Estimated blood loss can range from 150 ml (with a radius fracture) to 3,000 ml (in conjunction with a pelvic fracture), leading to hypovolemia and shock.

A pathologic fracture can produce painless swelling and generalized bone pain without swelling.

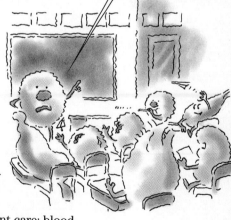

All right, people, let's get organized here. We've got a bone to form!

(Text continues on page 344.)

Understanding fractures

Fractures can occur in almost every part of every limb. Depending on where and how they occur, each brings with it specific complications and therapeutic interventions to be alert for. The chart below describes common fractures, their causes, signs and symptoms, interventions, and the possible complications associated with each type.

Fracture	Causes	Signs and symptoms
Clavicle	• Most common in pediatric patients • Fall on extended arm or shoulder • Direct blow to shoulder	• Pain in clavicle area • Swelling • Deformity • Bony crepitus • Patient can't or won't raise arm
Shoulder and humerus	• Fall on outstretched arm • Direct shoulder trauma from a fall or a blunt instrument	• Pain in shoulder area • Point tenderness • Posterior rotation • Inability to move affected arm • Adduction of the humerus • Abduction of humerus • Gross edema and discoloration that can extend to chest wall
Scapula	• Direct trauma; penetrating or blunt	• Pain on shoulder movement • Point tenderness • Arm held in adduction with resistance to abduction • Ecchymosis • Palpable bony displacement • Swelling
Upper arm	• Fall on arm or direct blow • Twisting or throwing of the arm	• Bony crepitus • Bruising • Inability to move arm • Pain • Point tenderness • Severe deformity • Swelling
Elbow	• Fall on extended arm • Fall on flexed elbow	• Severe pain • Point tenderness • Rapid swelling • Shortening of the arm • Delayed capillary refill

Interventions	Possible complications
Shoulder immobilization	• Brachial plexus injury • Ligament damage • Malunion • Subclavian vascular injury
Immobilization of arm in a sling or swath Surgery if fracture is impacted, comminuted, or displaced	• Laceration of the axillary artery • Brachial plexus injury • Avascular necrosis of the humeral head • Frozen shoulder syndrome • Nonunion
Immobilization of arm in a sling or swath Padding the axilla to avoid injury to the brachial plexus and artery	• Injury to the ribs • Pneumothorax • Hemothorax • Compression fractures of the spine
Immobilization of arm in a sling or swath Surgical intervention (for fracture that extends below the elbow, spiral fractures, or shaft fractures)	• Laceration or stretching of the radial nerve resulting in neuropraxia
Splint the arm "as it lies" Orthopedic consult Arteriogram to assess for vascular compromise	• Brachial artery laceration • Nerve damage • Volkmann's ischemic contracture

(continued)

Understanding fractures (continued)

Fracture	Causes	Signs and symptoms
Radius or ulna	• Fall on extended arm • Direct blow such as in "nightstick" fractures • Forced pronation of the forearm	• Pain • Point tenderness • Swelling • Deformity • Angulation • Shortening
Wrist	• Dorsiflexion, usually following a fall on an extended arm or open hand	• Pain • Snuff box tenderness • Swelling • Deformity • Limited range of motion • Numbness • Weakness
Hand and finger	• Forceful hyperextension • Direct trauma • Crush injury	• Pain • Point tenderness • Severe swelling • Deformity • Inability to use hand
Pelvis	• Motor vehicle collision • Fall from a height • Crush injury • Direct trauma	• Tenderness when iliac wings are compressed • Paraspinous muscle spasms • Sacroiliac joint tenderness • Hematuria • Pelvic ecchymosis • Groin pain • Blood at the urethral meatus • Perineal hematomas • Prostate displacement and loss of sphincter tone
Hip (acetabulum, greater trochanter, femoral head)	• Direct blow or fall • Common geriatric injury • Axial transmission of force from knees as in knee-to-dashboard injuries	• Pain in hip or groin area • Severe pain with movement • Inability to bear weight • External rotation of the affected hip and leg • Shortening of the affected limb

Interventions	Possible complications
Closed reduction Casting Referral to orthopedic surgeon Open reduction and internal fixation	• Paralysis of the radial nerve • Malunion • Volkmann's ischemic contracture
Closed reduction Rigid splint or a thumb spica cast Referral to orthopedic surgeon	• Rare aseptic necrosis
Closed reduction Finger traction Splinting distal phalanges with a padded aluminum guard Buddy taping an injured finger to an uninjured one Antibiotics for open fractures	• Malunion • Osteomyelitis • Subungual hematoma
Aggressive resuscitation (oxygen, crystalloids, blood transfusion) Immobilization of the spine and legs Pelvic stabilization (pneumatic antishock garment-abdominal section, pelvic binder, internal or external fixation) Pelvic computed tomography (CT) scan Abdominal CT scan Antibiotics	• Hemorrhage, shock, death • Bladder, genital, or lumbosacral trauma • Ruptured internal organs • Osteomyelitis • Compartment syndrome • Chronic pain • GI tract injury • Pulmonary or fat emboli
Immobilization in a comfortable position Traction Referral to an orthopedic surgeon Surgical intervention	• Avascular necrosis of the femoral head • Phlebitis of the femoral vein • Osteoarthritis • Sciatic nerve injury • Hypovolemic shock • Fat embolism syndrome

(continued)

Understanding fractures (continued)

Fracture	Causes	Signs and symptoms
Femur	• Indirect force upward through a flexed knee • Direct trauma • Falls • Gunshot wounds • Motor vehicle collision (especially vehicle-pedestrian collision)	• Angulation • Shortening of the limb • Severe muscle spasm • Bony crepitus • Severe pain • Swelling of the thigh • Hematoma in the thigh • Inability to bear weight on the affected leg
Knee	• High-velocity vehicle trauma • Pedestrian trauma (such as from a bumper or fender) • Fall from a height onto a flexed knee • Hyperabduction	• Bony crepitus • Tense swelling in the popliteal area • Hemarthrosis, swelling around the joint • Knee pain and tenderness • Inability to straighten or bend the knee
Patella	• Direct trauma (dashboard impact) or a fall • Indirect trauma (after quadriceps muscle pull or contraction)	• Knee pain • Hemarthrosis • Inability to extend the knee
Tibia and fibula	• Twisting or rotating forces • Direct trauma • Fall with compression forces • Fall with foot fixed in place such as in a ski injury	• Pain • Point tenderness • Swelling • Deformity • Bony crepitus
Ankle	• Direct trauma • Indirect trauma • Torsion, eversion, or inversion	• Popping sound at time of injury (torn ligaments) • Ecchymosis • Bony crepitus • Pain on ambulation or altered gait • Inability to bear weight if injury is unstable
Foot	• Similar to ankle injury • Athletic injuries • Direct trauma	• Deep pain • Point tenderness • Ecchymosis • Swelling • Subungual hematoma • Inability to bear weight • Deformity

Interventions	Possible complications
• Aggressive resuscitation (oxygen, crystalloids, blood transfusion) • Immobilization of the thigh with a traction splint • Referral to an orthopedic surgeon • Open reduction with internal fixation	• Hemorrhage • Severe muscle damage • Knee trauma (commonly overlooked)
• Non-weight bearing cast • Traction • Crutches • Referral to an orthopedic surgeon • Open reduction and internal fixation	• Popliteal nerve or artery injury • Fat emboli • Rotational deformities • Traumatic arthrosis
• Surgery for quadriceps repair	• Avascular necrosis
• Assessment for puncture wound associated with tibia (open fracture) • Wound debridement and irrigation • Casting • Crutches • Open reduction and internal fixation	• Compartment syndrome • Infection • Osteomyelitis • Nonunion
• Closed reduction • Posterior splint • Possible open reduction and internal fixation • Casting • Crutches	• Nonunion • Infection • Posttrauma arthritis
• Bulky dressing • Orthopedic shoe • Posterior splint • Cane or crutches	• Avascular necrosis • Malunion • Gait abnormalities

(continued)

Understanding fractures (continued)

Fracture	Causes	Signs and symptoms
Heel	• Fall from a height	• Increased pain with hyperflexion • Point tenderness • Pain in hindfoot • Soft tissue ecchymosis • Superficial skin blistering • Deformity
Toe	• Direct trauma (stubbing or kicking) • Crush injuries • Athletic injuries	• Subungual hematoma • Pain • Deformity • Discoloration

Signs and symptoms of stress fractures can vary depending on the area of injury. However, the patient's chief complaint is of pain that has been getting progressively worse over time during an activity.

What tests tell you

These tests help determine dislocation or fracture:
• Arteriograms are used with dislocations and fractures to assess associative vascular involvement.
• MRIs are most helpful with the diagnosis of tendon, ligament, and soft tissue injuries.
• CT scans can be used to evaluate a bone for a fracture, especially when serial radiography has been negative but the patient complains of persistent pain.
• X-rays provide evidence of most fractures. Some fractures will only show up after an extended time, so follow-up radiography is an important part of fracture management.

How it's treated

Fracture management is based on evaluation of the type and classification of the injury, and practitioner preference based on experience:
• Pain management is a primary concern for all dislocations and fractures.
• Splinting is the initial treatment for most fractures and is applied in the ED. Splints are used to prevent further soft tissue in-

Interventions	Possible complications
• Bulky and compression dressings • Ensuring non-weight-bearing or partial-weight-bearing • Crutches • Surgery (usually not scheduled for 2 days to 2 weeks following injury) • Closed reduction for displaced fractures • Assessment for associated trauma	• Chronic pain • Nerve entrapment
Compression bandage Buddy taping Orthopedic shoe Cane as needed	• None

jury from fracture fragments, to decrease pain by providing support and position of comfort, and to lower the risk of clinical fat emboli. (See *Common splint types.*)

• General indications for surgical treatment of fractures include displaced intra-articular fractures, associated arterial injury, when closed methods of treatment have failed, fractures through metastatic lesions, or for patients who can't be confined to bed. Postoperatively, a splint or cast is applied to maintain correct alignment.

• Closed reduction should be performed within 6 to 12 hours of the time of injury because swelling makes the procedure difficult.

Inspired casting

• Indications for applying a cast include pain relief, immobilization of a fracture to allow for healing, and stabilization of an unstable fracture. Casts are individually molded for the patient using plaster or fiberglass casting material. As a therapy, casts are generally reserved for application until swelling has resolved—approximately 3 to 5 days after the injury or surgery.

• Pathologic fractures are treated with immobilization and rest as well as pain control.

• Stress fracture treatment varies depending on severity and location, and is similar to the treatment of a sprain or strain. The injuring activity is limited or eliminated. Rest is one of the most important interventions for recovery. Treatment for stress fracture in the lower extremity involves crutches. The healing timeframe is approximately 4 to 6 weeks. The few cases in which casting treat-

Common splint types

Examples of commonly used splints include:
• the Hare traction and Sager splints for reduction and immobilization of femur fractures preoperatively
• prefabricated splints for immobilization and support of the wrist or ankle
• air splints used in the pre-hospital environment to provide immobilization to extremities
• fiberglass and plaster ready-to-mold splinting material in a variety of widths and lengths.

ment is preferred over splinting are usually managed by an orthopedist.
- Unstable fractures are treated surgically.

What to do

- Assess the patient's ABCs and ensure that the cervical spine has been cleared before addressing secondary findings.
- Assess for paresthesia.
- Assess the injured area for vascular stability, capillary refill, and pulses distal to the injury.
- Remove jewelry from or distal to affected area because it can act as a tourniquet if left in place.
- Evaluate the patient's tetanus status. Administer a booster if the patient hasn't had an immunization in the last 10 years, or if the wound is soiled and he hasn't had one in 5 years.
- Apply ice for 20-minute intervals to decrease swelling.
- Assist with splinting as appropriate.
- Cover open fractures with a moist, sterile dressing.
- Request and provide analgesia.
- Prepare the patient for admission if appropriate.
- Prepare the patient for the operating room if appropriate.

Pelvic plan

If the patient has a suspected pelvic fracture, follow these steps:
- Immobilize him by using a long spine board or pneumatic anti-shock garment.
- If not contraindicated, decrease pain by having the patient flex his knees.
- Monitor vital signs, including neurovascular assessment, every 5 minutes.
- If the pelvic fracture is unstable, initiate open trauma protocol.
- Administer fluids and antibiotics via a large-bore I.V. line (18G or larger) and administer supplemental oxygen. Expect and prepare the patient for peritoneal lavage.
- Prepare the patient for the operating room to receive definitive care.
- Prepare for and assist with moderate sedation.
- Administer blood products as ordered.

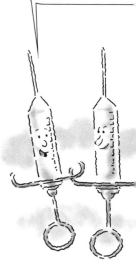

Don't forget about tetanus! Give your patient a booster if his last immunization was more than 10 years ago.

Puncture wounds

A *puncture wound* is a piercing of the skin by a foreign object, causing a hole in the skin and underlying tissues. Puncture wounds can be superficial and only involve the skin, or can extend through tissue and into the bone, depending on the mechanism of injury.

What causes it

Puncture wounds are caused by direct trauma. The possible mechanisms of injury are endless, but some examples include bites and foreign objects, such as nails, needles, pins, and knives.

What to look for

Assess the wound for signs and symptoms of infection and obvious presence of a retained foreign body.

What tests tell you

X-rays should be completed if the puncture wound is near a joint or bone to rule out underlying fracture and presence of some types of foreign bodies.

How it's treated

If the wound is uncomplicated and the patient is healthy, prophylactic antibiotics may not help; in fact, they may predispose the patient to superinfection of *Pseudomonas*. In many cases, cleaning and irrigating the wound is all that's necessary.

What to do

• Assess the patient's ABCs, and ensure cervical spine clearance before addressing secondary findings.
• Control bleeding with direct pressure and elevation; note the amount of blood loss from the wound. Notify the practitioner if blood loss is significant or bleeding doesn't stop within 10 minutes of applying pressure.
• Evaluate the patient's tetanus status. Administer a booster if the patient hasn't had an immunization in the last 10 years, or if the wound is soiled and he hasn't had one in 5 years.
• Irrigate the wound if it isn't associated with an underlying fracture.
• If the wound contains foreign matter, is associated with a fracture, or is more than 8 hours old, you may need to administer oral or I.V. antibiotics.
• Perform wound care and apply necessary dressings or immobilization devices.

Strains and sprains

Strain is the term used to describe a pulling apart of muscle fibers, while a *sprain* describes a pulling apart of the fibers within a ligament. Both can result from direct or indirect trauma.

What causes it

The most common cause of strains and sprains is sports-related trauma. Other common causes include motor vehicle collisions and falls.

How it happens

A strain is classified by degree and location of the muscle:

A *first-degree* strain is caused by a forceable overstretching of a muscle.

A *second-degree* strain is a disruption of more muscle fibers (more forceful contraction or stretch) than a first-degree strain.

A *third-degree* strain entails a complete disruption of the muscle fibers, and may be accompanied by a rupture of the overlying fascia or an avulsion fracture of the underlying bone.

Sprain, sprain, go away!

A sprain is also diagnosed by degree and location, but of ligaments (not muscle):

In a *first-degree* sprain, the involved ligament stretches without tearing—the joint remains stable and joint function remains normal.

A *second-degree* sprain involves stretching and tearing of the involved ligament, causing moderate function loss and mild to moderate joint instability.

A *third-degree* sprain is the most painful and physically limiting. It involves a complete disruption of the tendon, causing profound joint instability, moderate to severe loss of function, and an inability to hold an object (if located in the upper extremity) or bear weight (if located in the lower extremity).

What to look for

First- and second-degree strains are similar in presentation, therefore differentiation is based on the degree of loss of function and level of swelling. Characteristics of first- and second-degree strains include:

• mild localized swelling
• ecchymosis

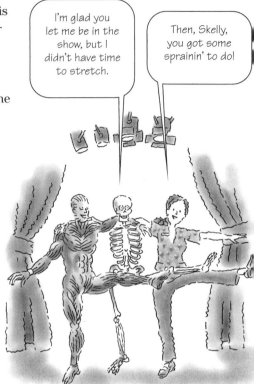

I'm glad you let me be in the show, but I didn't have time to stretch.

Then, Skelly, you got some sprainin' to do!

- mild spasms
- localized discomfort, possibly aggravated by movement or pressure
- minimal but transient loss of function and strength.
  Characteristics of a third-degree strain include:
- moderate to severe swelling with ecchymosis
- moderate to severe pain
- muscle spasm
- moderate to complete loss of function
- knotlike protrusion on the muscle at the injury site.

Any good chef will tell you that presentation is everything. That goes double when you're diagnosing strains and sprains.

Sprain symptoms

Patients with a first-degree sprain demonstrate:
- minimal swelling
- little or no joint instability
- mild discomfort.
  Symptoms of a second-degree sprain are more pronounced. They include:
- moderate to severe swelling
- ecchymosis
- moderate functional loss
- mild to moderate joint instability.
  A third-degree sprain causes:
- patient's inability to bear weight or hold an object
- moderate to severe swelling
- ecchymosis
- joint instability.

What tests tell you

Just like contusions, strains and sprains are diagnosed by clinical presentation. X-rays will only verify the lack of an underlying fracture. Thus, radiography isn't always needed before diagnosis. For example, if a patient has lower back pain and mild spasms but denies recent trauma such as a fall, then radiography isn't necessarily indicated.

How it's treated

Treatment depends on the injury's extent. All strains and sprains are treated with analgesia, ice, elevation, and immobilization on arrival at the ED. When a differential diagnosis has been made, treatment methods and recovery periods vary:
- *First-degree* strains and sprains are treated with ice and rest over a couple of days. Mild analgesics may be prescribed. Activity can be gradually resumed as tolerated.

• In addition to analgesia, rest, ice, and elevation, a *second-degree* strain or sprain is immobilized and all patient activity is restricted until swelling and pain subside. Use of immobilizers (for upper-extremity injuries) and crutches (for lower-extremity injuries) is common. Ice is applied for the first 24 to 48 hours, after which the use of heat is prescribed. Use of the injured muscle is gradual and stopped if pain is experienced. Slow and steady progression is the key to recovery. Returning to normal activity too soon will cause re-injury.

• A *third-degree* strain or sprain is initially treated in the same way as a second-degree strain: with analgesia, ice, elevation, and immobilization. After these interventions, the patient is referred to a specialist for further evaluation and treatment, which may include surgical repair. A more substantial analgesia medication may be required by these patients because of the injury's extent.

What to do

• Assess the patient's ABCs and manage his life-threatening concerns. The patient's ABCs and cervical spine should be cleared before addressing secondary findings.

• Immediately apply ice, provide support with a splint or other immobilization device, and elevate the area for comfort.

• Obtain a thorough history of the present illness, including precipitating factors. For example, a patient may have ankle pain as his chief complaint because that's what is bothering him now, but asking when the pain and swelling began may reveal that he fell down the steps. Further questioning may reveal that he actually had an episode of syncope while using the steps to get to his sublingual nitroglycerin medication.

• Remove jewelry from or distal to the affected area because it can act as a tourniquet if left in place.

• Request and administer analgesics.

• Assist the patient into a wheelchair or onto a stretcher, if appropriate, to prevent further injury from weight-bearing activity.

• Provide patient education. (See *Teaching about strains and sprains.*)

> There's often a lot more to a strain or sprain than meets the eye. Be sure to ask about precipitating factors.

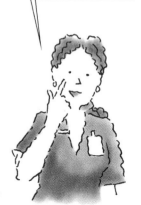

Education edge

Teaching about strains and sprains

Teaching about strains and sprains should include:
• explanation of the diagnosis
• information regarding prescribed medications
• instruction on use of supportive, immobilization, and assistive devices.
    In addition, follow these guidelines:
• The patient should be able to demonstrate his understanding of the use of the assistive devices provided.
• Emphasize applying ice and elevating and resting the affected area.
• Stress that use of the affected area shouldn't be initiated until all swelling and pain have subsided. When this occurs, the patient should begin progressively active exercises and perform them to the limit of pain.
• Instruct the patient to follow up with outside resources or return to the emergency department as directed.
• Explain the importance of follow-up care and the risks if follow-up care isn't completed.

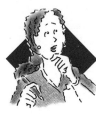

Quick quiz

1. If your patient can't move his right arm away from his side, you should document this as impaired:

    A.   supination.
    B.   abduction.
    C.   eversion.
    D.   adduction.

Answer: B. Abduction is the ability to move a limb away from the midline.

2. A condition in which increased pressure within a closed-tissue space compromises circulation to the capillaries, muscles, and nerves within that space is the definition of:

    A.   sprain.
    B.   strain.
    C.   compression fracture.
    D.   compartment syndrome.

Answer: D. Compartment syndrome is characterized by increased pressure within a closed-tissue space compromising circulation to its contents.

3. An injury that occurs at the articulation of two or more bones and causes the bones involved to be moved out of the anatomically correct position is the definition of a:

    A.   fracture.
    B.   sprain.
    C.   strain.
    D.   dislocation.

Answer: D. A dislocation is defined as an injury that occurs at the articulation of two or more bones, causing the bones involved to be moved out of the anatomically correct position.

Scoring

☆☆☆ If you answered all three questions correctly, way to go! You're a bred-in-the-bone musculoskeletal maven!

☆☆ If you answered two questions correctly, impressive! Make no bones about it, you have a mastery of musculoskeletal matters!

☆ If you answered fewer than two questions correctly, don't become unhinged! Just bone up a bit, and you'll be playing ball and socket with the big boys soon.

Genitourinary and gynecologic emergencies

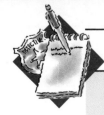

Just the facts

In this chapter, you'll learn:

♦ emergency assessment of the genitourinary (GU) and reproductive systems

♦ diagnostic tests and procedures for GU and gynecologic emergencies

♦ GU and gynecologic disorders and their treatments in the emergency department.

Understanding GU and gynecologic emergencies

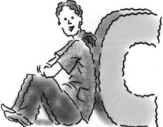

Compassion and comfort are two Cs that will put GU emergency patients right at ease.

The genitourinary (GU) and reproductive systems are closely related, and identifying subtle changes within them can mean the difference between effective and ineffective emergency care.

An emergency involving the urinary or reproductive system can have far-reaching consequences. In addition to affecting the system itself, it can trigger problems in other body systems and affect the patient's quality of life, self-esteem, and sense of well-being.

Despite these dangers, many patients are reluctant to discuss their problems with a nurse or have intimate areas of their bodies examined. Your challenge is to perform skilled, sensitive assessment. To do so, you must put the patient at ease; if you appear comfortable discussing the problem, the patient will feel encouraged to talk openly.

Assessment

When your patient comes to the emergency department (ED) with a GU or gynecologic emergency, your assessment can help determine whether the symptoms are related to a current medical problem or indicate a new one. You need to assess the patient thoroughly, always being alert for subtle changes that may indicate a potential deterioration in condition.

Unless the patient requires immediate stabilizing treatment, begin by taking a comprehensive patient history. Then probe further by conducting a thorough physical examination.

Peruse the record

If you can't interview the patient because of his condition, gather information from medical records. In some cases, you may need to ask the patient's family or the emergency medical response team that transported the patient to the ED.

Sex-specific

The urinary system consists of the kidneys, ureters, bladder, and urethra. Remember sex differences; for the male patient, the urethral meatus is also part of the reproductive system, carrying semen as well as urine. The male reproductive system also includes the penis, scrotum, testicles, epididymis, vas deferens, seminal vesicles, and prostate gland.

For the female patient, the reproductive system consists of the external genitalia (collectively called the *vulva*—mons pubis, labia majora, labia minora, clitoris, vagina, urethral meatus, and Skene's and Bartholin's glands) and the internal genitalia (vagina, uterus, ovaries, and fallopian tubes).

Health history

When gathering a health history, focus first on the patient's chief complaint, and then explore previous health status and sexual-reproductive history. Ask the patient to describe symptoms in his own words, encouraging free and open speech. As you obtain a history, remember that the patient may feel uncomfortable discussing urinary or reproductive problems. (See *Putting your patient at ease.*)

Chief complaint

Because the locations of the urinary and reproductive systems are so close, you and the patient may have trouble differentiating

Putting your patient at ease

Here are some tips for helping your patient feel more comfortable during the health history:
• Make sure that the room is private and that you won't be interrupted.
• Tell the patient that his answers will remain confidential, and phrase your questions tactfully.
• Start with less sensitive topic areas and work up to more sensitive areas such as sexual function.
• Don't rush or omit important facts because the patient seems embarrassed.
• Be especially tactful with older men, who may see a normal decrease in sexual prowess

as a sign of declining health and may be less willing to talk about sexual problems than younger men.
• When asking questions, keep in mind that the patient may view sexual problems as a sign of diminished masculinity or femininity. Phrase your questions carefully and offer reassurance as needed.
• Consider the patient's educational and cultural background. If he uses slang or euphemisms to talk about sexual organs or function, make sure you're both talking about the same thing.

signs and symptoms. Even if the patient's complaint seems minor, investigate it; ask about its onset, duration, aggravating factors, alleviating factors, severity, and the measures taken to treat it.

The most common complaints associated with GU problems involve output changes, such as polyuria, oliguria, and anuria. Patients also commonly report complaints related to voiding pattern changes, including:
• hesitancy
• frequency
• urgency
• dysuria
• nocturia
• incontinence
• urine color changes
• pain.

Common complaints associated with male reproductive problems include penile discharge, scrotal or inguinal masses, or pain and tenderness. For women, common reproductive complaints include vaginal discharge, abnormal uterine bleeding, and pruritus.

Current health status

Ask the patient about current problems and medications:
• Does he have diabetes (which increases the risk of urinary tract infection [UTI]), cardiovascular disease (which can alter kidney perfusion), or hypertension (which can contribute to renal failure and nephropathy)?

Be sure to weed out information about existing conditions, especially diabetes, cardiovascular disease, or hypertension.

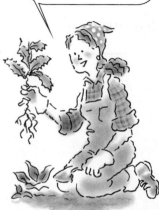

- Has the patient noticed a change in the color or odor of urine?
- Does he have pain or burning during urination or problems with incontinence or frequency?
- Does the patient have allergies? Allergic reactions can cause tubular damage; a severe anaphylactic reaction can cause temporary renal failure and permanent tubular necrosis.
- Make a list of all the prescribed medications the patient takes, including birth control and hormones, herbal preparations, and over-the-counter drugs. Some drugs can affect the appearance of urine; nephrotoxic drugs can alter urinary function.

Previous health status

Past illnesses and preexisting conditions can affect a patient's GU and reproductive health:
- Has the patient ever had a kidney or bladder infection or an infection of the reproductive system?
- Has the patient ever had kidney or bladder trauma, surgery, congenital problems, or kidney stones?
- Has he ever been catheterized?

Also ask about the patient's family history to get information about the risk of developing kidney failure or kidney disease.

Sexual-reproductive history

Many patients feel uncomfortable answering questions about their sexual health or reproductive history. To establish a rapport, begin with less personal questions.

Female patients

With a female patient, start by asking about her menstrual cycle. How old was she when she began to menstruate? In girls, menses generally starts by age 15. If it hasn't and if no secondary sex characteristics have developed, the patient should be evaluated by a practitioner.

How long does her menses usually last, and how often does it occur? When was her last menstrual period? The normal cycle for menstruation is one menses every 21 to 38 days. The normal duration is 2 to 8 days.

Does she have cramps, spotting, or an unusually heavy or light flow? Does she use tampons? Spotting between menses, or *metrorrhagia*, may be normal in patients taking low-dose hormonal contraceptives or progesterone; otherwise, spotting may indicate infection, cancer, or some other abnormality.

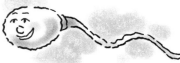

Talking about sexual-reproductive history should go swimmingly after you establish a rapport with your patient.

Comfort zone

When the patient seems comfortable, ask about:
• sexual practices
• number of current and past sexual partners
• whether she uses protection (contraception, condoms)
• pain with intercourse
• sexually transmitted disease (STD) history and precautions taken to prevent STD contraction
• human immunodeficiency virus status
• date of last intercourse
• date and results of last Papanicolaou (Pap) test
• vaginal discharge
• external lesions
• itching.

Pregnancy clues

Ask the patient if she has ever been pregnant. If so:
• How many times has she been pregnant and how many times did she give birth?
• Has she had any miscarriages or therapeutic abortions?
• Did she have a vaginal or cesarean birth?
• What kind of birth control, if any, does she use?
• Is she possibly pregnant now?

   If the patient is sexually active, talk to her about the importance of safer sex and the prevention of STDs.

   If your patient is postmenopausal, ask for the date of her last menses. To find out more about her menopausal symptoms, ask if she's having hot flashes, night sweats, mood swings, flushing, or vaginal dryness or itching.

Male patients

As with a female, ask the male patient about his sexual preferences and practices to assess risk-taking behaviors. Also ask about:
• number of current and past sexual partners
• STD history and precautions taken to prevent STD contraction
• HIV status (see *Don't forget to ask the elderly patient*)
• birth control measures.
   Also ask about his sexual health:
• Has he ever experienced trauma to his penis or scrotum?
• Was he ever diagnosed with an undescended testicle?
• Has he had a vasectomy?
• Has he ever been diagnosed with a low sperm count?
• If he participates in sports, how does he protect himself from possible genital injuries?

Ages and stages

Don't forget to ask the elderly patient

Elderly adults who are sexually active with multiple partners have as high a risk for developing a sexually transmitted disease as younger adults. However, because of decreased immunity, poor hygiene, poor symptom reporting and, possibly, several concurrent conditions, they may seek treatment for different symptoms.

Physical examination

Physical examination of the GU system usually includes inspection, auscultation, percussion, and palpation. (See *Percussing the kidney and bladder.*) Reproductive system examination involves inspection and palpation.

At ease, please

Before starting, explain the techniques you'll be using and warn the patient that some procedures may be uncomfortable. Perform the examination in a private, quiet, warm, well-lighted room.

Renal red flags

Begin the physical examination by assessing your patient's vital signs and mental status. These observations will provide clues about renal dysfunction. For example, a patient's vital signs might reveal hypertension, which can cause renal dysfunction if it isn't controlled.

Behavioral hints

Observing the patient's behavior can give you clues about mental status. Kidney dysfunction can cause such symptoms as trouble concentrating, memory loss, and disorientation. Progressive, chronic kidney failure can cause lethargy, confusion, disorientation, stupor, seizures, and coma.

It's in the skin

Observe the patient's skin. A person with decreased renal function may be pale because of a low hemoglobin level or may even have *uremic frost* (snow-like crystals on the skin from metabolic wastes). Also look for signs of fluid imbalance, such as dry mucous membranes, sunken eyeballs, edema, or ascites.

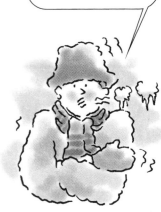

Uremic frost isn't cold, but that doesn't mean it's pleasant, either. It's a sign of decreased renal function.

Inspection

Inspection usually includes examination of the abdomen and external genitalia.

Leading off: The abdomen

Ask the patient to urinate; then help the patient into the supine position with arms at the sides. As you proceed, expose only the areas being examined.

First, inspect the patient's abdomen. When supine, the abdomen should be symmetrical and smooth, flat, or concave. The skin should be free from lesions, bruises, discolorations, and prominent veins.

Percussing the kidney and bladder

Percuss the kidneys and bladder using the techniques described here.

Kidney percussion

With the patient sitting upright, percuss each costovertebral angle (the angle over each kidney whose borders are formed by the lateral and downward curve of the lowest rib and the vertebral column). To perform mediate percussion, place your left palm over the costovertebral angle and gently strike it with your right fist. To perform immediate percussion, gently strike your fist over each costovertebral angle. Usually, the patient will feel a thudding sensation or pressure during percussion.

Bladder percussion

Using mediate percussion, percuss the area over the bladder, beginning 2″ (5 cm) above the symphysis pubis. To detect differences in sound, percuss toward the bladder's base. Percussion usually produces a tympanic sound. (Over a urine-filled bladder, it produces a dull sound.)

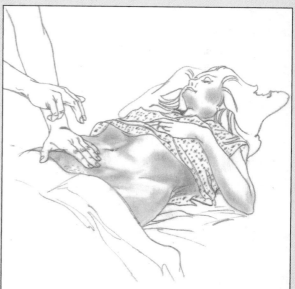

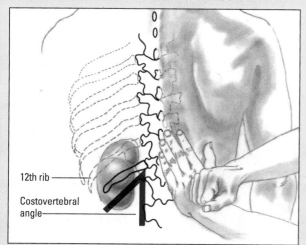

12th rib

Costovertebral angle

Watch for abdominal distention with tight, glistening skin and *striae*—silvery streaks caused by rapidly developing skin tension. These are signs of ascites, which may accompany nephrotic syndrome. This syndrome is characterized by edema, increased urine protein levels, and decreased serum albumin levels.

Lastly, inspect the external genitalia for inflammation or discharge from the urethral meatus.

Auscultation

Auscultate the renal arteries in the left and right upper abdominal quadrants by pressing the stethoscope bell lightly against the abdomen and instructing the patient to exhale deeply. Begin auscultating at the midline and work to the left; then return to the midline and work to the right. Listen for systolic bruits or other

Palpating the kidneys

To palpate the kidneys, first have the patient lie in a supine position. To palpate the right kidney, stand on his right side. Place your left hand under the back and your right hand on the abdomen.

Instruct the patient to inhale deeply, so the kidney moves downward. As he inhales, press up with your left hand and down with your right, as shown.

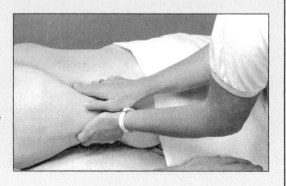

abnormal sounds, which may indicate a significant problem. For example, a systolic bruit may signal renal artery stenosis.

Percussion

Kidney percussion checks for costovertebral angle tenderness that occurs with inflammation. To percuss over the kidneys, ask the patient to sit up. Place the ball of your nondominant hand on his back at the costovertebral angle of the 12th rib. Strike the ball of that hand with the ulnar surface of your other hand; use just enough force to cause a painless but perceptible thud.

As you percuss the kidneys, check for pain or tenderness, which suggests a kidney infection. Remember to percuss both sides of the body to assess both kidneys.

Bladder up

To percuss the bladder, first ask the patient to empty it if he hasn't already. Then ask him to lie in the supine position. Start at the symphysis pubis and percuss upward toward the bladder and over it. You should hear tympany—a dull sound signals retained urine.

Palpation

Because the kidneys lie behind other organs and are protected by muscle, they normally aren't palpable unless they're enlarged. However, in very thin patients you may feel the lower end of the right kidney as a smooth round mass that drops on inspiration. (See *Palpating the kidneys.*)

Normally I hide behind other organs, but every once in a while I've got to stand up and be palpated!

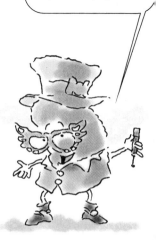

Diagnostic tests

Many tests provide information to guide your care of a GU or gynecologic emergency patient. Even if you don't participate in testing, you should know why the test was ordered, what the results mean, and what your responsibilities are before, during, and after the test.

Common diagnostic tests include blood studies, computed tomography (CT) scan, I.V. pyelography (IVP), kidney-ureter-bladder (KUB) radiography, laparoscopy, magnetic resonance imaging (MRI), percutaneous renal biopsy, renal angiography, renal scan, ultrasonography, and urine studies.

Blood studies

Blood studies used to diagnose and evaluate GU function include:
• complete blood count (CBC) to evaluate white blood cell (WBC) count, red blood cell (RBC) count, hemoglobin level, and hematocrit
• blood urea nitrogen (BUN) level
• electrolyte measurements to evaluate calcium, phosphorus, chloride, potassium, and sodium levels
• serum osmolality, creatinine clearance and urea clearance measurements, and serum creatinine, serum protein, and uric acid levels. (See *Interpreting blood studies*, page 362.)

Practice pointers

• Tell the patient that the test requires a blood sample.
• Check the patient's medication history for drugs that might influence test results.

CT scan

A CT scan may involve the abdomen or pelvis; in addition, a renal CT scan may be done. In a renal CT scan, the image's density reflects the amount of radiation absorbed by renal tissue, thus permitting identification of masses or other lesions. A CT scan may be done with or without a contrast medium, but use of a contrast medium is preferred unless the patient has an allergy or an increased BUN or creatinine level.

Interpreting blood studies

Here's how you may interpret the results of blood studies used in diagnosing problems of the genitourinary system.

Complete blood count

An increased white blood cell count may indicate urinary tract infection, peritonitis (in peritoneal dialysis patients), or kidney transplantation infection and rejection.

Red blood cell (RBC) count, hemoglobin level, and hematocrit (HCT) decrease in a patient with chronic renal insufficiency resulting from decreased erythropoietin production by the kidneys. HCT also provides an index of fluid balance because it indicates the percentage of RBCs in the blood.

Blood urea nitrogen

Increased blood urea nitrogen (BUN) levels may indicate glomerulonephritis, extensive pyogenic infection, oliguria (from mercuric chloride poisoning or posttraumatic renal insufficiency), tubular obstruction, or other obstructive uropathies. Because nonrenal conditions can also cause BUN levels to increase, interpret BUN levels in conjunction with serum creatinine levels.

Electrolytes

Because the kidneys regulate fluid and electrolyte balance, a critically ill patient with renal disease may experience significant serum electrolyte imbalances. The most commonly measured electrolytes are:

• *calcium and phosphorus*—Calcium and phosphorus levels have an inverse relationship; when one increases, the other decreases. In renal failure, the kidneys aren't able to excrete phosphorus, resulting in hyperphosphatemia and hypocalcemia.

• *chloride*—Chloride levels relate inversely to bicarbonate levels, reflecting acid-base balance. In renal disease, elevated chloride levels suggest metabolic acidosis. Hyperchloremia occurs in renal tubular necrosis, severe dehydration, and complete renal shutdown. Hypochloremia may also occur with pyelonephritis.

• *potassium*—Hyperkalemia occurs with renal insufficiency or acidosis. In renal shutdown, potassium may rapidly increase to life-threatening levels. Hypokalemia may reflect renal tubular disease.

• *sodium*—Sodium helps the kidneys regulate body fluid. Renal disease may result in the loss of sodium through the kidneys.

Serum creatinine

The serum creatinine level reflects the glomerular filtration rate (GFR). Renal damage is indicated more accurately by increases in serum creatinine than by the BUN level.

Serum osmolality

An increase in serum osmolality with a simultaneous decrease in urine osmolality indicates diminished distal tubule responsiveness to circulating antidiuretic hormone.

Serum proteins

Levels of the serum protein albumin may decline sharply from its loss in the urine during nephritis or nephrosis, which in turn causes edema. Nephrosis may also cause total serum protein levels to decrease.

Uric acid

Because uric acid clears from the body by glomerular filtration and tubular secretion, elevated levels may indicate impaired renal function; below-normal levels may indicate defective tubular absorption.

Creatinine clearance

Creatinine clearance indicates GFR. Typically, high creatinine clearance rates have little diagnostic value. Low creatinine clearance rates may indicate reduced renal blood flow (associated with shock or renal artery obstruction), acute tubular necrosis, acute or chronic glomerulonephritis, advanced bilateral chronic pyelonephritis, advanced bilateral renal lesions, or nephrosclerosis.

Urea clearance

While urea clearance is a less reliable measurement of GFR than creatinine clearance, it still provides a good measure of overall renal function. High urea clearance rates rarely have diagnostic value. Low urea clearance rates may reflect decreased renal blood flow, acute or chronic glomerulonephritis, advanced bilateral chronic pyelonephritis, acute tubular necrosis, nephrosclerosis, advanced bilateral renal lesions, bilateral ureteral obstruction, or dehydration.

Practice pointers

• Explain the procedure to the patient and tell him to lie still, relax, and breathe normally during the test. Explain that if the practitioner orders an I.V. contrast medium, he may experience discomfort from the needle puncture and a localized feeling of warmth on injection.
• Ascertain when the patient last ate or drank; restrict food and fluids as soon as possible, but continue any drug regimen as ordered.
• Confirm if the patient has an allergy to iodine or shellfish. If so, give him a pretest preparation kit containing prednisone (Prelone) and diphenhydramine (Benadryl) as ordered to reduce the risk of a dye reaction. Immediately report adverse reactions, such as nausea, vomiting, dizziness, headache, and urticaria.
• If the patient is on nothing-by-mouth status, increase the I.V. fluid rate as ordered after the procedure to flush the contrast medium from the system. Monitor serum creatinine and BUN levels for signs of acute renal failure, which may be caused by the contrast medium.

VP

After I.V. administration of a contrast medium, IVP, also known as *excretory urography,* allows visualization of the renal parenchyma, calyces, pelvises, ureters, bladder and, in some cases, the urethra. In the first minute after injection (the *nephrographic stage*), the contrast medium delineates the kidneys' size and shape. After 3 to 5 minutes (the *pyelographic stage*), the contrast medium moves into the calyces and pelvises, allowing visualization of cysts, tumors, and other obstructions.

Practice pointers

• Check the patient's history for hypersensitivity to iodine, iodine-containing foods, or contrast media containing iodine.
• Ensure that the patient is well-hydrated.
• Inform the patient that he may experience a transient burning sensation and metallic taste when the contrast medium is injected.

KUB radiography

KUB radiography, consisting of plain, contrast-free X-rays, shows kidney size, position, and structure. It can also reveal calculi and other lesions. Before performing a renal biopsy, the practitioner may use this test to determine kidney placement. For diagnostic

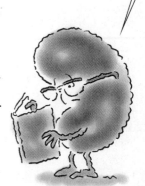

It says here that KUB radiography can show my size, position, structure, calculi, and lesions. Talk about scrutiny!

purposes, however, KUB radiography provides limited information.

Practice pointers

• KUB radiography requires no special pretest or posttest care. It's commonly a portable X-ray test performed at the bedside.
• Explain the procedure to the patient.

Laparoscopy

Laparoscopy allows the practitioner to inspect organs in the peritoneal cavity by inserting a *laparoscope* (small fiber-optic telescope) through the anterior abdominal wall. This test is used to:
• detect such abnormalities as cysts, adhesions, fibroids, and infection
• identify the cause of pelvic pain
• diagnose endometriosis, ectopic pregnancy, or pelvic inflammatory disease (PID)
• evaluate pelvic masses or the fallopian tubes of infertile patients
• stage cancer.
    This procedure may also be used therapeutically for analysis of adhesions, tubal sterilization, removal of foreign bodies, and fulguration of endometriotic implants.

Practice pointers

• Check the time the patient last ingested food or fluids; if possible, she should have nothing by mouth for approximately 8 hours before the test.
• Assure the patient that she'll receive a general anesthetic. Warn that she may experience pain at the puncture site and in the shoulders.
• Check the patient's history to make sure she isn't hypersensitive to the anesthetic. Make sure that all laboratory work is completed and results are reported before the test.
• Provide preoperative care.
• Explain that the patient will probably be transferred to the outpatient care unit after the procedure.

MRI

MRI provides tomographic images that reflect the differing hydrogen densities of body tissues. Physical, chemical, and cellular microenvironments modify these densities, as do the fluid characteristics of tissues. MRI can provide precise images of anatomic detail and important biochemical information about the tissue examined and can efficiently visualize and stage kidney, bladder, and prostate tumors.

Practice pointers

• Before the patient enters the MRI chamber, make sure that he has removed all metal objects, such as earrings, watches, necklaces, bracelets, and rings. Patients with internal metal objects, such as pacemakers and aneurysm clips, can't undergo MRI testing.
• If you're accompanying the patient, be sure to remove metal objects from your pockets, including scissors, forceps, penlights, metal pens, and credit cards (because the magnetic field will erase the numerical information in the code strips).
• Tell the patient to remain still throughout the test, which takes about 45 minutes, and that he will hear a loud thumping noise during the test. If the patient complains of claustrophobia, reassure him and provide emotional support.

Percutaneous renal biopsy

Histologic examination can help differentiate glomerular and tubular renal disease, monitor the disorder's progress, and assess the effectiveness of therapy. It can also reveal a malignant tumor such as Wilms' tumor.

Histologic studies can help diagnose:
• disseminated lupus erythematosus
• amyloid infiltration
• acute and chronic glomerulonephritis
• renal vein thrombosis
• pyelonephritis. (See *Assisting with percutaneous renal biopsy,* page 366.)

Practice pointers

• Check to ensure that the patient has had nothing by mouth for 8 hours before the test. Inform the patient that he'll receive a mild sedative before the test to aid relaxation.
• After the test, tell the patient that pressure will be applied to the biopsy site to stop superficial bleeding, and then a pressure dressing will be applied.
• Instruct the patient to lie flat on his back without moving for at least 6 hours after the biopsy to prevent bleeding.

Assisting with percutaneous renal biopsy

To prepare a patient for percutaneous renal biopsy, position him on his abdomen. To stabilize the kidneys, place a sandbag or rolled towels beneath his abdomen as shown.

After administering a local anesthetic, the practitioner instructs the patient to hold his breath and remain immobile. Then the practitioner inserts a needle with the obturator between the patient's last rib and the iliac crest as shown below. After asking the patient to breathe deeply, the practitioner removes the obturator and inserts cutting prongs, which gather blood and tissue samples. This test is commonly performed in the radiology department so that special radiographic procedures may be used to help guide the needle.

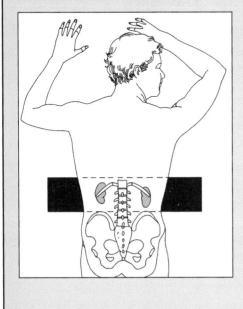

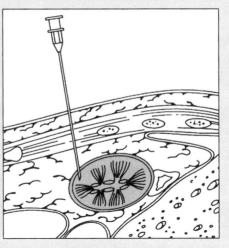

Renal angiography

Renal angiography is used to visualize the arterial tree, capillaries, and venous drainage of the kidneys. The test uses a contrast medium injected under fluoroscopy into a catheter in the femoral artery or vein.

On closer inspection

Renal arteriography (angiography of the arteries) may reveal:
- abnormal renal blood flow
- hypervascular renal tumors
- renal cysts
- renal artery stenosis

- renal artery aneurysms and arteriovenous fistulas
- pyelonephritis
- renal abscesses or inflammatory masses
- renal infarction
- renal trauma.

Practice pointers

- Explain the procedure to the patient and confirm that he isn't allergic to iodine or shellfish. A patient with these allergies may have an adverse reaction to the contrast medium. If he has a seafood or dye allergy, a pretest preparation kit with prednisone and diphenhydramine may be given.
- Preprocedure testing should include evaluation of renal function (serum creatinine and BUN levels) and the potential risk of bleeding (prothrombin time, partial thromboplastin time, and platelet count). Notify the practitioner if results are abnormal.
- Report adverse reactions, such as nausea, vomiting, dizziness, headache, and urticaria.
- Depending on the patient's renal status, the practitioner may order increased fluids after the procedure or an increased I.V. infusion rate to flush the contrast medium out of the patient's system.
- After the procedure, check the patient's serum creatinine and BUN levels to evaluate renal function (because contrast media can cause acute renal failure).

Renal scan

A radionuclide renal scan, which may be substituted for excretory urography in patients who are hypersensitive to contrast media, involves I.V. injection of a radionuclide, followed by scintigraphy. Observation of uptake concentration and radionuclide transit during the procedure allows assessment of renal blood flow, nephron and collecting system function, and renal structure.

Practice pointers

- Inform the patient that he'll be injected with a radionuclide and may experience transient flushing and nausea. Emphasize that it's only a small amount of radionuclide and is usually excreted within 24 hours.
- After the test, instruct the patient to flush the toilet immediately every time he urinates within the next 24 hours as a radiation precaution.

Ultrasonography

Ultrasonography uses high-frequency sound waves to reveal internal structures; it can involve the abdomen, pelvis, or specifically the renal structures. This test provides information about internal structures of the abdomen, pelvis and, more specifically, the kidney's size, shape, and position. It's also used to detect pregnancy.

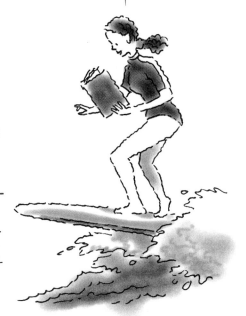

Whoa, dude! Ultrasonography uses high-frequency sound waves to reveal internal structures.

Practice pointers

• Tell the patient that he'll be prone (the renal examination position) or supine during the test.
• Explain that a technician will spread coupling oil or gel on his skin, and then move a probe or transducer against the skin and across the area being tested.
• If a pelvic ultrasound is being done, make sure that the patient has a full bladder, which is used as landmark for defining pelvic organs.

Urine studies

Urine studies, such as urinalysis and urine osmolality, can indicate acute renal failure, renal trauma, UTI, and other disorders. Urinalysis can indicate renal or systemic disorders, warranting further investigation. A random urine specimen is used. (See *What urinalysis findings mean.*)

Concentrate, concentrate

Urine osmolality is used to evaluate the diluting and concentrating ability of the kidneys and varies greatly with diet and hydration status. The ability to concentrate urine is one of the first functions lost in renal failure.

Practice pointers

• Before urinalysis, collect a random urine specimen from the indwelling urinary catheter. Send the specimen to the laboratory immediately.
• For urine osmolality testing, collect a random urine sample.

What urinalysis findings mean

Test	Normal values or findings	Abnormal findings	Possible causes of abnormal findings
Color and odor	• Straw color	Clear to black	Dietary changes; use of certain drugs; metabolic, inflammatory, or infectious disease
	• Slightly aromatic odor	Fruity odor	Diabetes mellitus, starvation, dehydration
	• Clear appearance	Turbid appearance	Renal infection
Specific gravity	• 1.005 to 1.030, with slight variations from one specimen to the next	Below-normal specific gravity	Diabetes insipidus, glomerulonephritis, pyelonephritis, acute renal failure, alkalosis
		Above-normal specific gravity	Dehydration, nephrosis
		Fixed specific gravity	Severe renal damage
pH	• 4.5 to 8.0	Alkaline pH (above 8.0)	Fanconi's syndrome (chronic renal disease), urinary tract infection (UTI), metabolic or respiratory alkalosis
		Acidic pH (below 4.5)	Renal tuberculosis, phenylketonuria, acidosis
Protein	• No protein	Proteinuria	Renal disease (such as glomerulosclerosis, acute or chronic glomerulonephritis, nephrolithiasis, polycystic kidney disease, and acute or chronic renal failure)
Ketones	• No ketones	Ketonuria	Diabetes mellitus, starvation, conditions causing acutely increased metabolic demands and decreased food intake (such as vomiting and diarrhea)
Glucose	• No glucose	Glycosuria	Diabetes mellitus
Red blood cells (RBCs)	• 0 to 3 RBCs/high-power field	Numerous RBCs	UTI, obstruction, inflammation, trauma, or tumor; glomerulonephritis; renal hypertension; lupus nephritis; renal tuberculosis; renal vein thrombosis; hydronephrosis; pyelonephritis; parasitic bladder infection; polyarteritis nodosa; hemorrhagic disorder
Epithelial cells	• Few epithelial cells	Excessive epithelial cells	Renal tubular degeneration

(continued)

What urinalysis findings mean (continued)

Test	Normal values or findings	Abnormal findings	Possible causes of abnormal findings
White blood cells (WBCs)	• 0 to 4 WBCs/high-power field	Numerous WBCs	UTI, especially cystitis or pyelonephritis
		Numerous WBCs and WBC casts	Renal infection (such as acute pyelonephritis and glomerulonephritis, nephrotic syndrome, pyogenic infection, and lupus nephritis)
Casts	• No casts (except occasional hyaline casts)	Excessive casts	Renal disease
		Excessive hyaline casts	Renal parenchymal disease, inflammation, glomerular capillary membrane trauma
		Epithelial casts	Renal tubular damage, nephrosis, eclampsia, chronic lead intoxication
		Fatty, waxy casts	Nephrotic syndrome, chronic renal disease, diabetes mellitus
		RBC casts	Renal parenchymal disease (especially glomerulonephritis), renal infarction, subacute bacterial endocarditis, sickle cell anemia, blood dyscrasias, malignant hypertension, collagen disease
Crystals	• Some crystals	Numerous calcium oxalate crystals	Hypercalcemia
		Cystine crystals (cystinuria)	Inborn metabolic error
Yeast cells	• No yeast cells	Yeast cells in sediment	External genitalia contamination, vaginitis, urethritis, prostatovesiculitis
Parasites	• No parasites	Parasites in sediment	External genitalia contamination
Creatinine clearance	• Males: 14 to 26 mg/kg/24 hours • Females: 11 to 20 mg/kg/24 hours	Above-normal creatinine clearance	Little diagnostic significance
		Below-normal creatinine clearance	Reduced renal blood flow (associated with shock or renal artery obstruction), acute tubular necrosis, acute or chronic glomerulonephritis, advanced bilateral renal lesions (as in polycystic kidney disease, renal tuberculosis, and cancer), nephrosclerosis, heart failure, severe dehydration

Treatments

GU and gynecologic emergencies present many treatment challenges because they stem from various mechanisms occurring separately or simultaneously. Common treatments include drug therapy and nonsurgical and surgical procedures.

Drug therapy

Ideally, drug therapy should be effective and not impair urologic function. However, because GU disorders can affect the chemical composition of body fluids and the pharmacokinetic properties of many drugs, standard regimens of some drugs may require adjustment. For example, dosages of drugs that are mainly excreted by the kidneys unchanged or as active metabolites may require adjustment to avoid nephrotoxicity.

Drug therapy for GU disorders can include:
- antibiotics
- urinary tract antiseptics
- diuretics.

In addition, electrolytes and replacements may be necessary depending on the underlying cause of the GU dysfunction.

Drug therapy for gynecologic disorders commonly includes antibiotics and analgesics for pain.

Nonsurgical procedures

Nonsurgical procedures employed to treat GU emergencies include calculi basketing, extracorporeal shock wave lithotripsy (ESWL), and urinary bladder catheterization.

Calculi basketing

When ureteral calculi are too large for normal elimination, removal with a basketing instrument is the treatment of choice and helps to relieve pain and prevent infection and renal dysfunction. In this technique, a basketing instrument is inserted through a cystoscope or ureteroscope into the ureter to capture the calculus and then withdrawn to remove it.

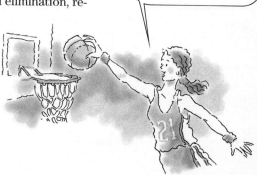

With calculi basketing, getting rid of the pain and infection risk associated with large ureteral calculi is a slam dunk!

Nursing considerations
- Tell the patient that after calculi removal, he'll have an indwelling urinary catheter in-

serted to ensure normal urine drainage. The catheter will probably remain in place for 24 to 48 hours.
• Tell the patient that he'll receive I.V. fluids during and immediately after the procedure to maintain urine output and prevent such complications as hydronephrosis and pyelonephritis.
• Administer fluids as ordered, usually to maintain a urine output of 3 to 4 L per day.

Basket boomerang

If the patient returns to the ED after the procedure, follow these steps:
• Observe the color of urine drainage from the indwelling urinary catheter; typically it's blood-tinged at first, with gradual clearing over 24 to 48 hours. Irrigate the catheter as ordered using sterile technique.
• Administer analgesics as ordered.
• Observe for and report signs or symptoms of septicemia, which may result from ureteral perforation during basketing.
• Assess for signs and symptoms of acute ureteral obstruction, such as severe pain and the inability to void.

ESWL

ESWL is a noninvasive technique for removing obstructive renal calculi. It uses high-energy shock waves to break up calculi and allow their normal passage.

Nursing considerations

• Tell the patient that he may receive a general or epidural anesthetic, depending on the type of lithotriptor and the intensity of shock waves needed.
• Insert an I.V. line if one isn't already in place.
• Inform the patient that he'll most likely have an indwelling urinary catheter in place after the procedure.
• Explain to the patient that, after the procedure, he'll be encouraged to ambulate as soon as possible and increase fluid intake as ordered to aid the passage of calculi fragments.
• If the patient returns to the ED after the procedure, strain all urine for calculi fragments and send these to the laboratory for analysis.
• Monitor the patient's urine for frank or persistent bleeding. Keep in mind that slight hematuria usually occurs for several days.
• Assess the patient for severe, unremitting pain, persistent hematuria, inability to void, fever and chills, or recurrent nausea and vomiting.

Patients are encouraged to ambulate as soon as possible after ESWL to aid the passage of calculi fragments. C'mon now, one foot in front of the other.

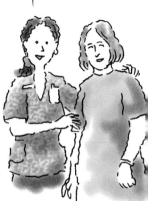

Urinary catheterization

Catheterization—the insertion of a drainage device into the urinary bladder—may be intermittent or continuous.

Intermittent catheterization drains urine remaining in the bladder after voiding. It's used for patients with urinary incontinence, urethral strictures, cystitis, prostatic obstruction, neurogenic bladder, or other disorders that interfere with bladder emptying. It may also be used postoperatively.

Indwelling urinary catheterization helps relieve bladder distention caused by such conditions as urinary tract obstruction and neurogenic bladder. It allows continuous urine drainage in patients with a urinary meatus swollen from local trauma or childbirth as well as from surgery. Catheterization can also provide accurate monitoring of urine output when normal voiding is impaired.

Nursing considerations

• Thoroughly review the procedure with the patient and reassure him that although catheterization may produce slight discomfort, it shouldn't be painful. Explain that you'll stop the procedure if he experiences severe discomfort.
• Assemble the necessary equipment, preferably a sterile catheterization package.
• Perform the catheterization; during catheterization, note difficulty or ease of insertion, patient discomfort, and the amount and nature of urine drainage.
• During urine drainage, monitor the patient for pallor, diaphoresis, and painful bladder spasms. If these occur, clamp the catheter tubing for 10 to 15 minutes. When symptoms resolve, resume drainage.

Fluid watch

• Frequently assess the patient's intake and output. Encourage fluid intake to maintain continuous urine flow through the catheter and decrease the risk of infection and clot formation.
• To help prevent infection, avoid separating the catheter and tubing unless absolutely necessary.
• Closely assess the patient for signs and symptoms of UTI and for signs of catheter obstruction.

Surgical procedures

Suprapubic catheterization surgery may be necessary when conservative measures fail to control the patient's problem.

Suprapubic catheterization

Suprapubic catheterization is a type of urinary diversion connected to a closed drainage system that involves transcutaneous insertion of a catheter through the suprapubic area into the bladder. Typically, suprapubic catheterization provides temporary urinary diversion after certain gynecologic procedures, bladder surgery, or prostatectomy and relieves obstruction from calculi, severe urethral strictures, or pelvic trauma. Less commonly, it may be used to create a permanent urinary diversion, thereby relieving obstruction from an inoperable tumor.

Nursing considerations

• Tell the patient that the practitioner will insert a soft plastic tube through the skin of the abdomen and into the bladder and then connect the tube to an external collection bag.
• Explain that the procedure is done under local anesthesia, causes little or no discomfort, and takes 15 to 45 minutes.
• Closely assess the insertion site.
• To ensure adequate drainage and tube patency, check the suprapubic catheter at least hourly for the first 24 hours after insertion. Make sure that the collection bag is below bladder level to enhance drainage and prevent backflow, which can lead to infection.
• Tape the catheter securely in place on the abdominal skin to reduce tension and prevent dislodgment. To prevent kinks in the tube, curve it gently but don't bend it.
• Assess dressings frequently and change as necessary. Observe the skin around the insertion site for signs of infection and encrustation.

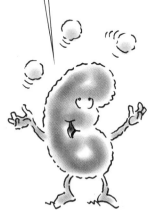

Suprapubic catheterization provides a temporary urinary diversion. Well, not THIS type of diversion.

Common disorders

GU and gynecologic disorders commonly encountered in the ED include kidney trauma, ovarian cyst, PID, pyelonephritis, renal calculi, sexual assault, testicular torsion, and UTI.

Kidney trauma

Kidney trauma can involve damage to minor tissues or, possibly, major vascular structures. Trauma to the kidney can be wide-ranging, from contusions and subcapsular hematomas to fractured kidney, renal artery thrombosis, or avulsion of the major renal artery or vein. Kidney trauma may be classified by severity using a grading scale of 1 to 5 or using the categories of minor, major, and critical trauma. (See *Staging kidney trauma*.)

Staging kidney trauma

This chart highlights the different classifications of kidney trauma, their locations and types, and associated signs and symptoms.

Classification grade and category	Location and type of trauma	Associated signs and symptoms
Grade: 1 Category: Minor	• Contusion (bruising of the renal parenchyma) • Superficial laceration of the renal cortex	• Microscopic or gross hematuria • Urologic studies within normal parameters • Flank tenderness
Grade: 2 Category: Minor	• Laceration of the renal parenchyma measuring less than 1 cm • Nonexpanding hematoma around the kidney	• Microscopic or gross hematuria • Urologic studies within normal parameters • Flank tenderness
Grade: 3 Category: Major	• Laceration of the parenchyma without involvement of the collecting system	• Hematuria • Flank pain • Possible hypotension
Grade: 4 Category: Major	• Major laceration involving the cortex and medulla with continuation through the renal capsule of the kidney—laceration involving the collecting system • Extravasation within and around the kidney • Thrombosis of a segment of the renal artery • Controlled bleeding involving the major renal artery or vein	• Hematuria • Flank pain • Possible hypotension
Grade: 5 Category: Critical	• Shattered kidney with injury and fragmentation (fracture) • Thrombosis of the main renal artery • Avulsion of the main renal artery or vein	• Severe blood loss • Hypovolemic shock

What causes it

Kidney trauma is commonly classified as *penetrating* or *blunt*, depending on the type of injury.

Penetrating kidney trauma involves an injury by a foreign object, such as a bullet (or a bullet fragment or effect of the blast) or knife. A gunshot wound involving the kidney typically results in a complex array of injuries.

Blunt kidney trauma is the cause of approximately 75% of all kidney injuries, most of which result from motor vehicle collisions. Other less common causes include sports injuries, occupational injuries, and assaults.

Kidney trauma may also result from iatrogenic causes. These causes may include percutaneous nephrostomy, renal biopsy, and ESWL.

How it happens

Three mechanisms are responsible for causing blunt kidney trauma:

 direct blow to the flank area

 laceration of the parenchyma from a fractured rib or vertebra

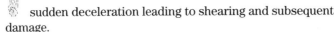 sudden deceleration leading to shearing and subsequent damage.

What to look for

Assessment findings may vary based on the type and extent of kidney trauma. One common finding is hematuria, which may be gross or microscopic. However, the degree of hematuria doesn't correlate with the severity of kidney trauma.

And that's not all

Additional findings may include:
- abdominal or flank pain
- tenderness along the back
- complaints of colicky pain with the passage of clots in the urine
- hematoma over the flank area, usually in the area of the 11th or 12th rib
- obvious wounds, bruises, or abrasions in the flank area or abdomen
- Turner's sign
- costovertebral angle pain or tenderness
- palpable mass in the flank or abdominal area
- signs and symptoms of hemorrhage and hypovolemic shock, such as pallor, diaphoresis, hypotension, tachycardia, and changes in mental status.

What tests tell you

Diagnostic testing depends on the patient's condition and extent of injuries. Some diagnostic tests may include:
- KUB radiography to identify the path and appearance of the object causing the penetrating trauma and to determine the outline or fragmentation of the kidney
- IVP to stage the degree of kidney injury
- ultrasound, CT scan, and MRI to evaluate kidney structure and identify hematomas, lacerations, and vascular disruptions

- renal angiography to detect arterial injury.
  Other tests include:
- arterial blood gas analysis to evaluate respiratory and acid-base status secondary to blood loss and shock
- CBC to evaluate the degree of blood loss
- coagulation studies to determine the patient's clotting ability
- serum electrolyte level to determine possible imbalances.

How it's treated

Treatment of blunt kidney trauma typically focuses on bed rest with frequent assessments and serial specimens for urinalysis. In addition, analgesics are used to manage pain. A penetrating kidney trauma, such as a laceration to the kidney, requires surgical intervention.

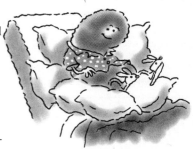

Blunt kidney trauma treatment focuses on bed rest. Sounds good to me!

Hemodynamics count

A kidney trauma patient who's hemodynamically stable requires close monitoring in the initial period after injury. Surgery is typically performed later, as indicated by the patient's condition.

For a patient who's hemodynamically unstable, has other associated trauma, or exhibits shock, treatment focuses on immediate stabilization; assessing and maintaining airway, breathing, and circulation (ABCs); assessing level of consciousness (LOC); and preparing the patient for transport. An exploratory laparotomy is performed immediately.

Wound care

If the patient has a wound, treatment may include controlling bleeding—usually by applying firm, direct pressure—and cleaning the wound. Pain medication and antibiotic therapy are instituted as indicated. In addition, I.V. therapy is started to ensure fluid balance and maintain the patient's hemodynamic status.

What to do

- Assess the patient's ABCs and initiate emergency measures if necessary; administer supplemental oxygen as ordered.
- Monitor the patient's vital signs and note significant changes.
- Assess oxygen saturation and cardiac rhythm for arrhythmias.
- Assess the patient's neurologic status, including LOC and pupillary and motor response.
- Obtain blood studies, including type and crossmatch.
- Insert two large-bore I.V. catheters and infuse normal saline or lactated Ringer's solution as ordered.
- Quickly and carefully assess for other areas of trauma.

- Institute complete bed rest with frequent assessments, such as every 15 to 30 minutes or as indicated by the patient's condition.
- Assess wounds and provide wound care as appropriate. Cover open wounds and control bleeding by applying pressure.

Watch for distention

- Assess for increased abdominal distention.
- Administer blood products as appropriate.
- Monitor for signs of hypovolemic shock.
- Provide pain medication, as appropriate.
- Prepare the patient and his family for diagnostic testing and possible surgery.
- Provide reassurance to the patient and his family.

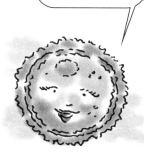

A funny thing happened on the way to the uterus...namely, a cyst. What type it is depends on its cause.

Ovarian cyst

An ovarian cyst refers to the development of a saclike structure on the ovary. The sac can contain fluid, semi-fluid, or solid material. Cysts may be categorized as *endometrial, follicular,* or *corpus luteal* depending on the underlying mechanism associated with their development.

What causes it

Ovarian cysts vary in size, consistency, and development. The underlying cause of the cyst identifies its type:
- *endometrial cyst*—results from an overgrowth of endometrial tissue such as endometriosis
- *follicular cyst*—results from failed follicular rupture from the ovary at ovulation
- *corpus luteal cyst*—results from the continued presence of a corpus luteum that has failed to atrophy.

How it happens

Within the ovary, the follicle develops because of hormonal influences. At the midpoint of a woman's menstrual cycle, a follicle, now mature, ruptures from the ovary (with follicular cysts, this rupture doesn't occur).

After ovulation, the follicle becomes the corpus luteum and travels to the fallopian tube where it may be fertilized by spermatozoa. If the corpus luteum isn't fertilized, it degenerates (with corpus luteal cysts, this degeneration doesn't occur).

Normally, endometrial tissue is located in the uterine cavity. However, for unknown reasons the tissue sometimes appears outside of the endometrial cavity, commonly around the ovaries. This tissue responds to estrogen and progesterone secretion and proliferates. Upon menstruation the tissue bleeds and becomes inflamed, leading to fibrosis.

What to look for

Most patients with ovarian cysts may be asymptomatic. Typically, they experience signs and symptoms when rupture, hemorrhage, or torsion (twisting) of a cyst occurs. Follicular cysts commonly rupture in the first half of the menstrual cycle with strenuous exercise or sexual intercourse, whereas corpus luteal cysts typically rupture in the last half of the cycle, usually in the weeks before the woman's menses.

> Diagnosing an ovarian cyst relies more on ruling out other conditions than on specific testing.

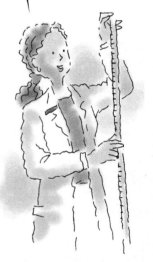

If the patient is experiencing symptoms, they may include:
- pressure or abdominal pain
- dull ache on the affected side
- prolonged menstruation
- mittelschmerz pain (pain with ovulation) with rupture of the cyst.

Pelvic examination may reveal ovarian tenderness and enlargement. With rupture, the patient may exhibit signs and symptoms of hypovolemic shock, especially with rupture of a blood-filled cyst such as a mature corpus luteal cyst. These symptoms may range from mild to severe, depending on the extent of blood loss.

What tests tell you

There's no specific test used to identify ovarian cysts. Usually, ultrasound is used to rule out other conditions, such as appendicitis, ectopic pregnancy, and intraperitoneal bleeding, which demonstrate similar symptoms. In addition, a pregnancy test is performed to rule out pregnancy. Routine diagnostic tests, such as CBC and urinalysis, are done to establish a baseline and rule out other possible disorders.

How it's treated

Treatment for an unruptured cyst includes analgesics for pain management and support for the patient. In most cases, nonopioids, such as nonsteroidal anti-inflammatory drugs (NSAIDs), are used. If necessary, opioids may be given for a short term.

Additional treatment may include:
- surgical excision of the endometrial cyst
- low-dose hormonal contraceptives for 6 to 12 weeks for follicular cysts
- low-dose hormonal contraceptives for 6 weeks for corpus luteal cysts
- pelvic rest if the patient is having moderate to severe pain.

Poly problems

If the patient has polycystic disease (multiple follicular cysts on both ovaries), clomiphene citrate (Clomid) may be used to induce ovulation; alternatively, a wedge resection of the ovary may be performed.

Typically, surgery isn't done unless the patient exhibits signs and symptoms of hypovolemic shock. Then treatment focuses on stabilizing the patient and preparing her for surgery as quickly as possible.

What to do

- Assess the patient's vital signs and be alert for signs and symptoms of hemorrhage (hypovolemic shock).
- Administer analgesics as ordered for pain management.
- Provide reassurance and support to the patient; explain that small cysts usually reabsorb on their own.
- Review the treatment plan for the patient, including drug therapy if ordered.
- Teach the patient about signs and symptoms of possible torsion.
- Prepare the patient for surgery if indicated.
   If the patient develops hypovolemic shock:
- Ensure ABCs.
- Initiate fluid therapy and start an I.V. line if one isn't already in place; administer fluids as ordered.
- Obtain a specimen for blood typing and crossmatching.

Pelvic inflammatory disease

PID refers to any acute, subacute, recurrent, or chronic infection of the oviducts and ovaries, with adjacent tissue involvement. It includes inflammation of the cervix (cervicitis), uterus (endometritis), fallopian tubes (salpingitis), and ovaries (oophoritis), which can extend to the connective tissue lying between the broad ligaments (parametritis). (See *Three types of PID*.)

Early diagnosis and treatment prevent damage to the reproductive system. Complications of PID include infertility and potentially fatal septicemia, pulmonary emboli, and shock. Untreated PID may be fatal.

What causes it

PID can result from infection with aerobic or anaerobic organisms. About 60% of cases result from overgrowth of one or more of the common bacterial species found in cervical mucus, including staphylococci, streptococci, diphtheroids, *Chlamydiae*, and

Three types of PID

This chart lists the types of pelvic inflammatory disease (PID), their signs and symptoms, and diagnostic test findings.

Type and signs and symptoms	Diagnostic test findings
Cervicitis	
• *Acute:* purulent, foul-smelling vaginal discharge; vulvovaginitis with itching or burning; red, edematous cervix; pelvic discomfort; sexual dysfunction; metrorrhagia; infertility; spontaneous abortion • *Chronic:* cervical dystocia, laceration or eversion of the cervix, ulcerative vesicular lesion (when cervicitis results from herpes simplex virus type 2)	• Cultures for *Neisseria gonorrhoeae* are positive; with chronic cervicitis, causative organisms are usually *Staphylococcus* or *Streptococcus*. • Cytologic smears may reveal severe inflammation. • If cervicitis isn't complicated by salpingitis, white blood cell (WBC) count is normal or slightly elevated; erythrocyte sedimentation rate (ESR) is elevated. • With acute cervicitis, cervical palpation reveals tenderness.
Endometritis (usually postpartum or postabortion)	
• *Acute:* mucopurulent or purulent vaginal discharge oozing from cervix; edematous, hyperemic endometrium, possibly leading to ulceration and necrosis (with virulent organisms); lower abdominal pain and tenderness; fever; rebound pain; abdominal muscle spasm; thrombophlebitis of uterine and pelvic vessels • *Chronic:* recurring acute episodes (usually from having multiple sexual partners and sexually transmitted infections)	• With severe infection, palpation may reveal boggy uterus. • Uterine and blood samples are positive for causative organism, usually *Staphylococcus*. • WBC count and ESR are elevated.
Salpingo-oophoritis	
• *Acute:* sudden onset of lower abdominal and pelvic pain, usually after menses; increased vaginal discharge; fever; malaise; lower abdominal pressure and tenderness; tachycardia; pelvic peritonitis • *Chronic:* recurring acute episodes	• WBC count is elevated or normal. • X-ray may show ileus. • Pelvic examination reveals extreme tenderness. • Smear of cervical or periurethral gland exudate shows gramnegative intracellular diplococci.

such coliforms as *Pseudomonas* and *Escherichia coli*. PID also results from infection with *Neisseria gonorrhoeae*. Finally, multiplication of typically nonpathogenic bacteria in an altered endometrial environment can cause PID. This multiplication occurs most commonly during parturition.

Upping the ante

These factors increase the patient's chances of developing PID:
• history of STDs

- more than one sexual partner
- conditions (such as uterine infection) or procedures (such as conization or cauterization of the cervix) that alter or destroy cervical mucus, allowing bacteria to ascend into the uterine cavity
- procedures that risk transfer of contaminated cervical mucus into the endometrial cavity by instrumentation, such as use of a biopsy curet or an irrigation catheter, tubal insufflation, abortion, or pelvic surgery
- infection during or after pregnancy
- infectious focus within the body, such as drainage from a chronically infected fallopian tube, a pelvic abscess, a ruptured appendix, or diverticulitis of the sigmoid colon.

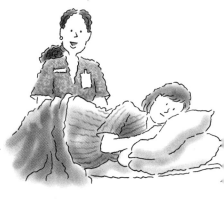

Infection during or after pregnancy is just one factor increasing a patient's risk of developing PID.

How it happens

Various conditions, procedures, or instruments can alter or destroy the cervical mucus, which usually serves as a protective barrier. As a result, bacteria enter the uterine cavity, causing inflammation of various structures.

What to look for

Signs and symptoms vary with the affected area and include:
- profuse, purulent vaginal discharge
- low-grade fever and malaise (especially if *N. gonorrhoeae* is the cause)
- lower abdominal pain
- extreme pain on movement of the cervix or palpation of the adnexa.

I'm glad to be cultured in this sense, and not in the sense that urethral and rectal secretions are.

What tests tell you

- Gram stain of secretions from the endocervix or cul-de-sac help identify the infecting organism.
- Culture and sensitivity testing aid selection of the appropriate antibiotic. Urethral and rectal secretions may also be cultured.
- Ultrasonography identifies an adnexal or uterine mass.
- Culdocentesis obtains peritoneal fluid or pus for culture and sensitivity testing.

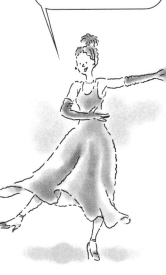

How it's treated

Effective management eradicates the infection, relieves symptoms, and leaves the reproductive system intact. It includes:

• aggressive therapy with multiple antibiotics beginning immediately after culture specimens are obtained.
• reevaluation of therapy as soon as laboratory results are available (usually after 24 to 48 hours)
• supplemental treatment, including bed rest, analgesics, and I.V. therapy
• adequate drainage if a pelvic abscess develops
• NSAIDs for pain relief (preferred treatment); opioids if necessary.

Additional considerations

Treatment for patients suffering from PID as a result of gonorrhea may include:
• I.V. doxycycline (Vibramycin) and I.V. cefoxitin (Mefoxin) followed by doxycycline (Vibra-Tabs) by mouth (P.O.)
• outpatient therapy of I.M. cefoxitin or P.O. amoxicillin (Amoxil) or ampicillin (Principen) (each with probenecid), followed by P.O. doxycycline
• therapy for syphilis.
   A total abdominal hysterectomy with bilateral salpingo-oophorectomymay be recommended for patients suffering from a ruptured pelvic abscess (a life-threatening complication).

What to do

• Institute aggressive antibiotic therapy as ordered.
• Position the patient with the head of the bed elevated approximately 30 to 45 degrees—this helps keep secretions pooled in the lower pelvic area.
• Administer analgesics as ordered for pain.
• Monitor vital signs for changes, especially in temperature.
• Assess the abdomen for rigidity and distention, which are possible signs of developing peritonitis.
• Provide frequent perineal care if vaginal drainage occurs.
• Support the patient and her family.
• Prepare the patient for possible surgery if a ruptured abscess is suspected.
• If the patient will be discharged, review the medication therapy regimen for outpatient therapy. Provide education related to recurrence prevention. (See *PID teaching tips.*)

Severe situation

If the patient's PID is considered severe, expect her to be admitted to the health care facility for I.V. antibiotic administration. Criteria for possible hospitalization include:
• child or adolescent age
• pregnancy or HIV infection

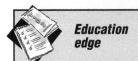

Education edge

PID teaching tips

If your patient has pelvic inflammatory disease (PID), cover these important points:
• To prevent recurrence, encourage compliance with treatment and explain the nature and seriousness of PID.
• Because PID may cause painful intercourse, advise the patient to consult with her practitioner about sexual activity.
• Stress the need for the patient's sexual partner to be examined and treated for infection.
• To prevent infection after minor gynecologic procedures, such as dilatation and curettage, tell the patient to immediately report fever, increased vaginal discharge, or pain. After such procedures, instruct her to avoid douching and intercourse for at least 7 days.

- suspected or positive evidence of a pelvic abscess or peritonitis
- temperature greater than 104° F (40° C)
- inability to eat or drink
- no response to outpatient therapy
- decreased resistance to infection because of her condition
- inability to confirm diagnosis
- lack of available follow-up
- noncompliance with outpatient treatment plan.

Pyelonephritis

One of the most common renal diseases, acute pyelonephritis is a sudden bacterial inflammation. It primarily affects the interstitial area, the renal pelvis and, less commonly, the renal tubules. With treatment and continued follow-up care, the prognosis is good; extensive permanent damage is rare. (See *Understanding chronic pyelonephritis.*)

What causes it

The two causes of pyelonephritis are:

 bacterial infection

 hematogenous or lymphatic spread.

Risk factors include:
- diagnostic and therapeutic use of instruments, such as in catheterization, cystoscopy, or urologic surgery
- inability to empty the bladder
- urinary stasis
- urinary obstruction
- sexual activity (in women)
- use of diaphragms and condoms with spermicidal gel
- pregnancy
- diabetes
- other renal diseases
- UTI.

How it happens

Typically, the infection spreads from the bladder to the ureters and then to the kidneys. Bacteria refluxed to intrarenal tissues may create colonies of infection within 24 to 48 hours.

What to look for

Signs and symptoms of pyelonephritis include:

Understanding chronic pyelonephritis

Chronic pyelonephritis, or persistent inflammation of the kidneys, can scar the kidneys and may lead to chronic renal failure. Its cause may be bacterial, metastatic, or urogenous. This disease occurs most commonly in patients who are predisposed to recurrent acute pyelonephritis such as those with urinary obstructions or vesicoureteral reflux.

Signs and symptoms
Patients with chronic pyelonephritis may have a childhood history of unexplained fevers or bed-wetting. Signs and symptoms include flank pain, anemia, low urine specific gravity, proteinuria, leukocytes in urine and, especially in late stages, hypertension. Uremia rarely develops from chronic pyelonephritis unless structural abnormalities exist in the urinary system. Bacteriuria may be intermittent. When no bacteria are found in the urine, diagnosis depends on excretory urography (where the renal pelvis may appear small and flattened) and renal biopsy.

Treatment
Treatment requires control of hypertension, elimination of the existing obstruction (when possible), and long-term antimicrobial therapy.

- urinary urgency and frequency
- pain over one or both kidneys
- burning during urination
- dysuria, nocturia, hematuria
- cloudy urine with an ammonia or fish odor
- temperature of 102° F (38.9° C) or higher
- shaking chills
- flank pain, including on palpation (costovertebral tenderness)
- anorexia
- general fatigue.

What tests tell you

- Urinalysis reveals pyuria and, possibly, a few RBCs; low specific gravity and osmolality; slightly alkaline pH; and, possibly, proteinuria, glycosuria, and ketonuria.
- Urine culture reveals more than 100,000 organisms/μl of urine.
- KUB radiography may reveal calculi, tumors, or cysts in the kidneys and the urinary tract.
- Excretory urography may show asymmetrical kidneys.

How it's treated

Therapy centers on antibiotic therapy appropriate to the specific infecting organism after it has been identified by urine culture and sensitivity studies. When the infecting organism can't be identified, therapy usually consists of a broad-spectrum antibiotic. If the patient is pregnant, antibiotics must be prescribed cautiously. Uri-

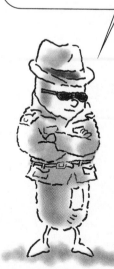

Even when the pyelonephritis perpetrator hasn't been identified, antibiotics usually take care of the problem.

nary analgesics, such as phenazopyridine (Pyridium), are also appropriate.

Antibiotic aid

Symptoms may disappear after several days of antibiotic therapy. Although urine usually becomes sterile within 48 to 72 hours, the course of such therapy is 10 to 14 days. Follow-up treatment includes reculturing urine 1 week after drug therapy stops and then periodically for the next year to detect residual or recurring infection. Most patients with uncomplicated infections respond well to therapy and don't suffer reinfection.

Infection from obstruction or vesicoureteral reflux may be less responsive to antibiotics. Treatment may then necessitate surgery to relieve the obstruction or correct the anomaly. Patients at high risk for recurring UTIs and kidney infections, such as those using an indwelling urinary catheter for a prolonged period and those on maintenance antibiotic therapy, require long-term follow-up care.

What to do

- Obtain a clean-catch urine specimen for culture and sensitivity.
- Monitor the patient's vital signs, especially temperature, and administer antipyretics for fever.
- Ensure adequate hydration with fluids. Encourage increased fluid intake to achieve a urine output of more than 2,000 ml/day. Don't encourage intake of more than 2 to 3 qt (2 to 3 L) because this amount of fluid intake may decrease the effectiveness of antibiotics. If the patient has difficulty with oral fluid intake, expect to administer I.V. fluids.
- Prepare the patient for discharge. Review the medication therapy regimen and teach recurrence prevention measures. (See *Acute pyelonephritis teaching tips.*)

Renal calculi

Renal calculi may form anywhere in the urinary tract, but usually develop in the renal pelvis or calyces. Such formation follows precipitation of substances normally dissolved in urine (calcium oxalate, calcium phosphate, magnesium ammonium phosphate or, occasionally, urate or cystine). Renal calculi vary in size and may be solitary or multiple. They may remain in the renal pelvis or enter the ureter and may damage renal parenchyma. Large calculi cause pressure necrosis. In certain locations, calculi cause obstruction (with resultant hydronephrosis) and tend to recur. (See *A close look at renal calculi*, page 388.)

Education edge

Acute pyelonephritis teaching tips

• Teach the patient about measures to reduce and avoid bacterial contamination, including using proper hygienic toileting practices such as wiping the perineum from front to back after bowel elimination.
• Teach the proper technique for collecting a clean-catch urine specimen. Tell the patient to be sure to refrigerate a urine specimen within 30 minutes of collection to prevent overgrowth of bacteria.
• Stress the need to complete the prescribed antibiotic therapy even after symptoms subside.
• Advise routine checkups for a patient with chronic urinary tract infections.
• Teach the patient to recognize signs and symptoms of infection, such as cloudy urine, burning on urination, and urinary urgency and frequency, especially when accompanied by a low-grade fever.
• Encourage long-term follow-up care for high-risk patients.

What causes it

Renal calculi may result from:
• dehydration. Decreased urine production concentrates calculus-forming substances.
• infection. Infected, damaged tissue serves as a site for calculus development. Infected calculi (usually magnesium ammonium phosphate or staghorn calculi) may develop if bacteria serve as the nucleus in calculus formation. Such infections may promote destruction of renal parenchyma.
• changes in urine pH. Consistently acidic or alkaline urine provides a favorable medium for calculus formation.
• obstruction. Urinary stasis (such as in immobility from spinal cord injury) allows calculus constituents to collect and adhere, forming calculi. Obstruction also promotes infection that, in turn, compounds the obstruction.
• diet. Increased intake of calcium or oxalate-rich foods encourages calculus formation.
• immobilization. Immobility from spinal cord injury or other disorders allows calcium to be released into the circulation and eventually filtered by the kidneys.
• metabolic factors. Hyperparathyroidism, renal tubular acidosis, elevated uric acid levels (usually with gout), defective metabolism of oxalate, genetically defective metabolism of cystine, and excessive intake of vitamin D, protein, or dietary calcium may predispose a patient to renal calculi.

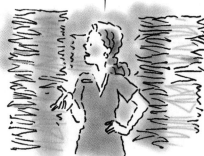

Renal calculi sure are calculating. Just look at all their possible causes!

A close look at renal calculi

Renal calculi vary in size and type. Small calculi may remain in the renal pelvis or pass down the ureter as shown below left. A staghorn calculus, shown below right, is a cast in the innermost part of the kidney—the calyx and renal pelvis. A staghorn calculus may develop from a calculus that stays in the kidney.

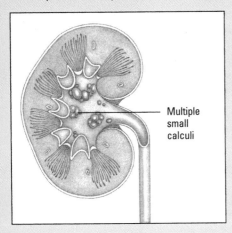

Multiple small calculi

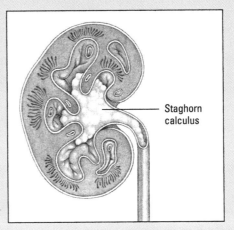

Staghorn calculus

How it happens

Calculi form when substances that normally dissolve in urine, such as calcium oxalate and calcium phosphate, precipitate. Large, rough calculi may occlude the opening to the ureteropelvic junction. The frequency and force of peristaltic contractions increase, causing pain.

What to look for

Clinical effects vary with size, location, and cause of the calculus. Pain is the key symptom. The pain of classic renal colic travels from the costovertebral angle to the flank, the suprapubic region, and the external genitalia. The pain fluctuates in intensity and may be excruciating at its peak. If calculi are in the renal pelvis and calyces, pain may be more constant and dull. Back pain occurs from calculi that produce an obstruction within a kidney. Nausea and vomiting usually accompany severe pain.

Other symptoms include:
- abdominal distention
- fever and chills
- hematuria, pyuria and, rarely, anuria
- restlessness
- inability to lie in a supine position.

What tests tell you

- KUB radiography reveals most renal calculi.
- Calculus analysis shows mineral content.
- Excretory urography confirms the diagnosis and determines the size and location of calculi.
- Renal ultrasonography may detect obstructive changes such as hydronephrosis.
- Urine culture of a midstream specimen may indicate UTI.
- Urinalysis results may be normal or may show increased specific gravity and acid or alkaline pH suitable for different types of calculus formation. Other urinalysis findings include hematuria (gross or microscopic), crystals (urate, calcium, or cystine), casts, and pyuria with or without bacteria and WBCs. A 24-hour urine collection is evaluated for calcium oxalate, phosphorus, and uric acid excretion levels.
- Other laboratory results support the diagnosis. Serial blood calcium and phosphorus levels detect hyperparathyroidism and show increased calcium levels in proportion to normal serum protein levels. Blood protein levels determine free calcium unbound to protein. Blood chloride and bicarbonate levels may show renal tubular acidosis. Increased blood uric acid levels may indicate gout as the cause.

> Vigorous hydration is a main component of renal calculi treatment—with enough hydration, the little suckers will eventually "go" with your flow.

How it's treated

Because 90% of renal calculi are smaller than 5 mm in diameter, treatment usually consists of measures to promote their natural passage. Along with vigorous hydration, such treatment includes antimicrobial therapy (varying with the cultured organism) for infection, analgesics such as ketorolac (Toradol) for pain, and diuretics to prevent urinary stasis and further calculus formation (because thiazide diuretics decrease calcium excretion into the urine, which reduces calculus formation).

Prophylaxis to prevent calculus formation includes a low-calcium diet for absorptive hypercalciuria, parathyroidectomy for hyperparathyroidism, allopurinol (Aloprim) for uric acid calculi, and daily administration of ascorbic acid by mouth to acidify the urine. A calculus that's too large for natural passage may require surgical removal, percutaneous ultrasonic lithotripsy and ESWL, or chemolysis.

What to do

- Promote sufficient intake of fluids to maintain a urine output of 3 to 4 L/day (urine should be very dilute and colorless). If the pa-

tient can't drink the required amount of fluid, supplemental I.V. fluids may be given.
• Strain all urine through gauze or a tea strainer and save the solid material recovered for analysis.
• Administer analgesics as ordered.
• Encourage ambulation if appropriate to aid in spontaneous passage of stones.
• Record intake, output, and weight to assess fluid status and renal function.
• If surgery is necessary, reassure the patient by supplementing and reinforcing what the surgeon has told him about the procedure. Explain preoperative and postoperative care.
• Prepare the patient for discharge, if appropriate. Assist him in arranging a follow-up visit with a urologist in 2 to 3 days. Provide discharge teaching and review the regimen, including how to strain urine for stones and dangerous signs and symptoms. (See *Renal calculi teaching tips.*)

Sexual assault

Sexual assault, commonly called *rape*, refers to sexual contact without the person's consent. It includes many behaviors—including physical and psychological coercion and force—that result in varying degrees of physical and psychological trauma.

Most information related to sexual assault is derived from statistics involving women who have been sexually assaulted. However, men and children can also be victims.

What's in a name?

Persons who have experienced sexual assault may be referred to as survivors or victims. Some health care practitioners use the term *survivor* because it's empowering and positive. Others use the term *victim* because it underscores the event's overwhelming severity and devastation. However, other health care practitioners feel that the term *victim* denotes hopelessness and helplessness.

Rape-trauma syndrome

Persons who have been sexually assaulted or have experienced an attempted sexual assault may develop rape-trauma syndrome. This syndrome involves the victim's short- and long-term reactions to the trauma and the methods used to cope with it. With support and counseling to help the patient deal with her feelings, the prognosis is good.

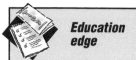

Education edge

Renal calculi teaching tips

• Before discharge, teach the patient and his family the importance of following the prescribed dietary and medication regimens to prevent recurrence of calculi.
• Encourage increased fluid intake.
• Tell the patient to immediately report symptoms of acute obstruction (such as pain and inability to void).
• Instruct the patient to return to the health care facility if he experiences fever, uncontrolled pain, or vomiting.

What causes it

Sexual assault is the result of a crime involving power, anger, and control. It isn't the result of wearing suggestive clothing, a secret desire to be raped, or a specific sexual orientation.

How it happens

The person committing the assault uses sex as a means to control and humiliate the victim. In this situation, all options for choice are removed from the victim. Subsequently, the attacker uses sexual contact forcibly and degradingly.

What to look for

Sexual assault is commonly characterized by:
- signs of physical trauma, including bruising, lacerations, abrasions, and avulsions
- clothing that's ripped, stained, or cut
- tearfulness, crying, and shaking
- withdrawal
- anxiety.

What tests tell you

Typically, several tests rule out possible STDs and pregnancy. Other tests may be done depending on the extent of the patient's injuries; for example, X-rays may be done to rule out fractures.

How it's treated

Treatment focuses on proper evidence collection, immediate care of apparent or life-threatening wounds or injuries, and medication therapy to prevent STDs and pregnancy.

Each institution or agency has a specific protocol for specimen collection in cases involving sexual assault. Specimens can be collected from many sources. Typically, they include blood, hair, nails, tissues, and body fluids, such as urine, semen, saliva, and vaginal secretions. In addition, evidence can be obtained via the results of diagnostic tests, such as CT scan and radiography. Regardless of the protocol or specimen source, accurate and precise specimen collection is essential in conjunction with thorough, objective documentation because, in many cases, this information will be used as evidence in legal proceedings.

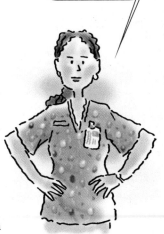

Sexual assault victims commonly display signs of withdrawal.

In good hands

Many institutions have a Sexual Assault Response Team, and may also have a Sexual Assault Nurse Examiner (SANE) available to care for sexual assault victims. SANEs are skilled rape-crisis professionals who can evaluate the victim and collect specimens. They may also be called upon at a later date to testify in legal proceedings.

What to do

When caring for the victim of a sexual assault, follow these steps:
• Stay with the patient at all times; offer comfort and support. Ask about calling a person for the patient who can also provide support, such as a friend, family member, or counselor.
• Develop a therapeutic relationship with the patient; make sure that she has given informed consent for testing that may be performed.
• Inform the patient of the facility's responsibility in reporting the assault; make sure that she understands this responsibility. Arrange for an advocate to talk with the patient about her choices and decision-making.
• Assist with history-taking and physical examination; obtain the following key information: date and time of the assault; where it occurred and the surroundings; body areas penetrated, including the use of foreign objects; and other sexual acts.
• Also ask about injuries occurring during the assault; actions after the assault, such as showering, urinating, douching, or changing clothing; recent gynecologic treatment or surgery; and history of sexual intercourse within the past 72 hours.

Collecting evidence

• Assist with evidence collection. (See *Collecting evidence in a sexual assault*.)
• Explain the specimens that are being taken and why; guide the patient through each step of the process.
• Make sure that the chain of custody for all evidence collected is maintained and logged according to the facility's protocol. Document all information completely, including the date and time that evidence was given to law enforcement officers. Include the names of the individuals in the patient's medical record.
• After the examination and evidence collection are completed, assist the patient with showering and donning clean clothing.

Medication and follow-up

• Administer medications as ordered to prevent STDs and pregnancy.
• Review instructions with the patient about medications and follow-up and what to expect physically and psychologically.
• Encourage the patient to have the support person accompany her home or to a safe place and stay with her.

Collecting evidence in a sexual assault

Accurate, precise specimen collection for evidence of a sexual assault is essential. Thorough, objective documentation with proper evidence collection is crucial because, in most cases, this information will be used as evidence in legal proceedings.

Although specific protocols and policies may vary among facilities, some general guidelines are listed here.

Guidelines for specimen collection

If you're responsible for collecting specimens in a sexual assault, follow these important guidelines:
• Be knowledgeable about your institution's policy and procedures for specimen collection in sexual assault cases.
• When obtaining specimens, be sure to collect them from the victim and, if possible, the suspect.
• Check with local law enforcement agencies regarding additional specimens that may be needed—for example, trace evidence, such as soot, grass, gravel, glass, or other debris.
• Wear gloves and change them frequently; use disposable equipment and instruments if possible.
• Avoid coughing, sneezing, or talking over specimens or touching your face, nose, or mouth when collecting specimens.
• Include the victim's clothing as part of the collection procedure.
• Place all items collected in separate paper bags.
• Never allow a specimen or item considered as evidence to be left unattended.
• Document each item or specimen collected; have another person witness each collection and document it.
• Obtain photographs of all injuries for documentation.

• Include written documentation of the victim's physical and psychological condition on the first encounter, throughout specimen collection, and afterward.

Patient preparation

• Assess the patient's ability to undergo the specimen collection procedure.
• Explain the procedures that the patient will undergo, what specimens will be collected and from where, and provide emotional support throughout.
• Obtain consent from the patient or her family for specimens to be obtained.
• Ask the patient if she would like someone—such as a family member, friend, or other person—to stay with her during the specimen collection.
• Ensure the patient's privacy throughout the collection procedure.

Specimen collection

When possible, obtain a special sexual assault evidence collection kit, which contains all the necessary items for specimen collection based on the evidence required by the local crime laboratory. In addition, the kit contains a form for the examiner to complete, sign, and date. Keep in mind that when collecting specimens for moist secretions, typically a one-swab technique is used; if secretions are dry, then a two-swab technique is used.

Clothing for specimen collection

• Ask the patient to stand on a clean piece of examination paper if she can stand. If the patient can't stand, then have her remain on the examination table or bed.
• Have the patient remove each article of clothing, one at a time, and place each article in a separate, clean paper bag.
• Fold the examination paper onto itself and place it into a clean paper bag. *(continued)*

Collecting evidence in a sexual assault *(continued)*

• Fold over, seal, label, and initial each bag.

Vaginal or cervical secretion collection
• Swab the vaginal area thoroughly with four swabs; swab the cervical area with two swabs, being sure to keep the vaginal swabs separate from the cervical swabs.
• Run the vaginal swabs over a slide (supplied in the kit) and allow the slide and swabs to air dry; do the same for the cervical swabs.
• Place the vaginal swabs in the swab container and close; place the slide in the cardboard sleeve, close it, and tape it shut; repeat for the cervical swabs.
• Place the swab container and cardboard sleeve into the envelope, and seal the envelope securely.
• Complete the information on the front of the envelope; if vaginal and cervical swabs are obtained, use a separate envelope for each.

Anal secretion collection
• Moisten a single swab with sterile water.
• Insert the swab gently into the patient's rectum approximately 1" to 1¼" (2 to 3 cm).
• Rotate the swab gently and then remove it.
• Allow the swab to air dry and then place it in an envelope.
• Seal and label the envelope appropriately.

Penile secretion collection
• Moisten a single swab with sterile water.
• Swab the entire external surface of the penis.
• Repeat this at least one more time (so that at least two swabs are obtained).
• Allow the swab to air dry and then place it in an envelope.
• Seal and label the envelope appropriately.

Pubic hair collection
• Use the comb provided in the kit and comb through the pubic hair.
• Collect approximately 20 to 30 pubic hairs and place them in the envelope.
• Alternatively, obtain 20 to 30 plucked hairs from the patient; allow the patient the option of plucking her pubic hair.

• Ensure that the patient has a follow-up appointment in 10 to 14 days with her health care practitioner or clinic and has the name and contact number of the rape crisis counselor.

Testicular torsion

Testicular torsion is the abnormal twisting of the spermatic cord that results from rotation of a testis or the *mesorchium*, a fold in the area between the testis and epididymis. It causes strangulation and, if untreated, eventual infarction of the testis.

This condition is almost always unilateral. Although it's most common between ages 12 and 18, it may occur at any age. The prognosis is good with early detection and prompt treatment.

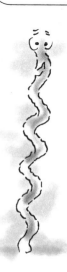

I happen to like my twisty figure, but I don't think a spermatic cord would share my opinion.

What causes it

Testicular torsion is caused in part by abnormalities inside or outside the *tunica vaginalis,* the serous membrane covering the internal scrotal cavity. Normally the tunica vaginalis envelops the testis and attaches to the epididymis and spermatic cord. Testicular torsion can be intravaginal or extravaginal.

Intra vs. extra

Intravaginal torsion is caused by:
• abnormality of the tunica vaginalis and the position of the testis
• incomplete attachment of the testis and spermatic fascia to the scrotal wall, leaving the testis free to rotate around its vascular pedicle.
    Extravaginal torsion is caused by:
• loose attachment of the tunica vaginalis to the scrotal lining, causing spermatic cord rotation above the testis
• sudden forceful contraction of the cremaster muscle due to physical exertion or irritation of the muscle.

How it happens

In testicular torsion, the testis rotates on its vascular pedicle and twists the arteries and vein in the spermatic cord. This twisting interrupts blood flow to the testis, resulting in vascular engorgement, ischemia, and scrotal swelling.

What to look for

Torsion produces excruciating pain in the affected testis or iliac fossa. Physical examination reveals tense, tender swelling in the scrotum or inguinal canal and hyperemia of the overlying skin. Scrotal swelling is unrelieved by rest or elevation of the scrotum.

What tests tell you

Doppler ultrasonography helps distinguish testicular torsion from strangulated hernia, undescended testes, or epididymitis. (See *Assessing Prehn's sign,* page 396.)

How it's treated

If manual reduction or detorsion is unsuccessful, torsion must be surgically corrected within 6 hours after the onset of symptoms to preserve testicular function (70% salvage rate). Treatment consists of immediate surgical repair by *orchiopexy* (fixation of a viable testis to the scrotum) or *orchiectomy* (excision of a nonviable

---

Assessing Prehn's sign

Differentiating between testicular torsion and epididymitis can be challenging. Follow these steps to elicit Prehn's sign to help determine which condition your patient has:
• Gently elevate the scrotum to the level of the symphysis pubis.
• Watch for changes in the patient's complaints of pain.
• Increased pain is associated with testicular torsion.
• Decreased pain is associated with epididymitis.

---

testis). Without treatment, the testis becomes dysfunctional and necrotic after 12 hours.

What to do

• Administer analgesics as ordered to aid pain relief.
• Assess vital signs and prepare the patient for surgery.
• Provide emotional support to the patient and his family.
• Perform preoperative teaching.
• Inform the patient and his family about transfer to the patient care unit after surgery.

Urinary tract infection

UTI typically refers to infection of the lower urinary tract. Lower UTIs commonly respond readily to treatment, but recurrence and resistant bacterial flare-up during therapy are possible. Lower UTIs are nearly 10 times more common in women than in men and affect 1 in 5 women at least once. Lower UTIs also occur in relatively large percentages in sexually active teenage girls. Lower UTIs fall into two types:

cystitis, which is an inflammation of the bladder that usually results from an ascending infection

urethritis, which is an inflammation of the urethra.

A large percentage of sexually active teenage girls contract UTIs.

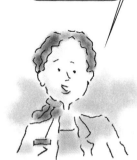

What causes it

UTI may be caused by:
• infection by gram-negative enteric bacteria, such as *E. coli*, *Klebsiella*, *Proteus*, *Enterobacter*, *Pseudomonas*, or *Serratia*
• simultaneous infection with multiple pathogens in a patient with neurogenic bladder
• indwelling urinary catheter

• fistula between the intestine and the bladder.

How it happens

Recent studies suggest that infection results from a breakdown in local defense mechanisms in the bladder that allows bacteria to invade the bladder mucosa and multiply. These bacteria can't be readily eliminated by normal micturition.

What to look for

Characteristic signs and symptoms include:
• urinary urgency and frequency
• dysuria
• bladder cramps or spasms
• itching
• feeling of warmth during urination
• nocturia
• possible hematuria
• fever
• urethral discharge in males.

Other common features include lower back pain, malaise, confusion, nausea, vomiting, abdominal pain or tenderness over the bladder, chills, and flank pain.

What tests tell you

• A clean-catch urinalysis reveals a bacteria count of 100,000/ml, confirming UTI. Lower counts don't necessarily rule out infection, especially if the patient is urinating frequently, because bacteria require 30 to 45 minutes to reproduce in urine. Culture and sensitivity testing determine the exact organism and the appropriate antimicrobial drug.
• A blood test or stained smear rules out STD.
• Voiding cystourethrography or excretory urography may detect congenital anomalies.

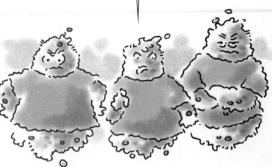

Looks like your bladder defenses broke down. Tough break; we're moving in and bringing a UTI with us.

How it's treated

A 7- to 10-day course of an appropriate antibiotic is usually the treatment of choice for an initial lower UTI. After 3 days of antibiotic therapy, urine culture should show no organisms. If the urine isn't sterile, bacterial resistance has probably occurred, making the use of a different antimicrobial necessary. Single-dose antibiotic therapy with amoxicillin or co-trimoxazole (Bactrim)

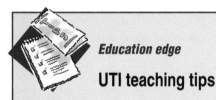

Education edge

UTI teaching tips

Follow these guidelines below when teaching your patient with a urinary tract infection (UTI):
• Explain the nature and purpose of antibiotic therapy. Emphasize the importance of completing the prescribed course of therapy and, with long-term prophylaxis, of adhering strictly to the ordered dosage.
• Urge the patient to drink plenty of water (at least eight glasses per day). Instruct the patient to avoid alcohol while taking antibiotics. Fruit juices, especially cranberry juice, and oral doses of vitamin C may help acidify urine and enhance the action of the medication.
• If therapy includes phenazopyridine (Pyridium), warn the patient that this drug may turn urine red-orange.
• Suggest warm sitz baths for relief of perineal discomfort. If baths aren't effective, apply heat sparingly to the perineum but be careful not to burn the patient.
• Teach the patient about general perineal hygiene measures, such as wiping from front to back, avoiding bubble baths and douching, and wearing cotton-lined underwear.

may be effective in women with acute uncomplicated UTI. A urine culture taken 1 to 2 weeks later indicates whether the infection has been eradicated.

Recurrent infections caused by renal calculi, chronic prostatitis, or a structural abnormality may require surgery. If there are no predisposing conditions, long-term, low-dose antibiotic therapy is preferred.

What to do

• Assess the patient's vital signs and obtain a clean-catch urine specimen for urinalysis and culture and sensitivity.
• Encourage fluid intake; if necessary, administer I.V. fluids.
• Initiate antimicrobial therapy as ordered.
• Provide comfort measures, such as a warm sitz bath and warm compresses.
• Prepare the patient for discharge. Instruct her about the medication regimen and measures to promote infection resolution and prevent recurrence. (See *UTI teaching tips.*)

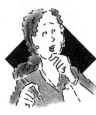

Quick quiz

1. When checking for costovertebral angle tenderness, where would you place the ball of your nondominant hand?
  A. At the symphysis pubis
  B. On the back at the level of the 12th rib
  C. On the abdomen just below the rib cage
  D. Just above the iliac crest

Answer: B. When checking costovertebral angle tenderness, place the ball of your nondominant hand on the back at the costovertebral angle of the 12th rib.

2. When assessing a patient for PID, which would you least expect to find?
  A. Profuse vaginal discharge
  B. Pain on palpation of the adnexa
  C. Fever greater than 104° F (40° C)
  D. Lower abdominal pain

Answer: C. A patient with PID typically has a low-grade fever with malaise, profuse purulent vaginal discharge, pain on palpation of the adnexa, and lower abdominal pain.

3. Which condition would you identify as a factor contributing to the development of renal calculi?
  A. Hypocalcemia
  B. Heart failure
  C. Hypothyroidism
  D. Changes in urine pH

Answer: D. Urine that's consistently acidic or alkaline provides a favorable medium for calculus formation.

4. When collecting evidence in a sexual assault, which action would be most appropriate?
  A. Placing all articles of clothing in one plastic, sealable bag
  B. Collecting secretion specimens primarily from the vagina
  C. Placing each item in a separate paper bag
  D. Telling the patient to shower before obtaining specimens

Answer: C. When evidence is collected from a survivor of sexual assault, it's important to place each item of evidence, including clothing, in a separate paper bag. Using plastic bags can promote faster deterioration of body fluids and other trace evidence.

Scoring

☆☆☆ If you answered all four questions correctly, get up and cheer! You're a GU and gynecologic genius!

☆☆ If you answered three questions correctly, pat yourself on the back! You're gearing up for GU success.

☆ If you answered fewer than three questions correctly, don't look grave. Just review the chapter and give it another go.

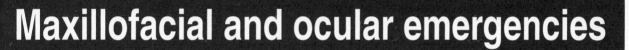

Maxillofacial and ocular emergencies

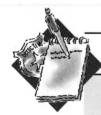

Just the facts

In this chapter, you'll learn:

♦ emergency assessment of the face and associated structures of the eyes, ears, nose, and mouth

♦ diagnostic tests and procedures for maxillofacial and ocular emergencies

♦ maxillofacial and ocular disorders in the emergency department and their treatments.

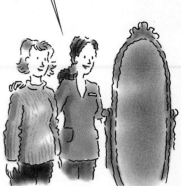

Maxillofacial and ocular emergencies can affect a patient's physical appearance as well as functional ability.

Understanding maxillofacial and ocular emergencies

The face consists of various structures that are closely related and, as such, an injury in one area can affect surrounding areas as well. Numerous bones and the organs of sight, hearing, taste, and smell are located on the face. In addition, the facial nerve (cranial nerve VII), its branches, and several other cranial nerves provide motor and sensory function for the face.

Maxillofacial and ocular emergencies typically involve some discomfort and pain. In addition, they may affect the patient's functional ability and physical appearance. Moreover, because of the proximity of the patient's airway to the structures of the face, there's always potential for the patient's airway to be compromised in some way, such as from edema or extension of the injury.

Quickness counts

When faced with a maxillofacial or an ocular emergency, you must assess the patient thoroughly and quickly, always staying alert for subtle changes that might indicate a potential deterioration in the patient's condition. A thorough assessment forms the basis for your interventions, which must be instituted quickly to minimize risks to the patient that can be life threatening. As with any emergency, the patient's airway, breathing, and circulation (ABCs) are priorities.

Assessment

Assessment of a patient's face and associated structures includes a health history and physical examination. If you can't interview the patient because of his condition, you may gather information from the patient's medical record. In some cases, you may need to ask his family or the emergency medical response team that transported the patient to the emergency department (ED) for information.

Health history

To obtain a health history, begin by introducing yourself and explaining what happens during the health history and physical examination. Use a systematic approach, focusing on one area of the face and then proceeding to another to gather information on the patient's chief complaint, past health status, family history, and cultural factors that may influence your assessment.

Chief complaint

When obtaining the patient's history, adapt the questions to the patient's specific complaints. Focus your questions on the onset, location, duration, and characteristics of the symptom as well as what aggravates or relieves it. Be sure to question the patient about complaints of pain or changes or loss of function in the area as well as the use of medications such as eyedrops.

Eye spy

Key questions related to the eye should address:
- routine problems with the eyes
- use of glasses or contact lenses and why
- problems with blurred vision or changes in the visual field
- history of eye surgery or injury, glaucoma, or cataracts
- medications to treat eye problems.

Earmark past problems

Key questions related to the ears, nose, and throat should address:
- changes in hearing, smell, or the ability to taste or swallow
- complaints of frequent headaches, nasal discharge, or postnasal drainage

> Frequent headaches can be symptoms of larger problems, so be sure to ask about them.

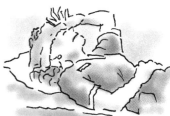

• history of ear infections, sinus infections, or nosebleeds.

Personal and family health and lifestyle

Next, question the patient about possible familial disorders related to the eyes, ears, nose, and throat. Also explore the patient's daily habits that might affect these structures. Appropriate questions may include:
• Does your occupation require intensive use of your eyes or require you to be exposed to loud noises or chemicals?
• Does the air where you work or live contain anything that causes you problems?
• Do you wear safety equipment, such as goggles and ear protection?

Physical examination

Maxillofacial and ocular emergencies affect people of all ages and can take many forms. To best identify abnormalities, use a consistent, methodical approach to the physical examination. Because of the emergency nature of the patient's condition, remember that you may need to limit your examination to specific problem areas or stop it entirely to intervene should the patient exhibit signs and symptoms of a deteriorating condition.

Examination of extraocular structures

Start by observing the patient's face. With the scalp line as the starting point, check that his eyes are in a normal position—about one-third of the way down the face and about one eye's width apart from each other. Then assess the eyelid, conjunctiva, cornea, anterior chamber, iris, and pupil.

Looking at lids

To examine the eyelid, follow these steps:
• Inspect the eyelids; each upper eyelid should cover the top quarter of the iris so the eyes look alike.
• Check for an excessive amount of visible sclera above the limbus (corneoscleral junction).
• Ask the patient to open and close his eyes to see if they close completely.
• If the downward movement of the upper eyelid in down gaze is delayed, the patient has a condition known as *lid lag*, which is a common sign of hyperthyroidism.
• Assess the lids for redness, edema, inflammation, or lesions.
• Check for a stye, or hordeolum, a common eyelid lesion. Also check for excessive tearing or dryness.

- The eyelid margins should be pink, and the eyelashes should turn outward.
- Observe whether the lower eyelids turn inward toward the eyeball (called *entropion*), or outward (called *ectropion*).
- Examine the eyelids for lumps.
- Put on examination gloves and gently palpate the *nasolacrimal sac*, the area below the inner canthus. Note any tenderness, swelling, or discharge through the lacrimal point, which could indicate blockage of the nasolacrimal duct.

Nice to meet ya, conjunctiva

Next, inspect the conjunctiva. To inspect the *bulbar conjunctiva* (the delicate mucous membrane that covers the exposed surface of the sclera), ask the patient to look up and gently pull his lower eyelid down. The bulbar conjunctiva should be clear and shiny; note excessive redness or exudate.

With the lid still secured, inspect the bulbar conjunctiva for color changes, foreign bodies, and edema. Also observe the sclera's color, which should be white. In a black patient, you may see flecks of tan. A bluish discoloration may indicate scleral thinning.

To examine the *palpebral conjunctiva* (the membrane that lines the eyelids), ask the patient to look down. Then lift the upper lid, holding the upper lashes against the eyebrow with your finger. The palpebral conjunctiva should be uniformly pink. In the patient with a history of allergies, the palpebral conjunctiva may have a cobblestone appearance.

Corneal matters

Examine the cornea by shining a penlight from both sides and then from straight ahead. The cornea should be clear without lesions. Test corneal sensitivity by lightly touching the cornea with a wisp of cotton. (See *Tips for assessing corneal sensitivity.*)

Observe the iris, which should appear flat, and the cornea, which should appear convex. The irises should be the same size, color, and shape.

Pupil examination

Each pupil should be round, equal in size, and about one-fourth the size of the iris in average room lighting. About one person in four has asymmetrical pupils without disease. Unequal pupils generally indicate neurologic damage, iritis, glaucoma, or therapy with certain drugs. A fixed pupil that doesn't react to light can be an ominous neurologic sign.

If these pupils fail my exam, it indicates a problem. The same goes for ocular pupils.

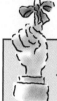

Tips for assessing corneal sensitivity

To test corneal sensitivity, touch a wisp of cotton from a cotton ball to the cornea, as shown below.

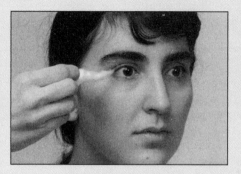

The patient should blink. If she doesn't, she may have suffered damage to the sensory fibers of cranial nerve V or to the motor fibers controlled by cranial nerve VI.

Keep in mind that people who wear contact lenses may have reduced sensitivity because they're accustomed to having foreign objects in their eyes.

Just a wisp
Remember that a wisp of cotton is the only safe object to use for this test. Even though a 4″ × 4″ gauze pad or tissue is soft, it can cause corneal abrasions and irritation.

> **Memory jogger**
>
> To make sure that your pupil assessment is complete, think of the acronym PERRLA.
>
> **P**upils
> **E**qual
> **R**ound
> **R**eactive
> **L**ight-reacting
> **A**ccommodation

Testing

Test the pupils for direct and consensual response. In a slightly darkened room, hold a penlight about 20″ (51 cm) from the patient's eyes, and direct the light at the eye from the side. Note the reaction of the pupil you're testing (direct response) and the opposite pupil (consensual response). They should both react the same way. Also, note sluggishness or inequality in the response. Repeat the test with the other pupil. *Note:* If you shine the light in a blind eye, neither pupil will respond. If you shine the light in a seeing eye, the pupils will respond consensually.

To test the pupils for accommodation, place your finger approximately 4″ (10 cm) from the bridge of the patient's nose. Ask the patient to look at a fixed object in the distance and then at your finger. His pupils should constrict and his eyes converge as he focuses on your finger.

Assessment of ocular muscle function

Evaluation of ocular muscle function involves assessing the corneal light reflex and the cardinal positions of gaze.

To assess the corneal light reflex, ask the patient to look straight ahead; then shine a penlight on the bridge of his nose from about 12″ to 15″ (30.5 cm to 38 cm) away. The light should fall at the same spot on each cornea. If it doesn't, the eyes aren't being held in the same plane by the extraocular muscles. This inequality commonly occurs in a patient who lacks muscle coordination, a condition called *strabismus* (cross-eye).

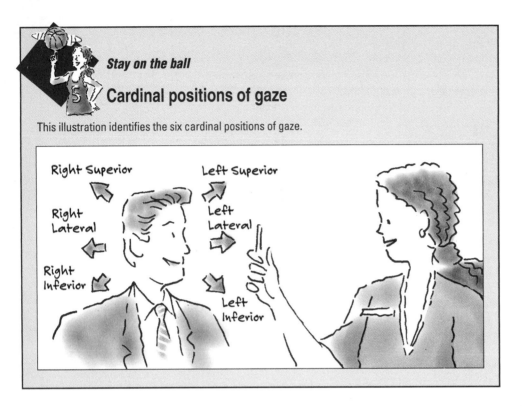

Stay on the ball

Cardinal positions of gaze

This illustration identifies the six cardinal positions of gaze.

Cardinal concerns

Cardinal positions of gaze evaluate the oculomotor, trigeminal, and abducent nerves as well as the extraocular muscles. To perform this test, ask the patient to remain still while you hold a pencil or other small object directly in front of his nose at a distance of about 18″ (46 cm). Ask him to follow the object with his eyes without moving his head. Then move the object to each of the six cardinal positions, returning to the midpoint after each movement. The patient's eyes should remain parallel as they move. Note abnormal findings, such as nystagmus and amblyopia (the failure of one eye to follow an object; also called *lazy eye*). (See *Cardinal positions of gaze.*)

Peek-a-boo!

If time and the patient's condition allow, you may perform the cover-uncover test. This test usually isn't done unless you detect an abnormality when assessing the corneal light reflex and cardinal positions of gaze.

Ask the patient to stare at a wall on the other side of the room. Cover one eye and watch for movement in the uncovered eye. Re-

> When testing with "cardinal" positions of gaze, make sure that the patient's head stays still.

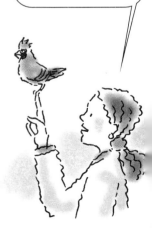

move the eye cover and watch for movement again. Repeat the test with the other eye.

Eye movement while covering or uncovering the eye is considered abnormal. It may result from weak or paralyzed extraocular muscles, which may be caused by cranial nerve impairment.

Visual acuity testing

Visual acuity testing is performed on the patient with an ocular emergency or who complains of eye or vision problems. In most cases, it's the first test performed; however, if the patient has experienced chemical exposure to the eyes, it follows eye irrigation.

very telling Snellen

To test your patient's far and near vision, use a Snellen chart and a near-vision chart. To test his peripheral vision, use confrontation. Before each test, ask the patient to remove corrective lenses if he wears them.

Have the patient sit or stand 20′ (6.1 m) from the chart, and then cover his left eye with an opaque object. Ask him to read the letters on one line of the chart and then to move downward to increasingly smaller lines until he can no longer discern all of the letters. Have him repeat the test covering his right eye. Lastly, ask him to read the smallest line he can read with both eyes uncovered to test his binocular vision.

If the patient wears corrective lenses, have him repeat the test wearing them. Record the vision with and without correction.

If a Snellen chart is unavailable, you can use other methods to assess the patient's visual acuity, including:
• using a pocket vision screener held 14″ (35.5 cm) from the patient's nose
• having the patient read newsprint
• asking the patient to identify the number of fingers being held up
• having the patient identify hand motion if he's unable to discern the number of fingers being held up.

With these methods, be sure to document the distance at which the patient identified or perceived it.

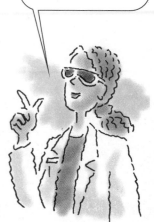

If your patient wears corrective lenses, have him repeat the Snellen test without them and record the difference.

for everyone else

Use the Snellen E chart to test visual acuity in a young child and a patient who can't read. Cover the patient's left eye to check the right eye; point to an E on the chart, and ask him to indicate which way the letter faces. Repeat the test on the other side. (See *Visual acuity charts*, page 408.)

If the test values between the two eyes differ by two lines—for example, 20/30 in one eye and 20/50 in the other—suspect an abnormality, such as amblyopia, especially in children.

Visual acuity charts

The most commonly used charts for testing vision are the Snellen alphabet chart (left) and the Snellen E chart (right), which is used for young children and adults who can't read. Both charts are used to test distance vision and measure visual acuity. The patient reads each chart at a distance of 20′ (6.1 m).

Recording results

Visual acuity is recorded as a fraction. The top number (20) is the distance between the patient and the chart. The bottom number is the distance from which a person with normal vision could read the line. The larger the bottom number, the poorer the patient's vision.

Age differences

In adults and children age 6 and older, normal vision is measured as 20/20. For children age 3 and younger, normal vision is 20/50; for children age 4, 20/40; and for children age 5, 20/30.

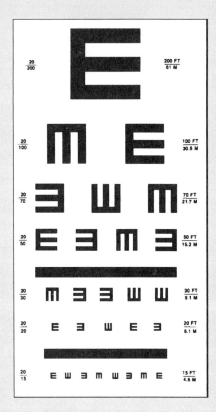

To test near vision, cover one of the patient's eyes with an opaque object and hold a Rosenbaum near-vision card 14″ from his eyes. Have him read the line with the smallest letters he can distinguish. Repeat the test with the other eye. If the patient wears corrective lenses, have him repeat the test while wearing them. Record the visual accommodation with and without lenses.

To assess peripheral vision, use a method known as *confrontation*. (See *Using confrontation.*)

Hearing acuity testing

Test your patient's gross hearing acuity. Ask him to occlude one ear, or occlude it for him. Then stand at a distance of 1′ to 2′ (30.5 to 61 cm) away, exhale fully, and whisper softly toward the unoccluded ear. Choose numbers or words that have two syllables that are equally accented such as "nine-four" or "baseball." If you note

Using confrontation

Follow these steps to assess peripheral vision with confrontation:
• Sit directly across from the patient and ask her to focus her gaze on your eyes.
• Place your hands on either side of the patient's head at ear level so that they're about 2′ (61 cm) apart (as shown).
• Tell the patient to focus her gaze on you as you gradually bring your wiggling fingers into her visual field.
• Instruct the patient to tell you as soon as she can see your wiggling fingers; she should see them at the same time you do.
• Repeat the procedure while holding your hands at the superior and inferior positions.

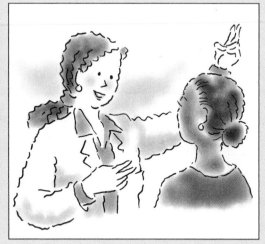

diminished hearing, perform tuning fork tests, such as the Weber's and Rinne tests.

Examination of the nose and sinuses

Begin by observing the patient's nose for position, symmetry, and color. Note such variations as discoloration, swelling, and deformity. Variations in size and shape are largely caused by differences in cartilage and in the amount of fibroadipose tissue.

Observe for nasal discharge or flaring. If discharge is present, note the color, quantity, and consistency; if you notice flaring, observe for other signs of respiratory distress.

Test nasal patency and olfactory nerve (cranial nerve I) function. Ask the patient to block one nostril and inhale a familiar aromatic substance through the other nostril. Possible substances include soap, coffee, citrus, tobacco, or nutmeg. Ask him to identify the aroma, and then repeat the process with the other nostril using a different aroma.

Now, inspect the nasal cavity. Ask the patient to tilt his head back slightly, and then push the tip of his nose up. Use the light from the otoscope to illuminate his nasal cavities. Check for severe deviation or perforation of the nasal septum. Examine the vestibule and turbinates for redness, softness, swelling, and discharge.

When life gives you lemons, use them to test cranial nerve I!

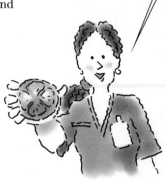

Upon closer inspection

Examine the nostrils by direct inspection, using a nasal speculum, a penlight or small flashlight, or an otoscope with a short, wide-tip attachment. Have the patient sit in front of you with his head tilted back. Put on gloves and insert the tip of the closed nasal speculum into one nostril to the point where the blade widens. Slowly open the speculum as wide as possible without causing discomfort. Shine the flashlight in the nostril to illuminate the area.

Observe the color and patency of the nostril, and check for exudate. The mucosa should be moist, pink to light red, and free from lesions and polyps. After inspecting one nostril, close the speculum, remove it, and inspect the other nostril. (See *Inspecting the nostrils.*)

Lastly, palpate the patient's nose and surrounding soft tissue with your thumb and forefinger, assessing for pain, tenderness, swelling, and deformity.

Face and sinuses

Next, examine the facial structures, using both hands and simultaneously palpating for irregularities and crepitus. Palpate in an upward fashion and then laterally. Observe the patient's face using a downward approach from the eyebrows to the chin. Then observe in the opposite manner to identify deformities.

Examine the sinuses. Remember, only the frontal and maxillary sinuses are accessible; you won't be able to palpate the ethmoidal and sphenoidal sinuses. Begin by checking for swelling around the eyes, especially over the sinus area. Then palpate the sinuses, checking for tenderness. To palpate the frontal sinuses, place your thumbs above the patient's eyes just under the bony ridges of the upper orbits, and place your fingertips on his forehead. Apply gentle pressure. Next, palpate the maxillary sinuses.

If the patient complains of tenderness during palpation, use transillumination to see if the sinuses are filled with fluid or pus. Transillumination can also help reveal tumors and obstructions. (See *Transilluminating the sinuses*, page 412.)

Examination of the mouth and throat

First, inspect the patient's lips. They should be pink, moist, symmetrical, and without lesions. A bluish hue or flecked pigmentation is common in dark-skinned patients.

Use a tongue blade and a bright light to inspect the oral mucosa. Have the patient open his mouth, and then place the tongue blade on top of his tongue. The oral mucosa should be pink, smooth, moist, and free from lesions and unusual odors. Increased pigmentation is seen in dark-skinned patients.

Inspecting the nostrils

This illustration shows the proper placement of the nasal speculum during direct inspection and the structures you should be able to see during this examination.

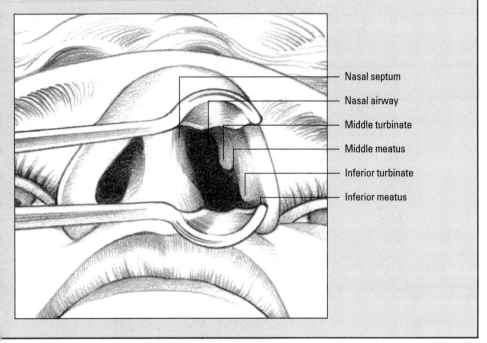

- Nasal septum
- Nasal airway
- Middle turbinate
- Middle meatus
- Inferior turbinate
- Inferior meatus

Gums...

Next, observe the gingivae, or gums; they should be pink, moist, and have clearly defined margins at each tooth. They shouldn't be retracted. Inspect the teeth, noting their number, condition, and whether any are missing or crowded. If the patient is wearing dentures, ask him to remove them so you can inspect the gums underneath. Ask the patient to open his jaw, and palpate the interior of the mouth while wearing gloves.

...and tongues

Lastly, inspect the tongue. It should be midline, moist, pink, and free from lesions. The posterior surface should be smooth, and the anterior surface should be slightly rough with small fissures. The tongue should move easily in all directions, and it should lie straight to the front at rest.

Ask the patient to raise the tip of his tongue and touch his palate directly behind his front teeth. Inspect the ventral surface of the tongue and the floor of the mouth. Next, wrap a piece of

Stay on the ball

Transilluminating the sinuses

Transillumination of the sinuses helps detect sinus tumors and obstruction, and requires only a penlight. Before you start, darken the room and have the patient close her eyes.

Frontal sinuses
Place the penlight on the supraorbital ring and direct the light upward to illuminate the frontal sinuses just above the eyebrow, as shown here.

Maxillary sinuses
Place the penlight on the patient's cheekbone just below her eye and ask her to open her mouth, as shown here. The light should transilluminate easily and equally.

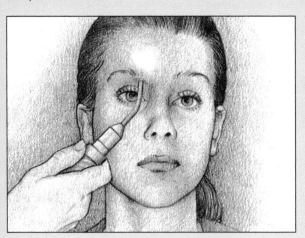

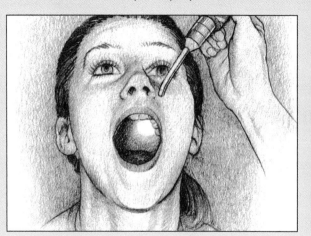

gauze around the tip of the tongue and move the tongue first to one side then the other to inspect the lateral borders. They should be smooth and even-textured.

Gag order

Inspect the patient's oropharynx by asking him to open his mouth while you shine the penlight on the uvula and palate. You may need to insert a tongue blade into the mouth and depress the tongue. Place the tongue blade slightly off center to avoid eliciting the gag reflex. The uvula and oropharynx should be pink and moist, without inflammation or exudate. The tonsils should be pink and shouldn't be hypertrophied. Ask the patient to say "Ahhh." Observe for movement of the soft palate and uvula.

Lastly, palpate the lips, tongue, and oropharynx. Note lumps, lesions, ulcers, or edema of the lips or tongue. Assess the patient's gag reflex by gently touching the back of the pharynx with a

cotton-tipped applicator or the tongue blade. This should produce
a bilateral response.

Diagnostic tests

Diagnostic tests include computed tomography (CT) scan, facial
X-rays, fluorescein angiography, fluorescein staining, and ultrasonography.

CT scan

A CT scan aids in diagnosing complex facial fractures. It's considered the standard for assessing soft tissue injury and provides useful information in identifying soft tissue injury involving the optic
nerve. It also confirms the diagnosis of cervical spine injury,
which may be present in a maxillofacial or ocular emergency patient.

It's orbital

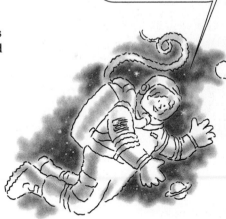

Orbital CT scan
reveals ocular
abnormalities that
standard X-rays
can't. Houston, we
have a hemangioma!

Performed specifically for an ocular emergency, an
orbital CT scan allows visualization of abnormalities
not readily seen on standard X-rays, such as size and
position delineation, and relationship to adjoining
structures. Contrast media may be used in orbital
CT scanning to define ocular tissues and help confirm a suspected circulatory disorder or hemangioma.

The application of CT scanning to ophthalmolo-
gy extends beyond the evaluation of the orbital and
adjoining structures; it also permits precise diagnosis of many intracranial lesions that affect vision.

Practice pointers

• Check the patient's history for hypersensitivity reactions to iodine, shellfish, or radiographic dyes.
• Tell the patient that he'll be positioned on an CT scan table and
that the table's head will be moved into the scanner, which will rotate around his head.
• If a contrast medium will be used, tell the patient that he may
feel flushed and warm and may experience a metallic taste and
nausea or vomiting after injection of the medium. Reassure him
that these reactions are typical.

Facial X-rays

Various types of X-rays may be used to determine maxillofacial injury. These include:
- *posteroanterior (Water's) view*, considered the most useful X-ray in helping to identify problems in the orbital rim and floor
- *Towne's view*, which detects problems in the mandibular condyles
- *anterior, posterior, and lateral views*, which provide information about the skull, sinuses, and roof of the orbit
- *submental vertex*, which provides information about the zygomatic arch and base of the skull
- *Anteroposterior and lateral oblique views* to detect injuries to the condylar and coronoid processes and the symphysis (of the mandible).

Practice pointers

- Prepare the patient for the X-ray to be performed; inform him of the reason for the X-ray.
- Verify that the X-ray order includes a pertinent history, such as trauma, and identifies the site of tenderness or pain.
- Make sure that the patient removes all jewelry from the head and neck area.

Fluorescein angiography

Fluorescein angiography records the appearance of blood vessels inside the eye through rapid-sequence photographs of the fundus (posterior inner part of the eye). The photographs, which are taken with a special camera, follow the I.V. injection of sodium fluorescein. This contrast medium enhances the visibility of microvascular structures of the retina and choroid, allowing evaluation of the entire retinal vascular bed, including retinal circulation.

Gesundheit! Sudden sneezing after contrast dye injection could mean hypersensitivity.

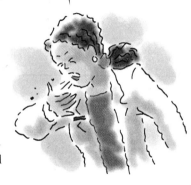

Practice pointers

- Check the patient's history for an intraocular lens implant, glaucoma, and hypersensitivity reactions, especially reactions to contrast media and dilating eyedrops.
- If miotic eyedrops are ordered, ask the patient with glaucoma if he has used eyedrops that day.
- Observe the patient for hypersensitivity reactions to the dye, such as vomiting, dry mouth, metallic taste, sudden increased salivation, sneezing, light-headedness, fainting, and hives. Rarely, anaphylactic shock may result.

• Explain that eyedrops will be instilled to dilate his pupils and that a dye will be injected into his arm. Remind him to maintain his position and fixation as the dye is injected. Tell him that he may briefly experience nausea and a feeling of warmth.
• Remind the patient that his skin and urine will be a yellow color for 24 to 48 hours after the test and that his near vision will be blurred for up to 12 hours.

Fluorescein staining

Fluorescein staining is used to evaluate ocular structures, specifically the cornea. It uses a stain that, when applied to the conjunctival sac, is distributed over the cornea. The cornea is then examined using a cobalt blue light; colors denote corneal irregularities. For example, corneal abrasions appear bright yellow like a highlighter, and loss of the protective conjunctiva appears as orange-yellow. Foreign bodies can vary in color depending on their material.

> Colorful AND informative! Fluorescein staining uses stain and a cobalt blue light to reveal corneal irregularities.

Practice pointers

• Explain the procedure and the reason for its use to the patient; make sure that he has removed his contact lenses if he wears them.
• Put on gloves and remove the strip from the package, being sure to keep the strip sterile.
• Moisten the strip with normal saline solution.
• Using your nondominant hand, gently pull down the eye's lower lid.
• Touch the tip of the fluorescein strip to the inner canthus of the lower lid. (See *Technique for fluorescein staining*, page 416.)
• Have the patient blink several times so that his tears can help transport the stain throughout the eye.
• Examine the patient's eye under cobalt blue light, looking for colored areas or spots.
• After completion, flush the patient's eye with normal saline solution to remove the stain.
• Instruct the patient to wait at least 1 hour before inserting his contact lenses.

Stay on the ball

Technique for fluorescein staining

When performing fluorescein staining, be sure to touch the dampened edge of the fluorescein strip to the conjunctiva at the inner canthus of the lower eyelid.

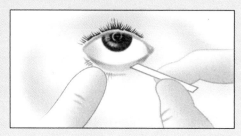

Ultrasonography

Ultrasonography involves the transmission of high-frequency sound waves. For ocular emergencies, the transmission of high-frequency sound waves through the eye are measured based on their reflection from ocular structures.

Illustrating the eyes' structures through ultrasound especially helps to evaluate a fundus clouded by an opaque medium, such as a cataract, or changes in density due to fractures. This test can identify pathologies that are normally undetectable through ophthalmoscopy. Ocular ultrasonography may also be performed before such surgeries as cataract removal or intraocular lens implantation.

Practice pointers

• Tell the patient that a small transducer will be placed on his closed eyelid and will transmit high-frequency sound waves that are reflected by the structures in the eye.
• Tell the patient that he may be asked to move his eyes or change his gaze during the procedure and that his cooperation is required to ensure accurate determination of test results.
• After the test, remove the water-soluble gel that was placed on the patient's eyelids.

Treatments

Treatments vary depending on the specific maxillofacial or ocular emergency. Common treatment measures include drug therapy, opthalmic agents, and surgery.

Drug therapy

Various drugs may be used in maxillofacial and ocular emergencies. Topical and systemic medications, including analgesic, antibiotic, and anti-inflammatory agents, are commonly employed.

Ophthalmic agents

Ophthalmic agents are usually administered in drop form but may also come in ointment form. Generally, ophthalmic agents fall into one of two groups:

 miotics

 mydriatics.

Miotics constrict the pupil; mydriatics dilate the pupil. In most cases, mydriatics are anticholinergic agents that also paralyze the muscle of accommodation (termed *cycloplegics*). (See *Examples of miotics and mydriatics*.)

Nursing considerations
• Administer the agent as ordered, making sure that the proper form is used.

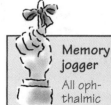

Memory jogger

All ophthalmic agents are manufactured in sterile, single-dose containers. To remember the action of mydriatics and miotics, just check the container's cap and ask, "Is it stop or go?" The caps are color-coded by the effect of the medication on the pupil. Mydriatics have a red cap (stop), and miotics have a green cap (go).

Examples of miotics and mydriatics

Commonly used miotics include:
• acetylcholine (Miochol)
• carbachol (Miostat)
• pilocarpine (Isopto Carpine)
• physostigmine (Isopto Eserine)
• betaxolol (Betoptic)
• levobunolol (Betagan Liquifilm)
• timolol (Timoptic).

Commonly used mydriatics include:
• atropine (Atrisol)
• cyclopentolate (Cyclogyl)
• epinephrine (Epifrin)
• homatropine (Isopto Homatropine)
• scopolamine (Isopto Hyoscine)
• tropicamide (Mydriacyl Ophthalmic).

Education edge

Instilling eye ointment and eyedrops

To teach about instilling eye ointment, instruct the patient to:
• Hold the tube for several minutes to warm the ointment.
• Squeeze a small amount of ointment—¼" to ½" (0.5 to 1.5 cm)—inside the lower lid.
• Gently close the eye and roll the eyeball in all directions with the eye closed.
• Wait 10 minutes before instilling other ointments.

To teach about instilling eyedrops, instruct the patient to:
• Tilt his head back and pull down on his lower lid.
• Drop the medication into the conjunctival sac.
• Apply pressure to the inner canthus for 1 minute after administration.
• Wait 5 minutes before instilling a second drop or other eye solutions.

• Instill topical agents appropriately, making sure you keep the tip of the applicator (eyedrop bottle or ointment tip) sterile.
• Provide patient teaching about the proper method for instilling eye ointment and eyedrops, especially if the patient is to continue the medication at home. (See *Instilling eye ointment and eyedrops.*)

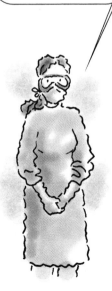

Safety first; laser surgery requires using lots of precautions—including eye protection—for everyone in the room.

Surgery

Surgery, such as laser surgery and scleral buckling, may be performed for ocular emergencies.

Laser surgery

Laser surgery is the treatment of choice for many ophthalmic disorders because it's relatively painless and especially useful for elderly patients, who may be poor risks for conventional surgery. Depending on the type of laser, the finely focused, high-energy beam shines at a specific wavelength and color to produce various effects. Laser surgery can be used to treat such ocular emergencies as retinal tears.

Nursing considerations

• Be aware that laser surgery requires safety precautions, including the use of eye protection for everyone in the room. Reflection of the laser beam from a smooth surface, such as a refractor, to a surface, such as a disposable drape, can start a fire.

Scleral buckling for retinal detachment

In scleral buckling, cryothermy (cold therapy), photocoagulation (laser therapy), or diathermy (heat therapy) creates a sterile inflammatory reaction that seals the retinal hole and causes the retina to re-adhere to the choroid. The surgeon then places a silicone plate or sponge—called an *explant*—over the site of reattachment and holds it in place with a silicone band. The pressure exerted on the explant indents (buckles) the eyeball and gently pushes the choroid and retina closer together.

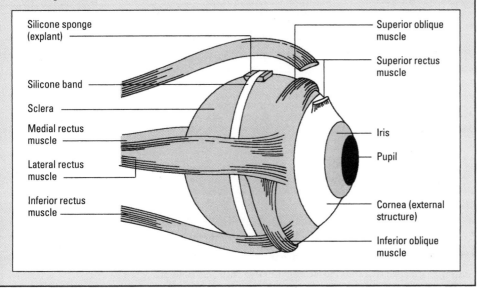

Silicone sponge (explant)

Superior oblique muscle

Superior rectus muscle

Silicone band

Sclera

Medial rectus muscle

Lateral rectus muscle

Iris

Pupil

Inferior rectus muscle

Cornea (external structure)

Inferior oblique muscle

• Advise the patient that he may experience some eye pain after the surgery. Encourage the use of ice packs as needed to help decrease the pain.

Scleral buckling

Used to repair retinal detachment, scleral buckling involves applying external pressure to the separated retinal layers, bringing the choroid into contact with the retina. Buckling (or *indenting*) brings the layers together so that an adhesion can form. It also prevents vitreous fluid from seeping between the detached layers of the retina and leading to further detachment and possible blindness. (See *Scleral buckling for retinal detachment*.)

Another method of reattaching the retina is pneumatic retinopexy. This procedure involves sealing the tear or hole with cryotherapy and introducing gas to provide a tamponade of the retina.

Nursing considerations

• Prepare the patient for surgery; depending on the patient's age and the surgeon's preference, advise him whether he'll receive a local or general anesthetic.
• Instruct the patient to report fever or eye pain that's sharp, sudden, or severe.

Common disorders

Common maxillofacial and ocular emergencies you're likely to "face" include:
• chemical burns to the eye
• corneal abrasion
• epistaxis
• facial fractures
• foreign body in the ear
• orbital fracture
• retinal detachment
• soft tissue facial injuries.

    Regardless of the disorder, the priorities are always to ensure vital functioning (the ABCs).

Chemical burns to the eye

Chemical burns to the eye can cause serious eye injury. These injuries may be work-related or may occur while using common household products.

What causes it

Chemical injury to the eye involves splashing or spraying hazardous materials into the eyes. It may also result from exposure to fumes or aerosols. Chemical burns may be caused by an acidic or alkaline substance or an irritant:
• Alkaline substances have a high pH and tend to cause the most severe ocular damage. Examples include lye, cement, lime, and ammonia.
• Acidic substances have a low pH and tend to cause less severe damage. (Even so, hydrofluoric acid, found in rust removers, aluminum brighteners, and heavy-duty cleaners, is an exception and causes severe burns.) An automobile battery explosion, causing a sulfuric acid burn, is the most common injury to the eye involving an acidic substance. Other common acids that can cause chemical burns include sulfurous acid, hydrochloric acid, nitric acid, acetic acid, and chromic acid.

• Irritant substances have a neutral pH and tend to cause discomfort, rather than ocular damage. Examples of irritants include pepper spray and many household detergents.

How it happens

The severity of chemical injury to the eye depends on the chemical's pH, the duration of contact with the chemical, the amount of chemical, and the chemical's ability to penetrate the eye.

Alkaline substances can penetrate the surface of the eye into the anterior chamber within 5 to 15 minutes, causing damage to such internal structures as the iris, ciliary body, lens, and trabecular network.

Acidic substances can't penetrate the corneal epithelial layer of the eye, which limits injury to superficial, nonprogressive damage. However, because hydrofluoric acid has properties similar to alkaline substances, it can cause more progressive and severe damage.

Household cleaning solutions carry with them a risk of eye irritation. As if you needed another excuse not to clean!

What to look for

• Obtain the patient's history; ask about a chemical spraying or splashing in the face or exposure to fumes or aerosols. Also ask about the use of cleaning solutions, solvents, or lawn and garden chemicals.
• Ask the patient about pain, irritation, inability to keep his eyes open, blurred vision, and a sensation of having something in the eye.
• Note patient complaints of severe pain and burning; observe for extreme redness, irritation, and excessive tearing.

What tests tell you

Chemical burns to the eye are an immediate threat to the patient's vision and are considered the most urgent of all ocular emergencies. Typically, no diagnostic tests are initially performed because eye irrigation takes priority.

How it's treated

The patient's eye is irrigated continuously with copious amounts of normal saline solution. Irrigation continues for at least 30 minutes and until the ocular pH reaches the desired level. Topical antibiotics, cycloplegic agents, and corticosteroids are ordered; opioid analgesia may also be ordered. Follow-up care with an ophthalmologist is essential.

Eye irrigation for chemical burns

The patient's eye may be irrigated using a Morgan lens or an I.V. tube.

Morgan lens

Connected to irrigation tubing, a Morgan lens permits continuous lavage and also delivers medication to the eye. Use an adapter to connect the lens to the I.V. tubing and the solution container. Begin the irrigation at the prescribed flow rate. To insert the device, ask the patient to look down as you insert the lens under the upper eyelid (as shown). Then have him look up as you retract and release the lower eyelid over the lens.

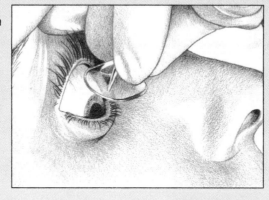

I.V. tube

If a Morgan lens isn't available, set up an I.V. bag and tubing without a needle. Direct a constant, gentle stream at the inner canthus so that the solution flows across the cornea to the outer canthus (as shown). Flush the eye for at least 15 minutes.

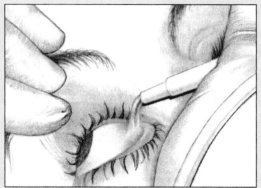

What to do

• Assess the patient's eye pH before irrigating the eye with sterile normal saline solution. Assessing the patient's visual acuity can be delayed until after irrigation.

• Flush the patient's eyes with large amounts of sterile isotonic saline solution for at least 30 minutes. Intermittently check the pH of the eye (because ocular pH may be increased if the offending chemical is alkaline, decreased if it's acidic, or neutral if it's an irritant). Continue to irrigate until the pH returns to a normal level (6.5 to 7.6). (See *Eye irrigation for chemical burns.*)

• After irrigation, inspect for conjunctival and scleral redness and tearing and corneal opacification.

• Prepare the patient for an ophthalmic examination.

• Provide analgesics as needed for pain.

- Administer other medications—topical or oral antibiotics, cycloplegics to prevent ciliary spasms and reduce inflammation, and topical lubricants—as ordered.
- Be prepared to administer beta-adrenergic blockers to lower intraocular pressure (IOP) if secondary glaucoma develops.
- If the patient has face burns from an alkaline substance, assess him for tracheal or esophageal burns; these burns can be life-threatening injuries.
- Because burns resulting from hydrofluoric acid may cause severe hypocalcemia, monitor serum calcium levels as ordered.
- Apply eye dressings or patches as needed to reduce eye movement.
- Teach the patient how to apply ophthalmic medications as necessary.
- Strongly advise patients to wear protective goggles or eyewear when working with toxic substances and to keep all toxic home products out of children's reach.

Corneal abrasion

A corneal abrasion is a scratch on the surface epithelium of the cornea. With treatment, prognosis is usually good.

What causes it

A corneal abrasion usually results from a foreign body—such as a cinder or a piece of dust, dirt, or grit—becoming embedded under the eyelid. Additional causes include small pieces of metal, improperly fitted contact lenses or falling asleep wearing hard contact lenses, or other items, such as a fingernail, piece of paper, or other organic substance.

How it happens

Small pieces of metal that get in the eyes of workers who don't wear protective glasses quickly form a rust ring on the cornea and cause corneal abrasion. Such abrasions are also common in the eyes of people who fall asleep wearing hard contact lenses or whose lenses aren't fitted properly. A corneal scratch caused by a fingernail, a piece of paper, or other organic substance may cause a persistent lesion. The epithelium doesn't always heal properly, possibly resulting in recurrent corneal erosion with delayed effects more severe than the original injury.

What to look for

• Reports of eye trauma or wearing contact lenses for a prolonged period
• Complaints of a sensation of something in the eye, sensitivity to light, decreased visual acuity (if the abrasion occurs in the pupillary region), and pain
• Redness, increased tearing
• Evidence of a foreign body on the cornea or eyelid

What tests tell you

Fluorescein staining confirms the diagnosis. The practitioner uses a cobalt-blue light and slit-lamp examination. The injured area appears yellow like a highlighter when examined.

How it's treated

If a foreign body is identified, the eye is irrigated and a topical anesthetic eyedrop is used. The practitioner uses a foreign body spud to remove a superficial foreign body. If the foreign body is a rust ring, it must be removed by the physician using an ophthalmic burr. When only partial removal is possible, reepithelialization lifts what remains of the ring to the surface so that removal can be completed the next day.

Brrr is for the cold, but a burr is for removing a rust ring from the eye.

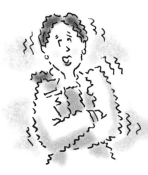

What to do

• Assist with the eye examination. Check visual acuity before beginning treatment.
• If a foreign body is visible, carefully irrigate the eye with normal saline solution.
• Instill topical anesthetic eyedrops in the affected eye before assisting the practitioner with removal.
• Instill broad-spectrum antibiotic eyedrops in the affected eye every 3 to 4 hours.
• Reassure the patient that the corneal epithelium usually heals in 24 to 48 hours.
• Provide tetanus prophylaxis.

To patch or not to patch

• If a patch is ordered, tell the patient to leave it in place for 6 to 12 hours. Warn him that a patch alters depth perception, and advise caution in performing daily activities, such as climbing stairs or stepping off a curb. (Patching is no longer routinely recommended in the treatment of corneal abrasions.)
• Stress the importance of instilling antibiotic eyedrops as ordered because an untreated corneal abrasion, if infected, can lead

Corneal ulceration

A major cause of blindness worldwide, corneal ulcers result in corneal scarring or perforation. They occur in the central or marginal areas of the cornea, vary in shape and size, and may be singular or multiple. Prompt treatment (within hours of onset) can prevent vision impairment.

Corneal ulcers generally result from bacterial, protozoan, viral, or fungal infections, but other causes may include ocular trauma, exposure, toxins, and allergens.

Signs and symptoms
Typically, corneal ulceration begins with pain (aggravated by blinking) and photophobia, followed by increased tearing. Eventually, central corneal ulceration produces pronounced visual blurring. The eye may appear red. Purulent discharge is possible if a bacterial ulcer is present.

Treatment
Prompt treatment is essential for all forms of corneal ulcer to prevent complications and permanent vision impairment. Treatment aims to eliminate the underlying cause of the ulcer and relieve pain.

A corneal ulcer should never be patched because patching creates the dark, warm, moist environment ideal for bacterial growth. However, it should be protected with a perforated shield. Antibiotics, antivirals, or antifungals are prescribed based on culture and sensitivity findings. Artificial tears and lubricating ointments may be prescribed as needed.

Nursing considerations
• Because corneal ulcers are quite painful, give analgesics as needed.
• Watch for signs of secondary glaucoma (transient vision loss and halos around lights).
• The patient may be more comfortable in a darkened room or when wearing dark glasses.

to a corneal ulcer and permanent vision loss. Teach the patient the proper way to instill eye medications. (See *Corneal ulceration*.)
• Advise the patient who wears contact lenses to abstain from wearing them until the corneal abrasion heals.
• Urge the patient to wear safety glasses to protect his eyes from flying fragments.
• Review instructions for wearing and caring for contact lenses to prevent further trauma.

Epistaxis

Epistaxis refers to a nosebleed. Such bleeding in children generally originates in the anterior nasal septum and tends to be mild. In adults, such bleeding most likely originates in the posterior septum and can be severe.

What causes it

Epistaxis may be a primary disorder or may occur secondary to another condition. It usually follows trauma from external or internal causes, such as a blow to the nose, nose picking, or insertion of a foreign body. Less commonly, it results from polyps, inhalation of chemicals that irritate the nasal mucosa, vascular abnormalities, or acute or chronic infections, such as sinusitis or rhinitis, that cause congestion and eventual bleeding from capillary blood vessels. Epistaxis may also follow sudden mechanical decompression (caisson disease) and strenuous exercise.

How it happens

A rich supply of fragile blood vessels makes the nose particularly vulnerable to bleeding. Air moving through the nose can dry and irritate the mucous membranes, forming crusts that bleed when they're removed. Dry mucous membranes are also more susceptible to infections, which can lead to epistaxis as well. In addition, trauma to the mucous membranes leads to bleeding.

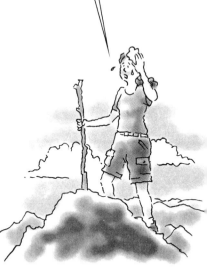

Life at a high altitude can predispose you to two things. One is yodeling. The other is epistaxis.

What to look for

The patient with epistaxis commonly comes to the ED holding bloody tissues, towels, or cloths. Bleeding from one or both nostrils is visible, and may range from a slow trickle to a profuse continuous flow. Unilateral bleeding is typical; bilateral bleeding suggests a blood dyscrasia or severe trauma.

Bright red blood oozing from the nostrils suggests anterior bleeding. Blood visible in the back of the throat originates in the posterior area and may be dark or bright red. It's commonly mistaken for hemoptysis because of expectoration.

The patient's history may reveal trauma to the nose or evidence of a predisposing factor, such as anticoagulant therapy, hypertension, chronic aspirin use, high altitudes and dry climate, sclerotic vessel disease, Hodgkin's disease, vitamin K deficiency, or blood dyscrasias.

What tests tell you

Diagnosis is determined by assessment findings. Facial X-rays may be done to determine if a fracture is present. If the patient's bleeding is severe, complete blood count and coagulation studies may be done to evaluate the patient's status. In addition, blood typing and crossmatching is done if the patient requires a transfusion because of blood loss.

How it's treated

The nose is cleared of blood clots by having the patient blow his nose or with suctioning via an 8 French or 10 French Frazier catheter. If the bleeding is anterior, treatment typically includes stopping the bleeding with topical vasoconstrictors, direct pressure for 5 to 10 minutes, cautery (chemical or electrical), and packing if needed. Nasal packing, which is coated with an antibiotic ointment before insertion, can be in the form of petroleum iodoform gauze, which requires removal in 24 to 72 hours, or commercial packing products that dissolve and don't require removal.

Posterior bleeding is treated with nasal packing in the form of nasal sponges, special epistaxis balloon devices, or a 12 French to 16 French urinary catheter (with the distal tip removed). This type of packing is usually removed in 2 to 3 days. Drug therapy to treat an underlying condition, such as hypertension, is ordered. If bleeding doesn't respond to treatment, surgery involving ligation or embolization may be necessary.

What to do

• Assess the patient's ABCs. If bleeding is severe or if there's associated trauma, institute emergency interventions as necessary, such as suctioning, oxygen saturation monitoring and oxygen therapy, I.V. therapy, and cardiac monitoring.
• Determine the location of the bleeding (anterior or posterior) and whether epistaxis is unilateral or bilateral. Inspect for blood seeping behind the nasal septum, in the middle ear, and in the corners of the eyes.
• Apply direct pressure to the soft portion of the nostrils against the septum continuously for 5 to 10 minutes. Maintain the patient in an upright position with his head tilted slightly downward as you compress the nostrils.
• Apply an ice collar or cold compresses to the nose. Bleeding should stop after 10 minutes.
• Assist with treatment for anterior bleeding, including the application of external pressure and a topical vasoconstrictor (such as a cotton ball saturated with 4% topical cocaine solution or a solution of 4% lidocaine and topical epinephrine at 1:10,000) to the bleeding site, followed by cauterization with electrocautery or a silver nitrate stick. If these measures don't control bleeding, petroleum gauze nasal packing may be needed. (See *Types of nasal packing*, page 428.)

Pack it up

• Assist with treatment for posterior bleeding, including the use of a nasal balloon catheter to control bleeding effectively, gauze

Types of nasal packing

Nosebleeds may be controlled with anterior or posterior nasal packing.

Anterior nasal packing

The practitioner may treat an anterior nosebleed by packing the anterior nasal cavity with an antibiotic-impregnated petroleum gauze strip (shown at right) or with a nasal tampon.

A nasal tampon is made of tightly compressed absorbent material with or without a central breathing tube. The practitioner inserts a lubricated tampon along the floor of the nose and, with the patient's head tilted backward, instills 5 to 10 ml of antibiotic or normal saline solution. This solution causes the tampon to expand, stopping the bleeding. The tampon should be moistened periodically, and the central breathing tube should be suctioned regularly.

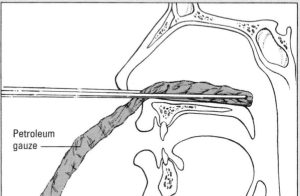

In a patient with blood dyscrasias, the practitioner may fashion an absorbable pack by moistening a gauzelike, regenerated cellulose material with a vasoconstrictor. Applied to a visible bleeding point, this substance will swell to form a clot. The packing is absorbable and doesn't need removal.

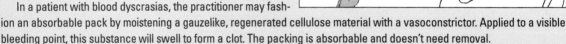

Posterior nasal packing

Posterior packing consists of a gauze roll shaped and secured by three sutures (one suture at each end and one in the middle) or a balloon-type catheter. To insert the packing, the practitioner advances one or two soft catheters into the patient's nostrils (shown at right). When the catheter tips appear in the nasopharynx, the practitioner grasps them with a Kelly clamp or bayonet forceps and pulls them forward through the mouth. He secures the two end sutures to the catheter tip and draws the catheter back through the nostrils.

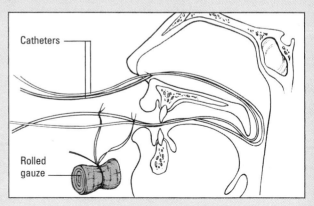

This step brings the packing into place with the end sutures hanging from the patient's nostril. (The middle suture emerges from the patient's mouth to free the packing, when needed.)

The practitioner may weight the nose sutures with a clamp. Then he'll pull the packing securely into place behind the soft palate and against the posterior end of the septum (nasal choana).

After the practitioner examines the patient's throat (to ensure that the uvula hasn't been forced under the packing), he inserts anterior packing and secures the whole apparatus by tying the posterior pack strings around rolled gauze or a dental roll at the nostrils (shown at right).

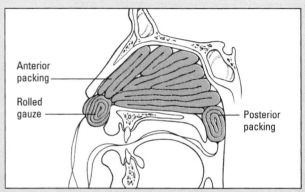

packing inserted through the nose, or postnasal packing inserted through the mouth, depending on the bleeding site.

• If local measures fail to control bleeding, assist with additional treatment, which may include supplemental vitamin K and, for severe bleeding, blood transfusions and surgical ligation or embolization of a bleeding artery.

• Monitor the patient's vital signs and skin color; record blood loss.

• Assess oxygen saturation levels via pulse oximetry and administer oxygen as needed.

• Tell the patient to breathe through his mouth and not to swallow blood, talk, or blow his nose.

• Keep vasoconstrictors, such as phenylephrine (Neo-Synephrine) nasal spray, on hand.

• Reassure the patient and his family that epistaxis usually looks worse than it is.

• Administer antibiotics as ordered if packing must remain in place for longer than 24 hours.

• If the bleeding is controlled effectively, prepare the patient for discharge; if the patient required posterior nasal packing, prepare him for admission. (See *Teaching tips for preventing epistaxis.*)

Education edge

Teaching tips to prevent epistaxis

Epistaxis can be a frightening experience for a patient, especially if he requires interventions other than just applying pressure to the nostril area. Therefore, educating the patient in measures to prevent epistaxis can help to alleviate his anxiety and decrease the risk of a recurrent episode. Be sure to include the following information in your discharge teaching:

• If the patient required anterior packing, instruct him to return to the emergency department (ED) or make an appointment with the practitioner for packing removal.

• Tell the patient to return to the ED if bleeding recurs or if packing becomes dislodged.

• Instruct the patient not to insert foreign objects into his nose and to avoid bending and lifting.

• Instruct the patient to sneeze with his mouth open.

• Emphasize the need for follow-up examinations and periodic blood studies after an episode of epistaxis. Advise the patient to seek prompt treatment for nasal infection or irritation.

• Suggest a humidifier if the patient lives in a dry climate or at a high elevation or if his home is heated with circulating hot air.

• Caution the patient against inserting cotton or tissues into his nose because these objects are difficult to remove and may further irritate nasal mucosa.

Facial fractures

A facial fracture refers to an injury that results in a broken bone or bones of the face. Facial fractures may involve damage to almost any of the bone structures of the face, including the nose, zygoma (cheekbone), mandible, frontal region, maxilla, and supraorbital rim. Nasal bone fractures are the most common type of facial fracture.

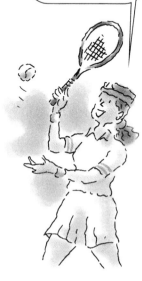

Watch that return! Sports-related injuries are a main facial-fracture culprit.

What causes it

Many facial fractures result from sports-related injuries. Other mechanisms of injury may include motor vehicle accidents, manual blows to the face, and falls.

How it happens

The amount of force necessary to fracture bones of the face varies depending on the bone. Nasal fractures require the least amount of force, whereas fractures of the supraorbital rim require the greatest amount of force.

What to look for

General findings related to facial fractures include:
- swelling
- displacement
- ecchymoses
- pain
- possible loss of function.
   Specific signs and symptoms vary depending on the areas and structures involved. (See *Assessing facial fractures.*)

What tests tell you

Typically, facial X-rays reveal the type of fracture and its location. CT scan may be used to determine the injury's extent.

How it's treated

Treatment of facial fractures involves stabilizing the patient's airway, including frequent suctioning if bleeding and secretions are profuse, and ruling out cervical spine injury. Orotracheal intubation is preferred for airway maintenance. Oxygen therapy and assisted ventilation are used as necessary. Hemorrhage is treated with direct pressure, ice packs, or an external compression dressing. Nasal fractures require splinting and setting of the bone.

Assessing facial fractures

When a patient experiences a facial fracture, signs and symptoms vary based on the area of injury. This chart highlights some of the common assessment and diagnostic test findings associated with various facial fracture areas.

Fracture area	Assessment findings	Diagnostic test findings
Nasal	• Pain • Changes in vision • Edema of the periorbital area and upper face • Ecchymosis • Epistaxis • Crepitus • Possible intracranial injuries	Facial computed tomography (CT) scan or nasal bone X-ray revealing disruption of the bone
Zygomatic arch	• Pain in the lateral cheek • Difficulty closing the jaw • Swelling and crepitus • Visible asymmetry	Facial X-ray or facial CT scan showing depressed arch
Mandibular	• Point tenderness • Crepitus • Trismus (tonic contracture of chewing muscles) • Asymmetrical facial appearance • Swelling • Ecchymosis • Malocclusion • Possible lower lip and chin paresthesia • Inability to grasp a tongue blade between his teeth	Facial X-ray or CT scan revealing displacement at the site of fracture (most commonly mandibular angle, condyle, molar, and mental areas)
Maxillary	• Severe facial pain • Lack of sensation or paresthesia of the upper lip • Vision changes • Severe facial edema and ecchymosis • Elongated facial appearance • Periorbital or orbital edema • Subconjunctival hemorrhage • Facial asymmetry • Malocclusion • Rhinorrhea • Moveable maxilla	Facial X-ray revealing displacement and site of fracture; CT scan identifying the extent and severity of the fracture

Surgery with open reduction and internal fixation or wiring is used to treat mandibular fractures.

What to do

• Because facial fractures typically involve structures located near the airway, immediately assess ABCs. If the patient has sustained severe facial trauma, oral airway insertion or endotracheal intubation and mechanical ventilation may be necessary.
• Immobilize the cervical spine until spinal injury is ruled out. Because of the force needed to cause a facial fracture, cervical spine injury may be present in 1% to 4% of those with facial fractures.
• Obtain facial X-rays and a CT scan of the face as ordered to locate the fracture and determine the level of severity.
• Initiate measures to reduce swelling and control bleeding (which may include elevating the patient's head if cervical spine injury has been ruled out); apply ice to the area.
• Administer analgesics and other medications as ordered, including tetanus prophylaxis.
• Prepare the patient for surgery as indicated.

Foreign body in the ear

Foreign body in the ear, as the name suggests, refers to any object in the ear canal that causes some obstruction. This problem is most commonly associated with children ages 9 months to 4 years.

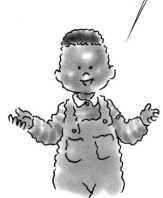

Little hands, big trouble! Children ages 9 months to 4 years are the usual suspects when it comes to foreign bodies in the ear.

What causes it

The most common cause of a foreign body in the ear is cerumen, commonly as a result of inserting cotton swabs into the ear and pushing cerumen further into the ear canal. Cerumen impaction is another cause, most commonly seen in the older adult. Other causes include insects and such objects as beads, small stones, beans, corn, and dry cereal.

How it happens

The object becomes lodged in the ear canal. Cerumen blocks the transmission of sound to the eardrum. Other objects, such as beans or insects, become lodged in the canal, leading to inflammation, pain, and possible infection.

What to look for

Typically, the patient reports a change in hearing. He may complain of ear pain or feelings of fullness. Signs and symptoms of ear infection or purulent foul-smelling drainage may be seen. If an insect is the cause, the patient commonly reports a feeling of buzzing or something moving in the ear.

What tests tell you

Gross hearing screening may be done to estimate the degree of hearing loss. Otoscopic examination reveals evidence of an obstruction.

How it's treated

Removal of the foreign body is key. This removal may be achieved with suctioning, irrigation, or special tools while directly visualizing the ear canal. These tools may include an ear curette, right-angle hook, Frazier suction catheter, funnel-tipped flexible catheter, or alligator forceps. Eardrops may be used to help soften impacted cerumen. If a patient has a live insect in his ear, mineral oil or 2% lidocaine may be used to kill the insect before its removal.

What to do

• Assess the patient's gross hearing acuity and determine evidence of obstruction.
• Prepare the patient for ear irrigation; provide comfort to the patient and his family.
• Explain procedures and treatments to the patient and family to help alleviate anxiety.
• If ordered, administer eardrops to soften cerumen or insert mineral oil or 2% lidocaine to kill a live insect.
• Irrigate the ear as ordered using warm tap water or a solution of 1:1 hydrogen peroxide and warm water; make sure that the solution is warmed to body temperature to prevent stimulating the inner ear, which could lead to dizziness, nausea, and vomiting. (See *Contraindications for irrigation.*)
• Assist with the instrument removal of a foreign object.

Ages and stages

Contraindications for irrigation

Remember that ear irrigation is contraindicated in patients:
• younger than 5 years old
• with a ruptured tympanic membrane
• with an ear infection
• with a vegetable or soft foreign body that would absorb water.

Orbital fracture

Orbital fracture refers to a break in the orbital floor and rim. This type of fracture is a serious condition and can lead to vision impairment or injury to the globe.

What causes it

Orbital fracture is usually caused by direct blunt trauma to the eye, such as from a motor vehicle collision, assault, or fall. A blowout fracture occurs when the direct injury causes such a significant increase in IOP that the floor of the orbit breaks.

How it happens

The direct force of the blunt trauma causes disruption to the orbital floor and rim. Fracture of the floor occurs when IOP rises significantly. Subsequently, the contents of the orbit can herniate into the maxillary and ethmoid sinuses. The inferior rectus muscle may also become trapped in the area.

What to look for

The patient with an orbital fracture typically reports some type of blunt trauma. Signs and symptoms may include:
- ecchymosis of the eyelid
- swelling
- pain
- difficulty blinking.

If the patient has a blowout fracture, the following may be present:
- periorbital ecchymosis
- sunken eye
- upward gazing
- diplopia.

Because of the close proximity of other facial structures and the location on the skull, there may be evidence of facial fractures or head trauma.

What tests tell you

Facial X-rays are used to determine the extent of the fracture and aid in the diagnosis of an orbital blowout fracture. CT scan helps to confirm entrapment of the inferior rectus and oblique extraocular muscles.

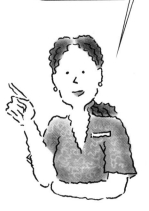

Eyelid ecchymosis, swelling, pain, and difficulty blinking all point to orbital fracture.

How it's treated

Treatment of an orbital fracture is conservative. If globe injury or muscle involvement hasn't occurred, the patient is referred to an ophthalmologist. If there's an associated nasal fracture, antibiotics are most likely ordered. Surgery for globe injury is typically postponed for approximately 2 weeks while swelling diminishes.

What to do

• Evaluate the patient's ABCs and intervene as necessary.
• Assess for evidence of associated trauma, including facial fractures and head trauma.
• Determine the type of injury, including the mechanism, time, force, and object causing the trauma.
• Assess visual acuity and perform an ophthalmic examination.
• Apply ice and elevate the patient's head.
• Provide reassurance to help alleviate anxiety.
• Refer the patient to an ophthalmologist as indicated.
• Advise the patient to avoid Valsalva's maneuver, coughing, and nose blowing; these activities can increase IOP, possibly leading to a blowout fracture.

Retinal detachment

Retinal detachment occurs when the outer retinal pigment epithelium splits from the neural retina, creating a subretinal space. This space then fills with fluid, called *subretinal fluid*.

Retinal detachment usually involves only one eye, but may later involve the other eye. Surgical reattachment is typically successful. However, the prognosis for good vision depends on which area of the retina has been affected.

What causes it

Predisposing factors include high myopia and cataract surgery. The most common causes are degenerative changes in the retina or vitreous humor. Other causes include:
• trauma or inflammation
• systemic diseases such as diabetes mellitus.

Retinal detachment is rare in children. However, it occasionally develops as a result of retinopathy of prematurity, tumors (retinoblastomas), trauma, or myopia, which tends to run in families.

How it happens

A retinal tear or hole allows the vitreous humor to seep between the retinal layers, separating the retina from its choroidal blood supply. Retinal detachment may also result from seepage of fluid into the subretinal space or from traction placed on the retina by vitreous bands or membranes. (See *Understanding retinal detachment.*)

What to look for

Signs and symptoms of retinal detachment include:
• floaters
• light flashes
• sudden, painless vision loss that may be described as a curtain that eliminates a portion of the visual field
• wavy or watery vision.

What tests tell you

Ophthalmoscopic examination through a well-dilated pupil confirms the diagnosis. It shows the usually transparent retina as gray and opaque; in severe detachment, it reveals folds in the retina and ballooning out of the area. Indirect ophthalmoscopy is also used to search the retina for tears and holes. Ocular ultrasonography may be necessary if the lens is opaque or if the vitreous humor is cloudy.

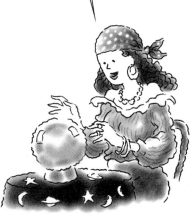

I see...a cloudy vitreous humor. I predict ocular ultrasonography in your future.

How it's treated

Treatment depends on the location and severity of the detachment:
• Eye movements are restricted through bed rest and sedation. If the patient's macula is threatened, his head may be positioned so the tear or hole is below the rest of the eye before surgical intervention.
• Bed rest is typically ordered with bilateral eye patching.
• A hole in the peripheral retina can be treated with cryotherapy; a hole in the posterior portion, with laser therapy.
• Retinal detachment rarely heals spontaneously. Surgery—including scleral buckling, pneumatic retinopexy, or vitrectomy (or a combination of these procedures)—can reattach the retina.

What to do

• Provide emotional support because the patient may be distraught about his vision loss.
• Maintain complete bed rest and instruct the patient to restrict eye movements until surgical reattachment is performed.

Understanding retinal detachment

Traumatic injury or degenerative changes cause retinal detachment by allowing the retina's sensory tissue layers to separate from the retinal pigment epithelium. This permits fluid—for example, from the vitreous humor—to seep into the space between the retinal pigment epithelium and the rods and cones of the tissue layers.

The pressure that results from the fluid entering the space balloons the retina into the vitreous cavity away from choroidal circulation. Separated from its blood supply, the retina can't function. Without prompt repair, the detached retina can cause permanent vision loss.

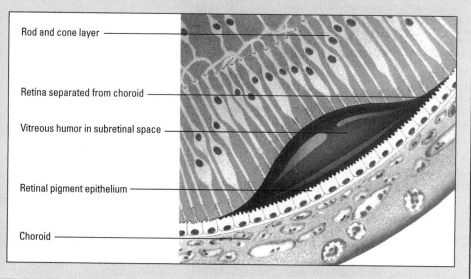

Rod and cone layer

Retina separated from choroid

Vitreous humor in subretinal space

Retinal pigment epithelium

Choroid

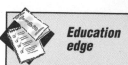

Teaching tips for the patient with retinal detachment

- Explain to the patient undergoing laser surgery that he may have blurred vision for several days afterward.
- Show the patient having scleral buckling how to instill eyedrops properly. Remind him to lie in the position recommended by the practitioner after surgery.
- Reinforce the need to rest and avoid driving, bending, heavy lifting, and other activities that affect intraocular pressure for several days after eye surgery. Discourage activities that could cause the patient to bump the eye.
- Review early symptoms of retinal detachment, and emphasize the need for immediate treatment.

- To avoid pressure to the globe of the eye, which could cause further extrusion of intraocular contents into the subretinal space, apply goggles or a metallic eye shield.
- Urge the patient to avoid activities in bed that could increase IOP, such as straining at stool, bending down, forceful coughing, sneezing, or vomiting.
- Prepare the patient for surgery; if indicated, wash the patient's face with no-tears shampoo. Give antibiotics and cycloplegic-mydriatic eyedrops.
- Provide preoperative and postoperative teaching, including care measures to avoid increased IOP. (See *Teaching tips for the patient with retinal detachment.*)

Soft tissue facial injuries

Soft tissue facial injuries include contusions, lacerations, abrasions, and friction injuries. These injuries are problematic because they can cause considerable upset or changes in physical appearance. Therefore, facial lacerations are typically repaired as soon as possible.

What causes it

Soft tissue facial injuries can be the result of numerous causes; motor vehicle collisions are a common one. Air bag deployment commonly causes minor abrasions of the face, neck, and upper chest.

Lacerations and contusions may result from blunt or penetrating trauma. Animal or human bites are a common cause of lacerations. Friction injuries, commonly called *road rash*, may be the result of a vehicle collision or, possibly, gunpowder fragments.

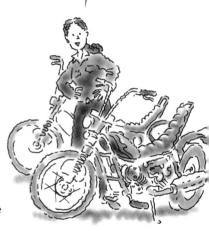

Skin plus asphalt equals shearing and abrasion. Bet I don't look too silly in these chaps now, huh?

How it happens

During the trauma, the skin of the face comes in contact with the offending cause. For example, in the case of a bite, the animal's teeth penetrate the outer layer of the skin, causing damage to the underlying tissue. Contact of skin with asphalt leads to shearing of the outer surface and abrasion.

What to look for

Signs and symptoms associated with soft tissue facial injuries may include:
- superficial to deep lacerations on any area of the face
- evidence of skin opening or revealing teeth marks
- epidermal staining (friction injuries)
- intraoral deformities, including lacerations and bleeding.
    If the patient sustains deep lacerations of the cheek, you may note:
- forehead asymmetry due to damage of the temporal branch of the facial nerve
- inability to close the eye on the affected side due to damage of the temporal or zygomatic branch of the facial nerve
- inability to purse lips due to damage to the buccal branch of the facial nerve
- elevation of the lower lip at rest with an inability to lower the lower lip from damage to the mandibular branch.

What tests tell you

Facial X-rays, CT scan, and magnetic resonance imaging aid in diagnosing the extent of injury and ruling out fractures.

How it's treated

Treatment of soft tissue facial injuries varies, depending on the type of injury and its severity. Regardless, bleeding is controlled and the wound area is cleaned and irrigated if necessary. In addition:
• superficial lacerations are sutured as soon as possible to minimize cosmetic disfigurement
• lacerations due to bites are thoroughly cleaned and irrigated; consultation with a plastic surgeon is recommended for the decision to close the wounds to minimize possible disfigurement. Animal bites require rabies evaluation and tetanus prophylaxis
• friction injuries are vigorously scrubbed with mild soap; dermabrasion may be needed
• surgical exploration and repair is conducted for large or deep lacerations
• debridement is conducted for wounds that are extensively contaminated
• antibiotic therapy is instituted to prevent and treat infection.

What to do

• Assess the patient's ABCs and intervene as necessary to stabilize him.
• Apply direct pressure to any openly bleeding wounds.
• Clean all wounds and irrigate as ordered; apply sterile dressings as appropriate.
• If the patient sustained an animal bite, question the patient about the animal and possible rabies.
• Prepare the patient for cleaning, debridement, suturing, or surgical exploration as appropriate.
• Provide comfort measures and support; patients may be anxious about how they may look after treatment.

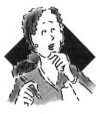

Quick quiz

1.   When preparing to assess a patient's corneal sensitivity, you should use:
    A.   a wisp of cotton.
    B.   a tissue.
    C.   a gauze pad.
    D.   ophthalmoscopy.

Answer: A. A wisp of cotton is the only safe object to use for assessing corneal sensitivity. Even though a gauze pad or tissue is soft, it can cause corneal abrasions and irritation.

2. Which cranial nerve would you expect to be possibly affected with a soft tissue injury of the face?
   A. IX
   B. VII
   C. II
   D. I

Answer: B. With a soft tissue facial injury, the most commonly affected cranial nerve would be cranial nerve VII, the facial nerve, because its branches are responsible for sensory and motor function of various facial structures.

3. Which drug should you identify as a mydriatic?
   A. pilocarpine
   B. epinephrine
   C. betaxolol
   D. timolol

Answer: B. Epinephrine is a mydriatic agent. Pilocarpine, betaxolol, and timolol are miotic agents.

Scoring

☆☆☆ If you answered all three questions correctly, give a big grin! You're tops when it comes to maxillofacial and ocular emergencies.

☆☆ If you answered two questions correctly, say "Eye caramba!" You're ahead of the competition in this emergency category.

☆ If you answered fewer than two questions correctly, don't frown. Keep your eyes on the prize as you look through the chapter again.

Environmental emergencies

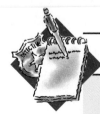

Just the facts

In this chapter, you'll learn:

♦ types of environmental emergencies

♦ assessment methods for environmental emergencies

♦ treatment for electrical shock

♦ treatment for snake bites

♦ antidotes for poisoning.

Understanding environmental emergencies

Environmental emergencies are emergencies that occur because of exposure to, or contact with, the environment. Environmental emergencies include injuries from fire, electricity, lightning, water, animals, insects, cold, and heat.

Assessment

Your environmental emergency assessment will depend on the type of injury and its location. First and foremost, assess the patient's airway, breathing and circulation (ABCs). (See *Primary survey*, page 442.)

Insects and lightning and fire—oh my! Environmental emergencies give new meaning to "the great outdoors!"

Primary survey

The primary survey consists of airway, breathing, circulation, and disability, or how alert and oriented the patient is.

A is for airway

Remember as you assess the airway of an environmental emergency patient to ensure cervical spine immobilization; any patient who has sustained a major trauma must be assumed to have a cervical spine injury until proven otherwise. The best way to achieve this is through the application of a cervical collar.

B is for breathing

The major trauma patient requires high-flow oxygen. If the patient doesn't have spontaneous respirations or has ineffective respirations, ventilate him using a bag-valve mask device until you can achieve intubation.

C is for circulation

All major trauma patients need two large-bore I.V. lines. Because these patients may require large amounts of fluids and blood, use a fluid warmer if possible. If external bleeding is present, apply direct pressure over the site.

If the patient has no pulse, cardiopulmonary resuscitation must be started. If there is a suspected injury to the heart (such as a gunshot or knife wound), the practitioner may elect to perform an emergency thoracotomy in the emergency department in an effort to repair the wound.

D is for disability

Assess the patient using the mnemonic AVPU:
- A stands for alert and oriented
- V stands for responds to voice
- P stands for responds to pain
- U stands for unresponsive.

If the patient isn't alert and oriented, conduct further assessments during the secondary survey.

Remember that ABCD is a rapid assessment designed to identify life-threatening emergencies. Treat any life-threatening emergencies before continuing your assessment.

Diagnostic tests

Diagnostic tests used to help assess environmental emergencies will also depend on the type and location of the injury and the emergency. They may include arterial blood gas (ABG) analysis to assess oxygenation and ventilation, electrocardiography to assess for possible cardiac arrhythmias, blood tests such as complete blood count (CBC), platelet count, clotting studies, liver function studies, and electrolyte, blood urea nitrogen (BUN), glucose, and creatinine levels. Bronchoscopy may be performed to visualize the condition of the trachea and bronchi in burn patients.

Practice pointers

- A practitioner, respiratory therapist, or specially trained emergency nurse draws samples for ABG analysis, usually from an arterial line if the patient has one.
- After obtaining the sample, apply pressure to the puncture site for 5 minutes and tape a gauze pad firmly in place. Regularly monitor the site for bleeding, and check the arm for signs of complications such as swelling, discoloration, pain, numbness, and tingling.

• Explain the procedure to the patient and that he may feel a needle stick with the venipuncture.
• Monitor cardiac status frequently for changes in heart rate or rhythm. Report tachycardia or evidence of an arrhythmia.
• After bronchoscopy, the patient is positioned on his side or may have the head of the bed elevated 30 degrees until the gag reflex returns. Assess respiratory status and monitor vital signs, oxygen saturation levels, and heart rhythm. Report signs and symptoms of respiratory distress, such as dyspnea, laryngospasm, or hypoxemia.
• If the patient isn't intubated, assess for return of the gag, cough, and swallow reflexes after bronchoscopy.

Treatments

Treatment for environmental emergencies may include cold application, a hypothermia-hyperthermia blanket, gastric lavage, or hemodialysis.

Temperature-related

Temperature-related treatments for environmental emergencies include cold application and use of a hyperthermia-hypothermia blanket.

Cold application

The application of cold constricts blood vessels; inhibits local circulation, suppuration, and tissue metabolism; relieves vascular congestion; slows bacterial activity in infections; reduces body temperature; and may act as a temporary anesthetic during brief, painful procedures.

Cold may be applied in dry or moist forms, but ice shouldn't be placed directly on a patient's skin because it may further damage tissue. Moist application is more penetrating than dry because moisture facilitates conduction. Devices for applying cold include an ice bag or collar, K pad (which can produce cold or heat), and chemical cold packs and ice packs. Devices for applying moist cold include cold compresses for small body areas and cold packs for large areas.

Nursing considerations
• Observe the site frequently for signs of tissue intolerance, such as blanching, mottling, cyanosis, maceration, and blisters. Also stay alert for shivering and complaints of burning or

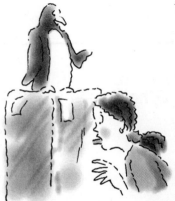

I don't think that this is what cold application is supposed to mean but, hey, you're the nurse!

numbness. If these signs or symptoms develop, discontinue treatment and notify the practitioner.
• Refill or replace the cold device as necessary to maintain the correct temperature. Change the protective cover if it becomes wet.
• Apply cold treatments cautiously on patients with impaired circulation, children, elderly patients, or patients with arthritis because of the risk of ischemic tissue damage.

Hyperthermia-hypothermia blanket

The hyperthermia-hypothermia blanket—which is actually a blanket-sized Aquamatic K pad—raises, lowers, or maintains body temperature through conductive heat or cold transfer between the blanket and the patient. It can be operated manually or automatically.

The blanket is used most commonly to reduce high fever when more conservative measures (such as baths, ice packs, and antipyretics) are unsuccessful. Its other uses include:
• maintaining normal temperature during surgery or shock
• inducing hypothermia during surgery to decrease metabolic activity and thereby reduce oxygen requirements
• reducing intracranial pressure
• controlling bleeding and intractable pain in patients with amputations, burns, or cancer
• providing warmth in cases of severe hypothermia.

Nursing considerations
• If the patient shivers excessively during hypothermia treatment, discontinue the procedure and notify the practitioner immediately; by increasing metabolism, shivering elevates body temperature.
• Avoid lowering the temperature more than 1 degree every 15 minutes to prevent premature ventricular contractions.
• Don't use pins to secure catheters, tubes, or blanket covers because an accidental puncture can result in fluid leakage and burns.

Other treatments

Other treatments for environmental emergencies include gastric lavage and hemodialysis.

Gastric lavage

After poisoning or a drug overdose, especially in patients who have central nervous system (CNS) depres-

> Be careful when you use cold treatments on children, elderly patients, or patients with arthritis. They run a high risk of ischemic tissue damage.

> If a patient shivers during hypothermia treatment, banish the blanket! His now-increasing metabolism will elevate body temperature without it.

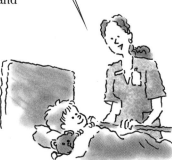

sion or an inadequate gag reflex, gastric lavage flushes the stomach and removes ingested substances through a gastric lavage tube. Gastric lavage can be continuous or intermittent. Typically, this procedure is performed in the emergency department (ED) or intensive care unit by a practitioner, gastroenterologist, or nurse; a wide-bore lavage tube is almost always inserted by a gastroenterologist.

Gastric lavage is contraindicated after ingestion of a corrosive substance (such as lye, petroleum distillates, ammonia, alkalis, or mineral acids) because the lavage tube may perforate the already compromised esophagus.

Correct lavage tube placement is essential for patient safety because accidental misplacement (in the lungs, for example) followed by lavage can be fatal. Other complications of gastric lavage include bradyarrhythmias and aspiration of gastric fluids.

Nursing considerations

• Never leave a patient alone during gastric lavage. Observe continuously for any changes in his level of consciousness (LOC), and monitor his vital signs frequently because the natural vagal response to intubation can depress his heart rate.
• If you need to restrain the patient, secure restraints on the same side of the bed or stretcher so you can free them quickly without moving to the other side of the bed.

Suck it up

• Remember to keep tracheal suctioning equipment nearby and watch closely for airway obstruction caused by vomiting or excess oral secretions. Throughout gastric lavage, you may need to suction the oral cavity frequently to ensure an open airway and prevent aspiration. For the same reasons, and if the patient doesn't exhibit an adequate gag reflex, he may require an endotracheal (ET) tube before the procedure.
• When aspirating the stomach for ingested poisons or drugs, save the contents in a labeled container to send to the laboratory for analysis along with a laboratory request form. If ordered after lavage to remove poisons or drugs, mix charcoal tablets with the irrigant (water or normal saline solution) and administer the mixture through the nasogastric (NG) tube. The charcoal will absorb remaining toxic substances. The tube may be clamped temporarily, allowed to drain via gravity, attached to intermittent suction, or removed.

Hemodialysis

The underlying mechanism in hemodialysis is differential diffusion across a semipermeable membrane. This diffusion extracts the by-products of protein metabolism (such as urea and uric acid) as well as creatinine and excess body water. This process restores or maintains the balance of the body's buffer system and electrolyte level. It's used in cases of acute poisoning such as barbiturate or analgesic overdose.

Nursing considerations

• Throughout hemodialysis, carefully monitor the patient's vital signs. Measure blood pressure at least hourly or as often as every 15 minutes if necessary.
• Perform periodic tests for clotting time on the patient's blood samples and on samples from the dialyzer.
• Continue necessary drug administration during dialysis unless the dialysate would remove the drug; if so, administer the drug after dialysis.

Common disorders

Common environmental emergencies include burns, caustic substance ingestion, hyperthermia, hypothermia, and poisoning.

Burns

A burn is a tissue injury resulting from contact with fire, a thermal chemical, or an electrical source. It can cause cellular skin damage and a systemic response that leads to altered body function.

What causes it

Thermal burns, the most common type of burn, typically result from residential fires, automobile collisions, playing with matches, improper handling of firecrackers, scalding and kitchen accidents (such as a child climbing on top of a stove or grabbing a hot iron), abuse (in children and elderly patients), and clothes catching on fire.

It's electric

Electrical burns usually result from contact with faulty electrical wiring or high-voltage power lines.

Scorching brews

Chemical burns result from contact, ingestion, inhalation, or injection of acids, alkalis, or vesicants.

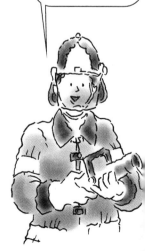

Thermal burn causes range from residential fires to kitchen accidents.

Visualizing burn depth

The most widely used system of classifying burn depth and severity categorizes burns by degree. However, it's important to remember that most burns involve tissue damage of multiple degrees and thicknesses. This illustration may help you visualize burn damage at the various degrees.

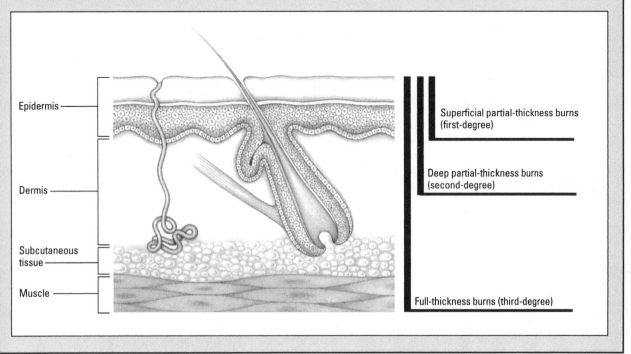

Epidermis

Dermis

Subcutaneous tissue

Muscle

Superficial partial-thickness burns (first-degree)

Deep partial-thickness burns (second-degree)

Full-thickness burns (third-degree)

How it happens

Specific pathophysiologic events depend on the cause and classification of the burn. (See *Visualizing burn depth.*) The injuring agent modifies the molecular structure of cellular proteins. Some cells die because of traumatic or ischemic necrosis. Loss of collagen cross-linking also occurs that moves intravascular fluid into interstitial spaces. Cellular injury triggers the release of mediators of inflammation, contributing to local and—in the case of major burns—systemic increases in capillary permeability.

Not just a matter of degrees anymore

Traditionally, burns were gauged only by degree. Today, however, most assessment findings use depth of tissue damage to describe a burn.

For your epidermis only

Superficial partial-thickness or first-degree burns are limited to the epidermis; these burns cause localized injury or destruction to the skin by direct or indirect contact. The barrier function of the skin remains intact.

Two differing degrees

Deep partial-thickness or second-degree burns involve destruction to the epidermis and some dermis. Pain and tactile responses remain intact, causing treatments to be very painful. The barrier function of the skin is lost.

In deep partial-thickness burns, destruction of the epidermis and dermis occur, producing blisters and mild to moderate edema and pain. The hair follicles remain intact. These burns are less painful than second-degree, superficial partial-thickness burns because the sensory neurons have undergone extensive destruction. The areas around the burn are sensitive to pain because the barrier function of the skin is lost.

Third layer, third degree

Full-thickness or third-degree burns extend through the epidermis and dermis and into the subcutaneous tissue layer. These burns may also involve muscle, bone, and interstitial tissues. Within hours, fluids and protein shift from capillary to interstitial spaces, causing edema.

What to look for

Assessment provides a general idea of burn severity. First, determine the depth of tissue damage; a partial-thickness burn damages the epidermis and part of the dermis, while a full-thickness burn also affects subcutaneous tissue.

Tracking burn traits

Signs and symptoms depend on the type of burn:
• *Superficial burn*—localized pain and erythema, usually without blisters in the first 24 hours
• *More severe superficial burn*—chills, headache, localized edema, and nausea and vomiting
• *Superficial partial-thickness burn*—thin-walled, fluid-filled blisters appear within minutes of the injury, with mild to moderate edema and pain
• *Deep partial-thickness burn*—white, waxy appearance to damaged area
• *Full-thickness burn*—white, brown, or black leathery tissue and visible thrombosed vessels due to destruction of skin elasticity, but without blisters (most commonly on the dorsum of the hand)

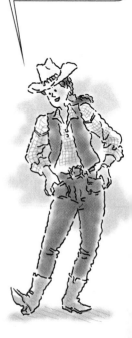

Whether white, brown, or black, full-thickness burn tissue tends to look as leathery as my boots here.

• *electrical burn*—silver-colored, raised or charred area, usually at the site of electrical contact.

Configure this

Inspection reveals the burn's location and the extent. Note its configuration:
• If the patient has a circumferential burn on an extremity, he runs the risk of edema occluding its circulation.
• If the patient has burns on his neck, he may suffer airway obstruction.
• Burns on the patient's chest can lead to restricted respiratory excursion.

More than just skin deep

Inspect the patient for other injuries that may complicate recovery, such as signs of pulmonary damage from smoke inhalation—singed nasal hairs, mucosal burns, voice changes, coughing, wheezing, soot in the mouth or nose, and darkened sputum.

What tests tell you

An assessment method that can be used to determine the size of a burn is the Rule of Nines chart, which determines the percentage of body surface area (BSA) covered by the burn. (See *Estimating burn size*, page 450.)

Burns may be classified into three categories:

 major

 moderate

minor.

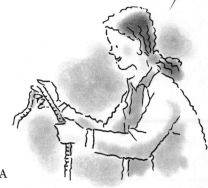

BSA coverage is the main factor used to determine burn category.

Paging Major Burns

Major burns include:
• full-thickness burns on more than 10% of BSA
• deep partial-thickness burns on more than 25% of BSA in adults and more than 20% in children
• burns on the hands, face, feet, or genitalia
• burns complicated by fractures or respiratory damage
• electrical burns
• any burn in a poor-risk patient.

Everything in moderation

Moderate burns include:
• full-thickness burns on 2% to 10% of BSA
• deep partial-thickness burns on 15% to 25% of BSA in adults and 10% to 20% of BSA in children.

Estimating burn size

Because body surface area (BSA) varies with age, two different methods are used to estimate burn size in adult and pediatric patients.

Rule of Nines

You can quickly estimate the extent of an adult patient's burn by using the Rule of Nines. This method quantifies BSA in multiples of 9 (thus, the name). To use this method, mentally transfer the burns on your patient to the body charts below. Add the corresponding percentages for each body section burned. Use the total—a rough estimate of burn extent—to calculate initial fluid replacement needs.

Lund and Browder Classification

The Rule of Nines isn't accurate for infants or children because their body shapes, and therefore BSA, differ from those of adults. For example, an infant's head accounts for about 17% of his total BSA, compared with 7% for an adult. Instead, use the Lund and Browder Classification to determine burn size for infants and children.

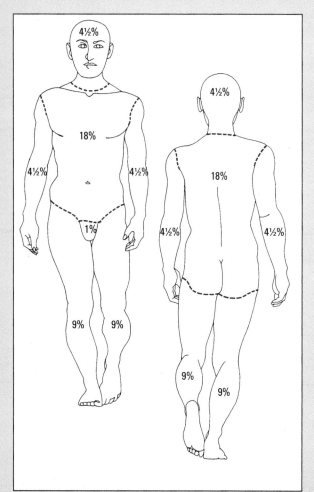

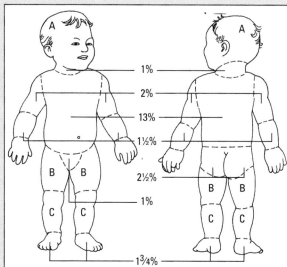

Percentage of burned body surface by age

	At birth	0 to 1 year	1 to 4 years	5 to 9 years	10 to 15 years	Adult
A: Half of head	9½%	8½%	6½%	5½%	4½%	3½%
B. Half of one thigh	2¾%	3¼%	4%	4¼%	4½%	4¾%
C. Half of one leg	2½%	2½%	2¾%	3%	3¼%	3½%

Minor yours?

Minor burns include:
• full-thickness burns on less than 2% of BSA
• deep partial-thickness burns on less than 15% of BSA in adults and less than 10% of BSA in children.

Meanwhile, back in the lab

Here are some additional diagnostic test results regarding burns:
• ABG levels may be normal in the early stages but reveal hypoxemia and metabolic acidosis later.
• Carboxyhemoglobin level may reveal the extent of smoke inhalation due to carbon monoxide presence.
• CBC may reveal a decreased hemoglobin level due to hemolysis, increased hematocrit (HCT) secondary to hemoconcentration, and leukocytosis resulting from a systemic inflammatory response or the possible development of sepsis.
• Electrolyte levels may show hyponatremia from massive fluid shifting and hyperkalemia from fluid shifting and cell lysis. Other laboratory tests may reveal elevated BUN level secondary to fluid loss or increased protein breakdown and decreased total protein and albumin levels resulting from plasma proteins leaking into the interstitial spaces.
• Creatine kinase (CK) and myoglobin levels may be elevated. Keep in mind that CK and myoglobin are helpful indicators of muscle damage; the higher the CK or myoglobin level, the more extensive the muscle damage. The presence of myoglobin in urine may lead to acute tubular necrosis.

How it's treated

Keep in mind that most EDs aren't equipped to handle full-thickness burns, and the patient will be transported to a burn center.

Initial burn treatments are based on the type of burn and may include:
• removing the source of the burn and items that retain heat, such as clothing and jewelry
• maintaining an open airway; assessing ABCs
• preparing for ET intubation if the airway is compromised
• administering supplemental humidified oxygen
• controlling active bleeding
• preventing further contamination of the burns by using sterile gloves
• covering deep partial-thickness burns that are over 30% of BSA or full-thickness burns that are over 5% of BSA with clean, dry, sterile bed sheets (because of the drastic

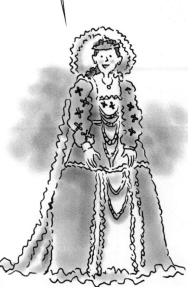

Pretty as it may be, all jewelry must be removed from burn patients because it retains heat. I guess this crown will have to go.

A closer look at fluid replacement

Fluid replacement is essential for the patient with burns because of the massive fluid shifts that occur. However, you must use extreme caution because of the risk of overreplacement.

How much?
Various formulas may be used to determine the amount of fluid replacement to be administered during the first 24 hours after a burn injury. Typically, these formulas use body weight and the percentage of body surface area (BSA) burned. One of the most common formulas used is the Parkland formula shown here:

2 to 4 ml of lactated Ringer's solution/kg
percentage of BSA burned

Over how long?
Typically, one-half of the calculated amount is administered during the first 8 hours after the injury. (Note that the time of injury—not the time of the patient's arrival in the emergency department—is used as the initial start time of the 8-hour duration.) The remaining one-half of the amount is then administered over the next 16 hours.

Which fluids?
During the first 24 hours, crystalloid solutions are commonly used because capillary permeability is greatly increased, allowing proteins to leak into the interstitial tissues. After the first 24 hours, colloid solutions can be included. Giving colloids before the initial 24-hour period would supply additional protein that could leak into the intersitial tissue.

Too much or too little?
During fluid replacement, always stay alert for indications of overreplacement and underreplacement. Signs and symptoms of heart failure and pulmonary edema suggest overreplacement. Assessment findings of hypovolemic shock suggest underreplacement.

reduction in body temperature, don't cover large burns with saline-soaked dressings)
• fluid replacement (see *A closer look at fluid replacement*)

After stabilization
• antimicrobial therapy (for all patients with major burns)
• pain medication as needed
• anti-inflammatory medications
• laboratory tests such as CBC; electrolyte, glucose, BUN, and serum creatinine levels; ABG analysis; typing and crossmatching; and urinalysis for myoglobinuria and hemoglobinuria
• close monitoring of intake, output, and vital signs
• surgical intervention, including skin grafts and thorough surgical debridement for major burns
• tetanus prophylaxis as ordered
• nutritional therapy.

Electrical burn care

Keep these tips in mind when caring for a patient with an electrical burn:
• Stay alert for ventricular fibrillation as well as cardiac and respiratory arrest caused by the electrical shock; begin cardiopulmonary resuscitation immediately.
• Get an estimate of the voltage that caused the injury.
• Tissue damage from an electrical burn is difficult to assess because internal destruction along the conduction pathway is usually greater than the surface burn would indicate.
• An electrical burn that ignites the patient's clothes may also cause thermal burns.

What to do

• Immediately assess the patient's ABCs. Institute emergency resuscitative measures as necessary. Monitor arterial oxygen saturation and serial ABG values and anticipate the need for ET intubation and mechanical ventilation if the patient's respiratory status deteriorates, especially with facial or neck burns.

Listen to the lungs

• Auscultate lung sounds for crackles, rhonchi, or stridor. Observe for signs of laryngeal edema or tracheal obstruction, including labored breathing, severe hoarseness, and dyspnea.
• Administer supplemental humidified oxygen as ordered.
• Perform oropharyngeal or tracheal suctioning as indicated by the patient's inability to clear his airway or evidence of abnormal breath sounds.
• Initiate continuous cardiac monitoring and monitor the patient's cardiac and respiratory status closely—at least every 15 minutes, or more frequently depending on his condition. Also monitor the patient for cardiac arrhythmias. Assess his LOC for changes, such as increasing confusion, restlessness, or decreased responsiveness. (See *Electrical burn care.*)

Minor burns

• Immerse the burned area in cool water (55° F [12.8° C]) or apply cool compresses.
• Cover the area with an antimicrobial agent and a nonstick bulky dressing after debridement.
• Provide a prophylactic tetanus injection as needed.

Moderate or major burns

• Provide 100% oxygen, and prepare for intubation and mechanical ventilation if necessary.

• If the patient has facial or neck burns, anticipate the need for early intubation to reduce the risk of airway obstruction.

Breathing room

• Place the patient in semi-Fowler's position to maximize chest expansion.
• Control active bleeding.
• Cover partial-thickness burns over 30% of BSA or full-thickness burns over 5% of BSA with a clean, dry, sterile bed sheet.
• Because of the drastic reduction in body temperature, don't cover large burns with saline-soaked dressings.
• Remove smoldering clothing (first soaking in saline solution if clothing is stuck to the patient's skin), rings, and other constricting items.
• Prepare the patient for emergency escharotomy of the chest and neck for deep burns or circumferential injuries to promote lung expansion.
• Assist with central venous or pulmonary artery catheter placement as needed.

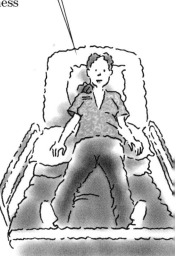

A dry, sterile bed sheet is the best thing to cover full- or partial-thickness burns.

In and out

• Insert an indwelling urinary catheter; monitor intake and output.
• Insert an NG tube to decompress the stomach and prevent aspiration of stomach contents.
• Maintain nothing-by-mouth (NPO) status.
• Watch for signs and symptoms of infection.
• For chemical burns, provide frequent wound irrigation with copious amounts of normal saline solution.
• Prepare the patient for surgical intervention, including skin grafts and more thorough surgical debridement for major burns.

Administration station

Expect to administer:
• pain medication and anti-inflammatories as needed
• analgesics I.V., rather than I.M., because tissue damage associated with the burn injury may impair absorption of the drug when given I.M.
• lactated Ringer's solution or a fluid replacement formula to prevent hypovolemic shock and maintain cardiac output
• antimicrobial therapy
• bronchodilators and mucolytics to aid in the removal of secretions.

Caustic substance ingestion

Caustic substances can be strong acids or strong bases. The most damaging substances are industrial products because they are highly concentrated. However, some common household products, including toilet bowl and drain cleaners as well as some dishwasher detergents, contain damaging caustic substances, such as sodium hydroxide and sulfuric acid.

Caustic substances are available as solids and liquids. The fact that solids stick to a moist surface (such as the lips) may prevent a person from consuming a large amount of a solid product. Because liquids don't stick, it's easier to consume more of the product and possibly damage the entire esophagus.

Regular offenders

Common acid-containing sources include:
- toilet bowl cleaning products
- automotive battery liquid
- rust-removal products
- metal-cleaning products
- cement-cleaning products
- drain-cleaning products
- soldering flux containing zinc chloride.
   Common alkaline-containing sources include:
- drain-cleaning products
- ammonia-containing products
- oven-cleaning products
- swimming pool cleaning products
- automatic dishwasher detergent
- hair relaxers
- Clinitest tablets
- bleaches
- cement.

What causes it

Ingestion of a caustic substance can be accidental, such as ingestion by a young child, or deliberate, as in an attempted suicide.

How it happens

The extent of the injury is determined by the amount of the ingested material, its concentration and form, and whether the patient has vomited or aspirated.
- After ingestion, an extreme inflammatory reaction occurs that results in erythema and edema of the superficial layers.

• Ingestion of caustic substances can cause esophageal stricture and laryngeal stenosis and can increase the risk of esophageal cancer.

• Alkaline cleaners, such as drain cleaner, are generally tasteless and odorless, allowing larger amounts to be ingested. These substances tend to cause injury to the mucosa and submucosa of the esophagus. Alkaline substances cause liquefication necrosis, a process in which necrosis continues from the superficial layers into the deeper tissues.

• Acidic cleaners, such as chlorinated household cleaners, undergo oxygenation reactions and form hydrochloric acid, which causes gastric injury if ingested. These agents cause coagulation necrosis, a process in which a protective layer forms at the site of the injury and limits its depth.

> Less odor equals more danger; because they're generally tasteless and odorless, alkaline cleaners can be ingested in large amounts.

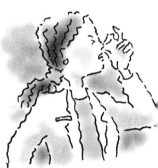

What to look for

• Abdominal pain or guarding
• Airway obstruction
• Altered mental status
• Burns around the mouth
• Diarrhea
• Drooling
• History of ingesting poisons
• Nausea and vomiting
• Odd breath odors (see *Identifying breath odor*)
• Respiratory distress
• Saliva or foaming at the mouth
• Unresponsiveness

What tests tell you

• pH testing of saliva determines whether the substance is an acid or base; however, a neutral pH can't rule out ingestion of a caustic substance. A pH of less than 2.0 (acidic substance) or greater than 12.5 (alkaline substance) indicates the potential for severe tissue damage.

• CBC and electrolyte, BUN, creatinine, and ABG levels evaluate the patient's renal status and acid-base balance as well as his blood oxygen ventilation status.

• Urinalysis can evaluate the patient's renal status because many toxic and caustic substances can be excreted through the kidneys.

• Ethanol and toxicologic screens rule out or confirm cases of suspected intentional ingestion by evaluating the levels of these substances in the blood.

• Chest X-ray may reveal mediastinitis, pleural effusions, pneumoperitoneum, and aspiration pneumonitis.

Identifying breath odor

The patient's breath odor may help determine what he ingested, especially if he arrives at the emergency department unconscious.

Breath odor	Possible substance
Alcohol	• Chloral hydrate • Ethanol • Phenols
Acetone	• Acetone • Isopropyl alcohol • Salicylates
Bitter almond	• Cyanide
Coal gas	• Carbon monoxide
Garlic	• Arsenic • Organophosphates • Phosphorus
Nonspecific	• Possible inhalant use
Wintergreen	• Methylsalicylates

• Abdominal X-ray may reveal pneumoperitoneum or ascites.

What to do

• Provide supplemental oxygen and prepare the patient for emergency ET intubation, cricothyroidotomy, or tracheostomy and mechanical ventilation if necessary.
• Initiate suicide precautions if necessary.
• Initiate NPO status.
• Obtain the patient's history, including the substance and the amount ingested.
• Assess the patient's LOC, airway, and rate, depth, and pattern of respirations.
• Auscultate the lung and heart sounds.
• Obtain the patient's vital signs, noting hypotension and fever; also observe the electrocardiogram tracing for arrhythmias.
• Don't induce emesis or perform gastric intubation and lavage, which may induce emesis; inducing emesis will reintroduce the caustic substances to the upper GI tract.

Call the pros

- Contact Poison Control or a toxicology center to get quick, accurate information, suggestions, and recommendations if necessary.
- Wash the mouth and face to remove any particles of the ingested substance.
- You may need to administer broad-spectrum antibiotics, antireflux medication, or sucralfate.

Look, listen, and ask

- Ask about chest pain.
- Inspect the oropharyngeal cavity for burns and injury.
- Observe for drooling and dysphagia.
- Ask about vomiting.
- Listen to the patient's voice to detect laryngitis, hoarseness, and dysphagia.
- Observe for stridor.
- Auscultate bowel sounds.
- Assess for abdominal pain; a boardlike, rigid abdomen; and other signs of peritonitis.
- Signs and symptoms of peritonitis, fever, chest pain, and hypotension suggest a full-thickness gastric injury or perforation, which requires immediate surgical intervention.
- Monitor serum electrolyte levels.
- Contact Child Protective Services if abuse or neglect is suspected.

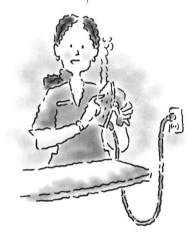

A stiff, boardlike abdomen is a sign of peritonitis.

Careful preparation

Prepare the patient for:
- flexible nasopharyngoscopy, laryngoscopy, or endoscopy to visualize the injuries
- chest X-ray to check the mediastinal width and detect free air in the mediastinum or abdomen
- neck X-ray if he has stridor
- surgical intervention, such as exploratory laparotomy or thoracotomy with possible esophagectomy, esophagogastrectomy, or gastrectomy for a full-thickness injury
- periodic esophagography with water-soluble contrast and possible esophageal stenting or dilatation with contrast to detect and correct dysphagia.

Hyperthermia

Hyperthermia, also known as *heat syndrome*, refers to an elevation in body temperature to more than 99° F (37.2° C). It may result from environmental or internal conditions that increase heat production or impair heat dissipation.

What causes it

Hyperthermia may result from excessive exercise, infection, and drug use such as amphetamines. It may also result from an impaired ability to dissipate heat. (See *Heatstroke in elderly patients.*) Factors that impair heat dissipation include:

- high temperatures or humidity
- lack of acclimatization
- excess clothing
- cardiovascular disease
- obesity
- dehydration
- sweat gland dysfunction
- drugs, such as phenothiazines and anticholinergics.

How it happens

Humans normally adjust to excessive temperatures with complex cardiovascular and neurologic changes that are coordinated by the hypothalamus. Heat loss offsets heat production to regulate body temperature. The body loses heat by the process of evapora-

---

Ages and stages

Heatstroke in elderly patients

With aging, an individual's thirst mechanism and ability to sweat decreases. These factors put the elderly patient at risk for heatstroke, especially during hot summer days. Heatstroke must be treated rapidly to prevent serious complications or death. To help prevent heatstroke, teach your older patient to follow these instructions:

- Reduce activity in hot weather, especially outdoor activity.
- Wear lightweight, loose-fitting clothing during hot weather; when outdoors, wear a hat and sunglasses, and avoid wearing dark colors that absorb sunlight.

- Drink plenty of fluids, especially water, and avoid tea, coffee, and alcohol because they can cause dehydration.
- Use air conditioning or open windows (making sure that a secure screen is in place) and use a fan to help circulate air. If the patient doesn't have air conditioning at home, suggest that, during periods of excessive heat, he go to community resources that have air conditioning, such as senior centers, libraries, and churches. Some community centers may even provide transportation for the patient.

Metabolism and increased body temperature

Central nervous system, cellular, and cardiac function are greatly affected by increased body temperature. For every 1° C (1.8° F) rise in body temperature, the body's metabolic rate increases by 13%. The body can't tolerate this level of increased metabolic rate for long, and death can quickly occur if the temperature isn't lowered.

Body temperature	Percentage of metabolic increase
38° C (100.4° F)	13
39° C (102.2° F)	26
40° C (104° F)	39
41° C (105.8° F)	52
42° C (107.6° F)	Cellular needs can't be met because of insufficient oxygen

From ENA: *Sheehy's Manual of Emergency Care,* 6th ed. Newberry, L. and Criddle, L. (eds), "Body Temperature and Metabolism," p. 505. © 2005, Reprinted with permission from Elsevier.

tion or vasodilation, which cools the body's surface by radiation, conduction, and convection. However, when heat loss mechanisms fail to offset heat production, the body retains heat.

Good-bye fluid, hello hypovolemic shock

If body temperature remains elevated, fluid loss becomes excessive and may lead to hypovolemic shock. If untreated, the patient's thermoregulatory mechanisms can fail.

Feeling hot, hot, hot

Hyperthermia occurs in varying degrees:
• Mild hyperthermia (heat cramps) occurs with excessive perspiration and loss of salt from the body.
• Moderate hyperthermia (heat exhaustion) occurs when the body is subjected to high temperatures and blood accumulates in the skin in an attempt to decrease the body's temperature. This accumulation causes a decrease in circulating blood volume, which decreases cerebral blood flow. Syncope then occurs.
• Critical hyperthermia (heatstroke) occurs when the body's temperature continues to rise and internal organs become damaged, eventually resulting in death. (See *Metabolism and increased body temperature.*)

Hyperthermia signs and symptoms

Hyperthermia, also known as *heat syndrome,* may be classified as mild (heat cramps), moderate (heat exhaustion), or critical (heatstroke). This table highlights the major assessment findings associated with each classification

Classification	Assessment findings
Mild hyperthermia (heat cramps)	• Mild agitation (central nervous system findings otherwise normal) • Mild hypertension • Moist, cool skin and muscle tenderness; involved muscle groups possibly hard and lumpy • Muscle twitching and spasms • Nausea, abdominal cramps • Report of prolonged activity in a very warm or hot environment without adequate salt intake • Tachycardia • Temperature ranging from 99° to 102° F (37.2° to 38.9° C)
Moderate hyperthermia (heat exhaustion)	• Dizziness • Headache • Hypotension • Muscle cramping • Nausea and vomiting • Oliguria • Pale, moist skin • Rapid, thready pulse • Syncope or confusion • Thirst • Weakness • Temperature elevated up to 104° F (40° C)
Critical hyperthermia (heatstroke)	• Atrial or ventricular tachycardia • Confusion, combativeness, delirium • Fixed, dilated pupils • Hot, dry, reddened skin • Loss of consciousness • Seizures • Tachypnea • Temperature greater than 106° F (41.1° C)

What to look for

Assessment findings vary with the degree of hyperthermia. (See *Hyperthermia signs and symptoms.*)

What tests tell you

No single diagnostic test confirms hyperthermia, but these test results may help support the diagnosis:
• ABG results may reveal respiratory alkalosis and hypoxemia.
• CBC may reveal leukocytosis and increased HCT secondary to hemoconcentration.
• Electrolyte levels may show hypokalemia. Other blood studies may reveal elevated BUN level, increased bleeding and clotting times, and fibrinolysis.
• Urinalysis may show concentrated urine with elevated protein levels, tubular casts, and myoglobinuria.

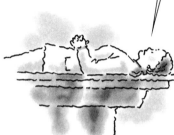

We could probably all use some rest in a cool environment, but for hyperthermia patients it's of the utmost importance.

How it's treated

Mild or moderate hyperthermia is treated by allowing the patient to rest in a cool environment. Oral or I.V. fluid and electrolyte replacement is administered as ordered.

Critical measures

Measures for treating critical hyperthermia include:
• removing the patient's clothing and applying cool water to the skin, and then fanning the patient with cool air
• controlling shivering by giving diazepam (Valium) or chlorpromazine (Thorazine)
• applying hypothermia blankets and ice packs to the groin and axillae if necessary
• continuing treatment until the patient's body temperature drops to 102.2° F (39° C).

In addition to the cool-down

Supportive measures for hyperthermia include:
• oxygen therapy
• central venous pressure and pulmonary artery wedge pressure monitoring
• ET intubation, if necessary.

What to do

• Assess the patient's ABCs and initiate emergency resuscitative measures as indicated. Remove as much of the patient's clothing as possible.
• Assess oxygen saturation and administer supplemental oxygen as indicated and ordered. Monitor the patient's pulmonary status closely, including respiratory rate and depth and lung sounds; anticipate the need for ET intubation and mechanical ventilation if respiratory status deteriorates.

• Monitor the patient's vital signs continuously, especially core body temperature. Although the goal is to reduce the patient's temperature rapidly, too rapid a reduction can lead to vasoconstriction, which can cause shivering. Shivering increases metabolic demand and oxygen consumption and should be prevented if possible.
• Employ external cooling measures, such as cool, wet sheets; tepid baths; and cooling blankets.
• Assess the patient's neurologic and cardiac status closely, including heart rate and rhythm. Institute continuous cardiac monitoring to evaluate for arrhythmias secondary to electrolyte imbalances. Monitor hemodynamic parameters; assess peripheral circulation, including skin color, peripheral pulses, and capillary refill.
• Monitor fluid and electrolyte balance and laboratory test results. Assess renal function studies to evaluate for rhabdomyolysis.

Hypothermia

Hypothermia is defined as a core body temperature below 95° F (35° C). It may be classified as:
• *mild*—89.6° to 95° F (32° to 35° C)
• *moderate*—86° to 89.6° F (30° to 32° C)
• *severe*—77° to 86° F (25° to 30° C), which can be fatal.

What causes it

Hypothermia commonly results from near drowning in cold water, prolonged exposure to cold temperatures, disease or debility that alters homeostasis, or administration of large amounts of cold blood or blood products.

Likely candidates

The risk of serious cold injury, especially hypothermia, is higher in patients who are:
• young
• elderly
• lacking in insulating body fat
• wearing wet or inadequate clothing
• abusing drugs or alcohol or smoking
• suffering from cardiac disease
• fatigued
• malnourished with a depletion of calorie reserves.

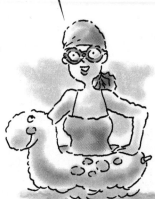

Hypothermia can result from near drowning in cold water—I may look silly, but at least I'm not taking any chances!

How it happens

In hypothermia, metabolic changes slow the functions of most major organ systems, resulting in decreased renal blood flow and decreased glomerular filtration. Vital organs are physiologically affected. Severe hypothermia results in depression of cerebral blood flow, diminished oxygen requirements, reduced cardiac output, and decreased arterial pressure.

What to look for

Obtaining the history of a patient with a cold injury may reveal:
• cause of hypothermia
• temperature to which the patient was exposed
• length of exposure.

Temperature dependent

Assessment findings in a patient with hypothermia vary with the patient's body temperature:
• Mild hypothermia includes severe shivering, slurred speech, and amnesia.
• Moderate hypothermia includes unresponsiveness, peripheral cyanosis, and muscle rigidity. If the patient was improperly rewarmed, he may show signs of shock.
• Severe hypothermia includes absence of palpable pulses, no audible heart sounds, dilated pupils, and a rigor mortis-like state. In addition, ventricular fibrillation and a loss of deep tendon reflexes are common. (See *Clinical findings and body temperature.*)

What tests tell you

• Technetium 99m pertechnetate scanning shows perfusion defects and deep tissue damage and can be used to identify nonviable bone.
• Doppler and plethysmographic studies help determine pulses and the extent of frostbite after thawing.

How it's treated

Treatment for hypothermia consists of supportive measures and specific rewarming techniques, including:
• passive rewarming (when the patient rewarms on his own)
• active external rewarming with heating blankets, warm water immersion, heated objects such as water bottles, and radiant heat
• active core rewarming with heated I.V. fluids, genitourinary tract irrigation, extracorporeal rewarming, hemodialysis, and peritoneal, gastric, and mediastinal lavage.

Clinical findings and body temperature

A patient's signs and symptoms can change, depending on his core body temperature. This chart lists body temperature ranges and their associated signs and symptoms.

Body temperature	Signs and symptoms
96° to 99° F (35.6° to 37.2° C)	• Loss of manual coordination • Shivering
91° to 95° F (32.8° to 35° C)	• Amnesia • Violent shivering • Slurred speech
86° to 90° F (30° to 32.2° C)	• Decreased shivering • Cyanosis • Muscular rigidity
< 86° (< 30° C)	• Atrial fibrillation • Rewarming shock
81° to 85° F (27.2° to 29.4° C)	• Patient is irrational • Stupor • Decreased pulse and respirations
78° to 80° F (25.6° to 26.7° C)	• Erratic heartbeat • Coma
< 81° F (< 27.2° C)	• Ventricular fibrillation
< 78° F (< 25.6° C)	• Cardiopulmonary arrest

From ENA: *Sheehy's Manual of Emergency Care,* 6th ed. Newberry, L. and Criddle, L. (eds), "Clinical Manifestations of Hypothermia," p. 503. © 2005, Reprinted with permission from Elsevier.

Cardiac concerns

Arrhythmias that develop usually convert to normal sinus rhythm with rewarming. If the patient has no pulse or respirations, cardiopulmonary resuscitation (CPR) is needed until rewarming raises the core temperature to at least 89.6° F (32° C).

Monitoring dependent

The administration of oxygen, ET intubation, controlled ventilation, I.V. fluids, and treatment for metabolic acidosis depend on test results and careful patient monitoring.

What to do

• Assess the patient's ABCs and initiate CPR as appropriate. Keep in mind that hypothermia helps protect the brain from anoxia, which normally accompanies prolonged cardiopulmonary arrest. Therefore, even if the patient has been unresponsive for a long time, CPR may resuscitate him, especially after a cold water near drowning.
• Administer supplemental oxygen, and prepare for ET intubation and mechanical ventilation if necessary.
• Initiate continuous cardiac monitoring.
• Initiate CPR if necessary.
• Assist with rewarming techniques as necessary. (In moderate to severe hypothermia, only experienced personnel should attempt aggressive rewarming.)
• During rewarming, provide supportive measures as ordered, including mechanical ventilation and heated, humidified therapy to maintain tissue oxygenation, and I.V. fluids that have been warmed with a warming coil to correct hypotension and maintain urine output.
• Continuously monitor the patient's core body temperature and other vital signs during and after initial rewarming. Continuously monitor his cardiac status, including continuous cardiac monitoring, for evidence of arrhythmias.
• If using a hyperthermia blanket, discontinue the warming when core body temperature is within 1° to 2° F (0.6° to 1.1° C) of the desired temperature. The patient's temperature will continue to rise even when the device is turned off.

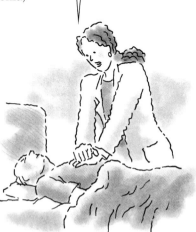

CPR is a-OK for hypothermia victims. Even when they've been unresponsive for a while, their lack of brain anoxia provides a chance for survival.

As time goes by

• If the patient has been hypothermic for longer than 45 to 60 minutes, administer additional fluids as ordered to compensate for the expansion of the vascular space that occurs during vasodilation in rewarming. Monitor the patient's heart rate and hemodynamic parameters closely to evaluate fluid needs and response to treatment.
• Monitor the patient's hourly output, fluid balance, and serum electrolyte levels, especially potassium. Stay alert for signs and symptoms of hyperkalemia. If hyperkalemia occurs, administer calcium chloride, sodium bicarbonate, glucose, and insulin as ordered. Anticipate the need for sodium polystyrene sulfonate

(Kayexalate) enemas. If his potassium level is extremely elevated, prepare the patient for dialysis.

Poisoning

Poisoning refers to inhalation, ingestion, and injection of, or skin contamination from, any harmful substance. It's a common environmental emergency. In the United States, about 1 million people are poisoned annually—800 of them fatally. The prognosis depends on the amount of poison absorbed, its toxicity, and the time interval between poisoning and treatment. (See *Poisoning facts*.)

What causes it

Because of their curiosity and ignorance, children are the most common poison victims. In fact, accidental poisoning (usually from the ingestion of salicylates [aspirin], cleaning agents, insecticides, paints, cosmetics, and plants) is the fourth leading cause of death in children.

In adults, poisoning is most common among chemical company employees—particularly those in companies that use chlorine, carbon dioxide, hydrogen sulfide, nitrogen dioxide, and ammonia—and in companies that ignore safety standards. Other causes of poisoning in adults include improper cooking, canning, and storage of food; ingestion of or skin contamination from plants (for example, dieffenbachia, mistletoe, azalea, and philodendron); and accidental or intentional drug overdose (usually barbiturates) or chemical ingestion.

How it happens

The pathophysiology of poisons depends on the substance that's inhaled or ingested. The extent of damage depends on the pH of the substance, the amount ingested, its form (solid or liquid), and the length of exposure to it.

Substances with an alkaline pH cause tissue damage by liquefaction necrosis, which softens the tissue. Acids produce coagulation necrosis. Coagulation necrosis denatures (changes the molecular composition of) proteins when the substance contacts tissue. This limits the extent of the injury by preventing penetration of the acid into the tissue.

The mechanism of action for inhalants is unknown, but they're believed to act on the CNS similarly to a very potent anesthetic. Hydrocarbons sensitize the myocardial tissue and allow it to be sensitive to catecholamines, resulting in arrhythmias.

Ages and stages

Poisoning facts

Adolescents tend to overdose on over-the-counter drugs instead of prescription drugs. Elderly patients who overdose do so usually because of polypharmacy, improper use of their prescribed medication, improper storage of the medication (not in its original container), or mistaking the identity of the medication.

It doesn't look tasty to me, but household plant ingestion is one of the most common poisoning sources in children.

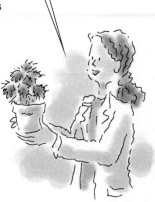

Pinpointing poison's effects

Review the assessment findings and possible toxins listed below to help determine what type of poison is causing your patient's signs and symptoms.

Agitation, delirium
Alcohol, amphetamines, atropine, barbiturates, neostigmine (Prostigmin), scopolamine (Scopace)

Coma
Atropine, barbiturates, bromide, carbon monoxide, chloral hydrate, ethanol, paraldehyde, salicylates, scopolamine

Constricted pupils
Barbiturates, chloral hydrate, morphine, propoxyphene

Diaphoresis
Alcohol, fluoride, insulin, physostigmine

Diarrhea, nausea, vomiting
Alcohol (ethanol, methanol, ethylene glycol), cardiac glycosides, heavy metals (lead, arsenic), morphine and its analogues, salicylates

Dilated pupils
Alcohol, amphetamines, belladonna alkaloids (such as atropine and scopolamine), botulinum toxin, cocaine, cyanide, ephedrine, glutethimide, meperidine (Demerol), parasympathomimetics

Dry mouth
Antihistamines, belladonna alkaloids, botulinum toxin, morphine, phenothiazines, tricyclic antidepressants

Extrapyramidal tremor
Phenothiazines

Hematemesis
Fluoride, mercuric chloride, phosphorus, salicylates

Kussmaul's respirations
Ethanol, ethylene glycol, methanol, salicylates

Partial or total blindness
Methanol

Pink skin
Atropine (flushed, dry skin), carbon monoxide, cyanide, phenothiazines

Seizures
Alcohol (ethanol, methanol, ethylene glycol), amphetamines, carbon monoxide, cholinesterase inhibitors, hydrocarbons, phenothiazines, propoxyphene, salicylates, strychnine

What to look for

The patient's history should reveal the poison's source and form of exposure (ingestion, inhalation, injection, or skin contact). Assessment findings vary with the poison. (See *Pinpointing poison's effects*.)

What tests tell you

• Toxicology studies (including drug screens) of poison levels in the mouth, vomitus, urine, stool, or blood, or on the victim's hands or clothing, confirm the diagnosis. If possible, have the family or patient bring the container holding the poison to the ED for comparable study.
• In inhalation poisoning, chest X-rays may show aspiration pneumonia. In petroleum distillate inhalation, they may show pulmonary infiltrates or edema. Abdominal X-rays may reveal iron pills or other radiopaque substances.

Common antidotes used in the ED

Here are some common antidotes used in the emergency department (ED) to treat accidental or intentional poisoning.

Poison	Antidote
Acetaminophen	acetylcysteine (Mucomyst)
Arsenic, mercury, and lead	dimercaprol (BAL)
Benzodiazepines	flumazenil (Romazicon)
Beta-adrenergic blockers and calcium channel blockers	glucagon
Cardiac glycosides	digoxin immune FAB (Digibind)
Iron	deferoxamine (Desferal)
Lead	edetate calcium disodium (EDTA [Calcium Disodium Versenate])
Methanol	folic acid (Folate) or leucovorin
Methanol and ethylene glycol	ethanol
Organophosphates and carbamates	atropine

Adapted from Jenkins, J., and Braen, G. *Manual of Emergency Medicine,* 5th ed. Philadelphia: Lippincott Williams & Wilkins, 2005.

• ABG analysis, serum electrolyte levels, and CBC are used to evaluate oxygenation, ventilation, and the metabolic status of seriously poisoned patients.

What to do

• Initial treatment includes emergency resuscitation, support of the patient's ABCs, and prevention of further poison absorption. Secondary treatment consists of continuing supportive or symptomatic care and, when possible, administration of a specific antidote. (See *Common antidotes used in the ED.*)
• A poisoning victim who exhibits altered LOC routinely receives oxygen, glucose, and naloxone (Narcan). Activated charcoal is effective in eliminating many toxic substances. Specific treatment depends on the poison.

- Carefully monitor the patient's vital signs and LOC. If necessary, begin CPR.
- Depending on the poison, prevent further absorption by administering activated charcoal, inducing emesis, or by administering gastric lavage and cathartics (magnesium sulfate). For specific treatment, contact the poison center (local or national). The treatment's effectiveness depends on the speed of absorption and the time elapsed between ingestion and removal.

Emesis nemesis

- Never induce emesis if you suspect corrosive acid poisoning, if the patient is unconscious or has seizures, or if the gag reflex is impaired, even in a conscious patient. Instead, neutralize the poison by instilling the appropriate antidote by an NG tube. Common antidotes include milk, magnesium salts (Milk of magnesia), activated charcoal, or other chelating agents, such as deferoxamine and edetate disodium.
- When possible, add the antidote to water or juice.
- To perform gastric lavage, instill 30 ml of fluid by NG tube, and then aspirate the liquid; repeat until the aspirate is clear. Save vomitus and aspirate for analysis. (To prevent aspiration in the unconscious patient, an ET tube should be in place before lavage.)

Enter the I.V.

- If several hours have passed since the patient ingested the poison, use large quantities of I.V. fluids to force the poison through the kidneys to be excreted. The kind of fluid you use depends on the patient's acid-base balance and cardiovascular status and on the flow rate necessary for effective diuresis of poison.
- If ingested poisoning is severe and requires peritoneal dialysis or hemodialysis, assist as necessary.

Give him some air

- To prevent further absorption of inhaled poison, remove the patient to fresh or uncontaminated air. Provide supplemental oxygen and, if needed, intubation. To prevent further absorption from skin contamination, remove the clothing covering the contaminated skin and immediately flush the area with large amounts of water.
- If the patient is in severe pain, give analgesics as ordered; frequently monitor fluid intake and output, vital signs, and LOC.

• Keep the patient warm and provide support in a quiet environment.
• If the poison was ingested intentionally, refer the patient for
counseling to help prevent future attempts at suicide.

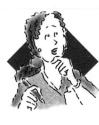

Quick quiz

1. Your patient has partial- and full-thickness burn injuries to
his anterior chest, anterior abdomen, and entire right arm. Using
the Rule of Nines, the percent of total body surface area involved
can be estimated at:
    A.   18%.
    B.   27%.
    C.   45%.
    D.   50%.

Answer: B. The anterior chest and abdomen constitute 18% of
the BSA, and the entire right arm is 9%, for a total of 27%.

2. A patient admitted to the ED is suspected of taking an overdose of atropine. Which clinical finding would you look for?
    A.   Kussmaul's respirations
    B.   Diarrhea and nausea and vomiting
    C.   Flushed, dry skin
    D.   Extrapyramidal tremors

Answer: C. A patient who has overdosed on atropine will have
flushed, dry skin and dilated pupils.

3. Your patient has a core body temperature of 80° F (26.7° C).
Which classification of hypothermia is this?
    A.   Low
    B.   Mild
    C.   Moderate
    D.   Severe

Answer: D. Severe hypothermia is a core body temperature of
77° to 86° F (25° to 30° C).

4. An unconscious patient is admitted to the ED with a very
strong wintergreen odor on his breath. What might he have
ingested?
    A.   Ethanol
    B.   Acetone
    C.   Methylsalicylates
    D.   Cyanide

Answer: C. If a patient has ingested methylsalicylates, his breath will have a wintergreen odor.

Scoring

☆☆☆ If you answered all four questions correctly, stop and smell the roses! You're quite erudite when it comes to environmental emergencies.

☆☆ If you answered three questions correctly, breathe in the smell of success! Hopefully lightning will strike again for you in the next chapter.

☆ If you answered fewer than three questions correctly, don't let it rain on your parade. Review the chapter again and give it another try.

Shock and multisystem trauma emergencies

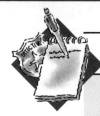

Just the facts

In this chapter, you'll learn:

♦ emergency assessment of the patient experiencing shock and multisystem trauma

♦ diagnostic tests and procedures for shock and multisystem trauma

♦ shock disorders and multisystem trauma in the emergency department and their treatments.

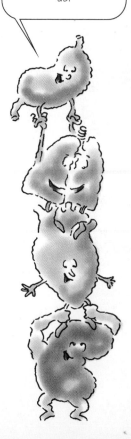

You hurt one of us, you hurt all of us!

Understanding shock and multisystem trauma emergencies

Shock and multisystem trauma are emergencies that can affect the control of every system in the body. Due to their wide-ranging effects, these conditions are commonly life-threatening.

Truly shocking effects

Shock involves a disruption in the components responsible for maintaining normal circulation and cell perfusion. These components include adequate circulating volume, cardiac output, and peripheral vascular resistance. Blood pressure also plays a role. With shock, oxygenation and perfusion of the cells are altered.

Shock is typically categorized by the underlying mechanism affected. Types of shock include:

• hypovolemic
• cardiogenic
• distributive (which includes neurogenic, septic, and anaphylactic)
• obstructive.

Here, there, and everywhere

Multisystem trauma involves injury or damage in more than one body area or organ system. Consequently, it can cause widespread dysfunction.

Assessment

When faced with an emergency involving shock or multisystem trauma, assess the patient quickly yet thoroughly, always being alert for subtle changes that might indicate a potential deterioration in the patient's condition. Patients with shock or multisystem trauma require immediate attention because of possible wide-ranging effects on one or more body systems; prompt attention to the patient's vital functions is essential. Perform a primary and then a secondary assessment; you may need to intervene at any time.

When you've completed the assessment and the patient is stabilized, obtain a patient history. If you can't interview the patient because of his condition, gather history information from his medical record. In some cases, you may need to ask the patient's family or the emergency medical response team that transported him to the emergency department (ED).

Primary assessment

A primary survey consists of assessing the patient's airway (ensuring cervical spine immobilization), the patient's breathing (all major trauma patients require high-flow oxygen; the patient may need ventilation), the patient's circulation (the patient may require large amounts of fluids; cardiopulmonary resuscitation may be required), and disability (assess the patient's alertness and orientation and if he responds to voices or pain).

Secondary assessment

Secondary assessment involves a more in-depth evaluation of the patient's status after the ABCs have been maintained. Typically, this survey includes vital signs, history, head-to-toe physical examination, and inspection of the patient's posterior surfaces.

When the secondary assessment is complete, you can start on a more focused assessment of each body system. (See previous body-system chapters for specific assessment information.)

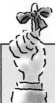

Memory jogger

In the secondary survey, continue the alphabet from the primary survey to guide your assessment and care. After primary survey (*ABCD*) comes:

E: Expose and Environment

• Remove the patient's clothing to assess for obvious injuries or problems.

• Provide blankets or warming lights to prevent chilling.

F: Full vitals, Five interventions, Family presence

• Obtain a complete set of vital signs.

• Anticipate the need for five interventions—pulse oximetry, cardiac monitoring, urinary catheterization, gastric intubation, laboratory tests.

• Facilitate family presence.

G: Giving comfort

• Provide verbal reassurance as warranted.

• Use touch to help alleviate anxiety and fear.

• Manage pain.

H: Head-to-toe assessment

• Complete a head-to-toe assessment.

• Observe for wounds, ecchymosis, deformities, and impaired movement or function.

I: Inspection of posterior

• Log roll the patient to his side.

• Inspect the posterior areas for wounds, bruising, and deformities.

• Palpate areas for tenderness and pain.

From *Trauma Nursing Core Course,* 5th ed. Des Plaines, Ill.: Emergency Nurses Association. © 2000, Reprinted with permission from the Emergency Nurses Association.

Diagnostic tests

Numerous diagnostic tests may be performed, depending on the patient's underlying condition and overall status. Blood studies and radiologic and imaging studies are commonly performed.

Additional tests may be used based on facility policy and body area or systems affected. For example, angiography may be done to evaluate for vessel injury; more specifically, cerebral angiography may be used to evaluate cerebral blood flow. Cardiac monitoring and hemodynamic monitoring may be used to evaluate the patient's cardiac function and overall hemodynamic status.

Blood studies

Although specific blood studies may vary among facilities, some more common studies ordered for patients with shock or multisystem trauma include:
- complete blood count (CBC)
- electrolytes
- coagulation studies, such as prothrombin time (PT) and partial thromboplastin time (PTT)
- serum amylase, lipase, and lactate
- liver function tests
- blood cultures.

Less common but important

In addition, arterial blood gas (ABG) analysis is commonly performed to evaluate the patient's acid-base balance. In trauma situations, a blood type and cross match is done in anticipation of the need for a blood and blood products transfusion.

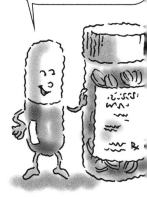

Some medications may influence blood test results, so be sure to check your patient's medication history.

Practice pointers

- Tell the patient that the test requires a blood sample.
- Check the patient's medication history for medications that might influence test results.

Radiologic and imaging studies

Specific radiologic and imaging studies completed for these patients depend on the underlying mechanism causing the shock and the body areas or organs affected by the trauma. The most common studies include X-rays of the chest, pelvis, cervical spine, thoracic and lumbar spine, and extremities. In addition, computed tomography (CT) scan of the head and abdomen may be performed.

Practice pointers

- Prepare the patient for the X-ray or CT scan to be performed, including the reason for the study.
- Verify that the order includes pertinent history, such as trauma, and identifies sites of injury, tenderness, or pain.
- Make sure that all jewelry is removed from the patient.

Treatments

Treatments vary depending on the specific type of shock or the areas of injury with multisystem trauma. Common treatment measures include blood transfusion therapy, drug therapy, and surgery.

Other treatments relate to the organ system affected. For example, diagnostic peritoneal lavage may be used to evaluate abdominal trauma. Oxygen therapy and ventilatory support may be required to ensure adequate respiratory function and oxygenation and treat respiratory associated injuries. Fluid replacement therapy is initiated to restore fluid and electrolyte balance.

I know that "packed" RBCs are highly valued for transfusions, but this seems a little extreme.

Blood transfusion therapy

Blood transfusions treat decreased hemoglobin (Hb) level and hematocrit (HCT). A whole blood transfusion replenishes the circulatory system's volume and oxygen-carrying capacity by increasing the mass of circulating red blood cells (RBCs). It's usually used in cases of hemorrhage.

Packed RBCs, a blood component from which 80% of the plasma has been removed, are transfused to restore the circulatory system's oxygen-carrying capacity. Packed RBCs are used when the patient has a normal blood volume to avoid possible fluid and circulatory overload. (See *Guide to whole blood and cellular products*, pages 478 to 481.)

Whole blood and packed RBCs contain cellular debris, requiring in-line filtration during administration. Washed packed RBCs, commonly used for patients previously sensitized to transfusions, are rinsed with a special solution that removes white blood cells and platelets, thus decreasing the chance of a transfusion reaction.

It may be hard to stomach, but the patient's right of self-determination means he can choose to refuse a blood transfusion.

Refusin' transfusion

In some cases, a patient may refuse a blood transfusion; for example, a Jehovah's Witness may refuse one because of his religious beliefs. A competent adult has the right to refuse treatment. You may be able to use other treatment options if the patient refuses the blood transfusion, such as providing erythropoietin, iron, and folic acid supplements before and after surgery. Using available alternative treatments supports the patient's right of self-determination and honors his wishes. A court order requiring the patient to undergo transfusion therapy can be obtained when the patient's mental competency is questionable.

Nursing considerations
• Verify the practitioner's orders and signed consent.

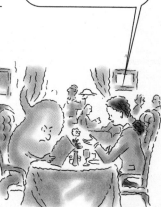

(Text continues on page 480.)

Guide to whole blood and cellular products

This chart lists blood components along with indications for their use and nursing considerations.

Blood component	Indications
Whole blood	
Complete (pure) blood	• To treat symptomatic chronic anemia • To prevent morbidity from anemia in patients at greatest risk for tissue hypoxia • To control active bleeding with signs and symptoms of hypovolemia • To aid preoperatively; hemoglobin less than 9 g/dl with possibility of major blood loss • To treat sickle cell disease
Packed red blood cells (RBCs)	
Same RBC mass as whole blood with 80% of the plasma removed	• To treat symptomatic chronic anemia • To prevent morbidity from anemia in patients at greatest risk for tissue hypoxia • To control active bleeding with signs and symptoms of hypovolemia • To aid preoperatively; hemoglobin less than 9 g/dl with possibility of major blood loss • To treat sickle cell disease
Leukocyte-poor RBCs	
Same as packed RBCs except 70% of the leukocytes are removed	• To treat symptomatic anemia • To prevent morbidity from anemia in patients at greatest risk for tissue hypoxia • To control active bleeding with signs and symptoms of hypovolemia • To aid preoperatively; hemoglobin less than 9 g/dl with possibility of major blood loss • To treat sickle cell disease • To prevent febrile reactions from leukocyte antibodies • To treat immunosuppressed patients • To restore RBCs to patients who have had two or more nonhemolytic febrile reactions

Nursing considerations

Compatibility is ABO identical.
Group A receives A; group B receives B; group AB receives AB; group O receives O. Rh type must match.
Use blood administration tubing. You can infuse rapidly in emergencies, but adjust the rate to the patient's condition and the transfusion order, and don't infuse over more than 4 hours.
Whole blood is seldom administered other than in emergency situations because its components can be extracted and administered separately.
Warm blood if giving a large quantity.
Use only with normal saline.
Monitor the patient's volume status for fluid overload.

Compatibility: Group A receives A or O; group B receives B or O; group AB receives AB, A, B, or O; group O receives O. Rh type must match.
Use blood administration tubing to infuse over more than 4 hours.
Packed RBCs shouldn't be used for anemic conditions correctable by nutrition or drug therapy.
Use only with normal saline.

• Compatibility: Group A receives A or O; group B receives B or O; group AB receives AB, A, B, or O; group O receives O. Rh type must match.
• Use blood administration tubing. May require a microaggregate filter (40-micron filter) for hard-spun, leukocyte-poor RBCs.
• Cells expire 24 hours after washing.
• Leukocyte-poor RBCs shouldn't be used for anemic conditions correctable by nutrition or drug therapy.

(continued)

Guide to whole blood and cellular products *(continued)*

Blood component	Indications
White blood cells (WBCs, leukocytes)	
Whole blood with all the RBCs and 80% of the plasma removed	• To treat sepsis that's unresponsive to antibiotics (especially if the patient has positive blood cultures or a persistent fever exceeding 101° F [38.3° C]) and life-threatening granulocytopenia (granulocyte count less than 500/µl)
Platelets	
Platelet sediment from RBCs or plasma	• To treat bleeding due to critically decreased circulating platelet counts or functionally abnormal platelets • To prevent bleeding due to thrombobytopenia • To treat a patient with a platelet count less than 50,000/µl before surgery or a major invasive procedure

• Obtain baseline vital signs and start an I.V. line if one isn't already started. Use a 20G or larger-diameter catheter.

• Identify the patient and check the blood bag identification number, ABO blood group, Rh compatibility, and blood product expiration date. This step should be confirmed by another licensed professional. Follow your facility's policy for blood administration.

• Obtain the patient's vital signs after the first 15 minutes and then every 30 minutes (or according to your facility's policy) for the remainder of transfusion therapy.

• Record the date and time of the transfusion (time started and completed); the type and amount of transfusion product; the type and gauge of the catheter used for infusion; the patient's vital signs before, during, and after transfusion; a verification check of all identification data (including the names of individuals verifying the information); and the patient's response.

• Obtain follow-up laboratory tests as ordered to determine the effectiveness of therapy.

• For rapid blood replacement, use a pressure bag or rapid transfusion device if necessary. Be aware that excessive pressure may develop, leading to broken blood vessels and extravasation with

Nursing considerations

• Compatibility: Group A receives A or O; group B receives B or O; group AB receives AB, A, B, or O; group O receives O. Rh type must match. WBCs are preferably human leukocyte antigen (HLA)-compatible, although compatibility isn't necessary unless the patient is HLA-sensitized from previous transfusions.
• Use blood administration tubing. One unit daily is given for 4 to 6 days or until infection clears.
• WBC infusion may induce fever and chills. To prevent this reaction, the patient is premedicated with antihistamines, acetaminophen (Tylenol), or steroids. If fever occurs, give an antipyretic, but don't stop the transfusion. Reduce the flow rate for the patient's comfort.
• Because reactions are common, administer slowly over 2 to 4 hours. Check the patient's vital signs and assess him every 15 minutes throughout the transfusion.
• Give the transfusion with antibiotics to treat infection.

• Compatibility: ABO should be identical. Rh-negative recipients should receive Rh-negative platelets.
• Use a blood filter or leukocyte-reduction filter. Don't use a microaggregate filter.
• Platelet transfusions aren't usually indicated for thrombocytopenic autoimmune thrombocytopenia or thrombocytopenia purpura unless the patient has a life-threatening hemorrhage.
• Patients with a history of platelet reaction require premedication with antipyretics and antihistamines.
• Use single donor platelets if the patient has a need for repeated transfusions.

hematoma and hemolysis of the infusing RBCs. Large-gauge catheters and central lines are preferred for rapid and pressured transfusions.
• If administering platelets or fresh frozen plasma, administer each unit immediately after obtaining it. Although some microaggregate filters can be used for up to 10 units of blood, always replace the filter and tubing if more than 1 hour elapses between transfusions. When administering multiple units of blood under pressure, use a blood warmer to avoid hypothermia.
• Document the patient's transfusion reaction and the treatment required (if any).
• Notify the practitioner if the patient refuses the blood transfusion.

Drug therapy

Drug therapy for shock and multisystem trauma also varies depending on the patient's underlying condition. For example, antibiotics may be used to treat septic shock or multisystem trauma, while vasopressors may be considered to treat the various forms of shock.

In cases of shock and multisystem trauma, drugs are commonly required to support blood flow to the vital organs, such as the heart and brain. These drugs include:

- epinephrine (Adrenalin)
- vasopressin (Pitressin)
- norepinephrine (Levophed)
- dopamine
- dobutamine (Dobutrex)
- inamrinone
- milrinone (Primacor)
- calcium
- cardiac glycosides
- nitroglycerin (Nitro-Bid)
- sodium nitroprusside (Nitropress).

Surgery

Surgery also depends on the patient's underlying condition. For example, surgery may be indicated to repair a laceration of a wound or organ, repair a fracture, insert pins or a fixation device to stabilize bone, or incise and drain an abscess. Exploratory surgery may be necessary to identify the source of hemorrhage in a patient experiencing hypovolemic shock.

Common disorders

In the ED, you're likely to encounter patients with anaphylactic shock, cardiogenic shock, hypovolemic shock, neurogenic shock, septic shock, or multisystem trauma. Regardless of the disorder, your first priority is to ensure ABCs.

Anaphylactic shock

Anaphylactic shock, also called *anaphylaxis*, is an acute, potentially life-threatening type I (immediate) hypersensitivity reaction marked by the sudden onset of rapidly progressive *urticaria* (vascular swelling in skin accompanied by itching) and respiratory distress.

What causes it

Anaphylaxis usually results from ingestion of, or other systemic exposure to, sensitizing drugs or other substances. Such substances may include:

- serums (usually horse serum)
- vaccines
- allergen extracts
- enzymes, such as L-asparaginase
- hormones
- penicillin or other antibiotics (which induce anaphylaxis in 1 to 4 of every 10,000 patients treated, most likely after parenteral administration or prolonged therapy and in patients with an inherited tendency to food or drug allergy)
- sulfonamides
- local anesthetics
- salicylates
- polysaccharides
- diagnostic chemicals, such as sulfobromophthalein, sodium dehydrocholate, and radiographic contrast media
- food proteins, such as those in legumes, nuts, berries, seafood, and egg albumin
- food additives containing sulfite
- insect venom.

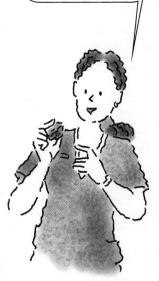

For some, it's a healthy snack; for others, it brings on an attack. In other words, nuts contain food proteins that cause anaphylaxis in some patients.

All about speed

With prompt recognition and treatment, the prognosis for anaphylaxis is good. However, a severe reaction may precipitate vascular collapse, leading to systemic shock and, sometimes, death. The reaction typically occurs within minutes but can occur up to 1 hour after exposure to an antigen.

How it happens

Anaphylaxis requires previous sensitization or exposure to the specific antigen, resulting in immunoglobulin (Ig) E production by plasma cells in the lymph nodes and enhancement by helper T cells. IgE antibodies then bind to basophils and membrane receptors on mast cells in connective tissue.

Here it comes again!

Upon exposure, IgM and IgG recognize the antigen and bind to it. Activated IgE on the basophils promotes the release of histamine, serotonin, and leukotrienes. An intensified response occurs as venule-weakening lesions form. Fluid then leaks into the cells, resulting in respiratory distress. Further deterioration occurs as the body's compensatory mechanisms fail to respond. (See *Understanding anaphylaxis*, pages 484 and 485.)

(Text continues on page 486.)

Understanding anaphylaxis

An anaphylactic reaction occurs after previous sensitization or exposure to a specific antigen. The sequence of events in anaphylaxis is described here.

Response to the antigen
Immunoglobulin (Ig) M and IgG recognize the antigen as a foreign substance and attach to it. Destruction of the antigen by the complement cascade begins but remains unfinished because of insufficient amounts of the protein catalyst or the antigen inhibits certain complement enzymes. The patient has no signs or symptoms at this stage.

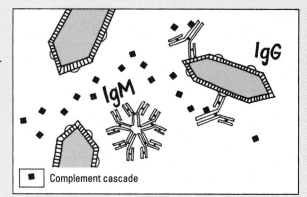

Complement cascade

Released chemical mediators
The antigen's continued presence activates IgE on basophils. The activated IgE promotes the release of mediators, including histamine, serotonin, and leukotriene. The sudden release of histamine causes vasodilation and increases capillary permeability. The patient begins to have signs and symptoms, including sudden nasal congestion; itchy, watery eyes; flushing; sweating; weakness; and anxiety.

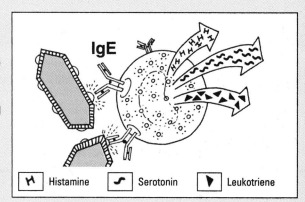

Histamine   Serotonin   Leukotriene

Intensified response
The activated IgE also stimulates mast cells in connective tissue along the venule walls to release more histamine and eosinophil chemotactic factor of anaphylaxis (ECF-A). These substances produce disruptive lesions that weaken the venules. Red, itchy skin; wheals; and swelling appear, and signs and symptoms worsen.

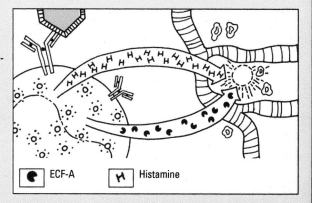

ECF-A   Histamine

Understanding anaphylaxis *(continued)*

Distress

In the lungs, histamine causes endothelial cells to burst and endothelial tissue to tear away from surrounding tissue. Fluids leak into the alveoli, and leukotriene prevents the alveoli from expanding, thus reducing pulmonary compliance. Tachypnea, crowing, use of accessory muscles, and cyanosis signal respiratory distress. Resulting neurologic signs and symptoms include changes in level of consciousness, severe anxiety and, possibly, seizures.

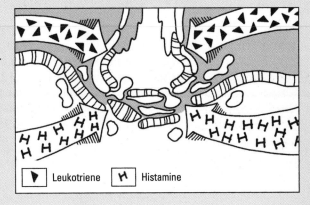

Leukotriene | Histamine

Deterioration

Basophils and mast cells begin to release prostaglandins and bradykinin along with histamine and serotonin. These substances increase vascular permeability, causing fluids to leak from the vessels. Shock; confusion; cool, pale skin; generalized edema; tachycardia; and hypotension signal rapid vascular collapse.

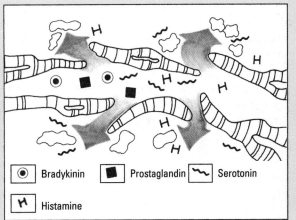

Bradykinin | Prostaglandin | Serotonin

Histamine

Failed compensatory mechanisms

Damage to the endothelial cells causes basophils and mast cells to release heparin. Additional substances are also released to neutralize the other mediators; eosinophils release arylsulfatase B to neutralize leukotriene, phospholipase D to neutralize heparin, and cyclic adenosine monophosphate and the prostaglandins E_1 and E_2 to increase the metabolic rate. These events can't reverse anaphylaxis. Hemorrhage, disseminated intravascular coagulation, and cardiopulmonary arrest result.

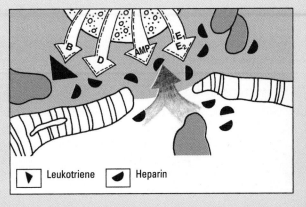

Leukotriene | Heparin

What to look for

An anaphylactic reaction produces sudden physical distress within seconds or minutes after exposure to an allergen. A delayed or persistent reaction may occur up to 24 hours later. The severity of the reaction is inversely related to the interval between exposure to the allergen and the onset of symptoms. The patient, a relative, or another responsible person will report the patient's exposure to an antigen.

Immediately after exposure, the patient may complain of feeling impending doom or fright, weakness, sweating, sneezing, dyspnea, nasal pruritus, and urticaria. He may appear extremely anxious. Keep in mind that the sooner signs and symptoms begin after exposure to the antigen, the more severe the anaphylaxis.

It's in the skin

On inspection, the patient's skin may display well-circumscribed, discrete cutaneous wheals with erythematous, raised, indented borders and blanched centers. They may coalesce to form giant hives. Angioedema may cause the patient to complain of a lump in his throat, or you may hear hoarseness or stridor. Wheezing, dyspnea, and complaints of chest tightness suggest bronchial obstruction. These signs and symptoms are early indications of impending, potentially fatal respiratory failure.

Other effects may follow rapidly. The patient may report GI and genitourinary effects, including severe stomach cramps, nausea, diarrhea, and urinary urgency and incontinence. Neurologic effects include dizziness, drowsiness, headache, restlessness, and seizures. Cardiovascular effects include hypotension, shock, and cardiac arrhythmias, which may precipitate vascular collapse if untreated.

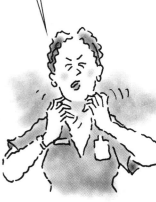

Giant hives are a possible anaphylaxis symptom. Somebody draw me an oatmeal bath!

What tests tell you

No single diagnostic test can identify anaphylaxis. It can be diagnosed by the rapid onset of severe respiratory or cardiovascular symptoms after ingestion or injection of a drug, vaccine, diagnostic agent, food, or food additive or after an insect sting. If these symptoms occur without a known allergic stimulus, other possible causes of shock (such as acute myocardial infarction [MI], status asthmaticus, or heart failure) must be ruled out.

These test results may provide some clues to the patient's risk for anaphylaxis:
- skin tests showing hypersensitivity to a specific allergen
- elevated serum IgE levels.

How it's treated

Treatment focuses on maintaining a patent airway, ensuring adequate oxygenation, restoring vascular volume, and controlling and counteracting the effects of the chemical mediators released. Treatment includes:

• immediate administration of epinephrine (Adrenalin) 1:1,000 aqueous solution to reverse bronchoconstriction and cause vasoconstriction—I.M., subcutaneously if the patient hasn't lost consciousness and is normotensive, or I.V. if the reaction is severe (repeating dosage every 5 to 20 minutes as needed)
• tracheostomy or endotracheal (ET) intubation and mechanical ventilation to maintain a patent airway
• oxygen therapy to increase tissue perfusion
• longer-acting epinephrine, corticosteroids, and diphenhydramine (Benadryl) and famotidine (Pepcid)—histamine blockers—to decrease circulating histamine levels to reduce the allergic response (long-term management)
• albuterol (Proventil) nebulizer treatment
• aminophylline (Truphylline) to treat bronchospasm
• volume expanders to maintain and restore circulating plasma volume
• I.V. vasopressors, such as norepinephrine (Levophed) and dopamine, to stabilize blood pressure
• cardiopulmonary resuscitation (CPR) to treat cardiac arrest.

What to do

• Administer epinephrine as ordered. (See *Giving epinephrine*, page 488.)
• Assess the patient's ABCs. If the patient is in cardiac arrest, begin CPR and provide appropriate care.
• To reverse hypoxemia, administer supplemental oxygen as ordered at appropriate concentrations (usually starting at 6 L/minute) to maintain partial pressure of arterial oxygen (PaO_2).
• Assess the patient's vital signs and respiratory status initially every 5 to 15 minutes and then less frequently as the patient's condition improves. Note continued evidence of hypotension and notify the practitioner immediately. Auscultate the lungs for decreased adventitious breath sounds.
• Be alert for decreased wheezing, which may signal an improvement in the patient's airflow. However, it could also indicate worsening of bronchoconstriction and obstruction. To determine what's happening, auscultate air movement throughout the lung fields. If decreased wheezing is a result of worsening bronchoconstriction, airflow will decrease.

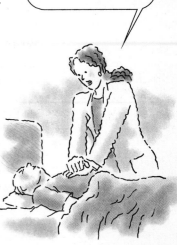

If an anaphylaxis patient is in cardiac arrest, begin CPR right away.

Stay on the ball

Giving epinephrine

When giving epinephrine to a patient with anaphylaxis, do the following:
• Check the patient's history for medication use. Epinephrine may be ineffective in patients taking beta-adrenergic blockers. Instead, anticipate administering glucagon as I.V. bolus as ordered.
• When administering epinephrine I.M., expect to repeat after 5 to 10 minutes if no improvement is seen.
• Remember that I.V. administration of epinephrine is limited to profound, immediately life-threatening situations (such as the patient who's in shock or experiencing airway obstruction). In these cases, expect to give a dose I.V. over 5 minutes. If the patient is in cardiac arrest, give high-dose epinephrine I.V. push and repeat every 3 to 5 minutes.

Looking at ABG

• Observe for a positive response to oxygen therapy, such as improved breathing, color, oximetry, and ABG values.
• Monitor oxygen saturation levels and ABG values for changes. Anticipate the need for ET intubation and mechanical ventilation if Pao_2 continues to fall or partial pressure of arterial carbon dioxide ($Paco_2$) rises.
• Expect ET intubation if the patient exhibits hoarseness, lingual edema, or posterior or oropharyngeal swelling. However, keep in mind that ET intubation may be difficult or impossible because it can result in increased laryngeal edema, bleeding, and further narrowing of the glottic opening. Fiber-optic ET intubation, needle cricothyrotomy (followed by transtracheal ventilation), or cricothyrotomy may be necessary.
• Institute continuous cardiac monitoring to identify and treat arrhythmias as ordered.
• Assist with insertion of a central venous or pulmonary artery catheter for hemodynamic monitoring if indicated. Monitor parameters at least every 15 to 30 minutes initially, and then every hour as the patient's condition improves.

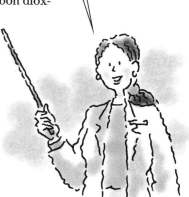

Watch the ABGs, because falling Pao_2 means you may need to intubate.

Eyeing the I.V.

• Begin I.V. fluid replacement therapy with crystalloids, such as lactated Ringer's or normal saline solution, and colloids, such as albumin and plasma protein fraction, as ordered. Monitor the patient's hemodynamic status for changes indicating improved cardiac output.

• Assess the patient closely for signs and symptoms of fluid overload, such as crackles, S₃ heart sounds, jugular vein distention, and increases in hemodynamic parameters.
• If the patient doesn't respond to fluid replacement therapy, expect to administer vasopressors to raise blood pressure.
• Monitor intake and output closely, checking urine output every hour. Insert an indwelling urinary catheter as indicated and ordered to ensure accurate measurements. Notify the practitioner if urine output is less than 30 ml/hour.
• Administer additional pharmacotherapy as ordered, including antihistamines such as diphenhydramine, H_2 antagonists such as cimetidine (Tagamet), inhaled beta-adrenergic agonists such as albuterol (Proventil), and high-dose corticosteroids. If the patient's history reveals use of beta-adrenergic blockers, anticipate administration of an inhaled anticholinergic agent (such as ipratropium [Atrovent]) instead of a beta-adrenergic agonist.

Perfusion pointers

• Monitor level of consciousness (LOC) for changes indicating decreased cerebral perfusion.
• Evaluate peripheral tissue perfusion, including skin color, temperature, pulses, and capillary refill.
• Institute measures to control itching, such as cool compresses, avoidance of scratching, and using finger pads instead of nails.
• Reassure the patient and stay with him; help him relax as much as possible.

Ages and stages

Cardiogenic shock and children

Although cardiogenic shock is uncommon in children, it may occur after cardiac surgery. It can also occur in children with acute arrhythmias, heart failure, or cardiomyopathy.

Cardiogenic shock

Sometimes called *pump failure*, cardiogenic shock is a condition of diminished cardiac output (CO) that severely impairs tissue perfusion. Cardiogenic shock occurs as a serious complication in nearly 15% of patients who are hospitalized with acute MI. (See *Cardiogenic shock in children.*)

It typically affects patients whose area of infarction involves 40% or more of left ventricular muscle mass; in such patients, mortality may exceed 85%. Most patients with cardiogenic shock die within 24 hours of onset. The prognosis for those who survive is poor.

What causes it

Cardiogenic shock can result from any condition that causes significant left ventricular dysfunction with reduced CO, such as MI (the most common cause), myocardial ischemia, papillary muscle dysfunction, and end-stage cardiomyopathy.

I feel so guilty—cardiogenic shock kills most patients within 24 hours of onset, and the prognosis for survivors is poor.

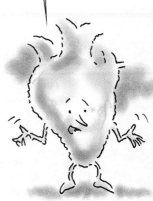

Other causes include myocarditis and depression of myocardial contractility after cardiac arrest and prolonged cardiac surgery. Mechanical abnormalities of the ventricle, such as acute mitral or aortic insufficiency or an acutely acquired ventricular septal defect or ventricular aneurysm, may also result in cardiogenic shock.

How it happens

Regardless of the cause, left ventricular dysfunction initiates a series of compensatory mechanisms that increases heart rate, strengthens myocardial contractions, promotes sodium and water retention, and causes selective vasoconstriction. These mechanisms attempt to increase CO and maintain vital organ function.

Stable, but brief

However, these mechanisms also increase myocardial workload and oxygen consumption, thus reducing the heart's ability to pump blood, especially if the patient has myocardial ischemia. As CO falls, aortic and carotid baroreceptors activate sympathetic nervous responses. These compensatory responses further increase heart rate, left ventricular filling pressure, and peripheral resistance to flow in order to enhance venous return to the heart. These actions initially stabilize the patient but later cause deterioration with rising oxygen demands on the compromised myocardium.

CO cycle

These events constitute a vicious cycle of low CO, sympathetic compensation, myocardial ischemia, and even lower CO. Consequently, blood backs up, resulting in pulmonary edema. Eventually, CO falls and multisystem organ failure develops as the compensatory mechanisms fail to maintain perfusion.

What to look for

Typically, the patient's history includes a disorder (such as MI or cardiomyopathy) that severely decreases left ventricular function. A patient with underlying cardiac disease may complain of anginal pain because of decreased myocardial perfusion and oxygenation. Urine output is usually less than 20 ml/hour. Inspection typically reveals pale skin, decreased sensorium, and rapid, shallow respirations. Palpation of peripheral pulses may detect a rapid, thready pulse. The skin feels cold and clammy.

Auscultation of blood pressure usually discloses a mean arterial pressure (MAP) of less than 60 mm Hg and a narrowing pulse pressure. In a patient with chronic hypotension, the MAP may fall below 50 mm Hg before the patient exhibits signs of shock. Auscultation of the heart detects gallop rhythms, faint heart sounds and, possibly (if shock results from rupture of the ventricular septum or papillary muscles), a holosystolic murmur.

Although many of these clinical features also occur in heart failure and other shock syndromes, they're usually more profound in cardiogenic shock. Patients with pericardial tamponade may have distant heart sounds.

Compensation clues

The patient's signs and symptoms may also provide clues to the stage of shock. For example, in the compensatory stage of shock, signs and symptoms may include:
• tachycardia and bounding pulse due to sympathetic stimulation
• restlessness and irritability related to cerebral hypoxia
• tachypnea to compensate for hypoxia
• reduced urine output secondary to vasoconstriction
• cool, pale skin associated with vasoconstriction; warm, dry skin in septic shock due to vasodilation.

That's progress for ya

In the progressive stage of shock, signs and symptoms may include:
• hypotension as compensatory mechanisms begin to fail
• narrowed pulse pressure associated with reduced stroke volume
• weak, rapid, thready pulse caused by decreased CO
• shallow respirations as the patient weakens
• reduced urine output as poor renal perfusion continues
• cold, clammy skin caused by vasoconstriction
• cyanosis related to hypoxia.

No going back

In the irreversible stage, clinical findings may include:
• unconsciousness and absent reflexes caused by reduced cerebral perfusion, acid-base imbalance, or electrolyte abnormalities
• rapidly falling blood pressure as decompensation occurs
• weak pulse caused by reduced CO
• slow, shallow or Cheyne-Stokes respirations secondary to respiratory center depression
• anuria related to renal failure.

What tests tell you

• Pulmonary artery pressure (PAP) monitoring reveals increased PAP and pulmonary artery wedge pressure (PAWP), reflecting a

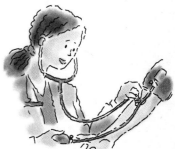

In a patient with chronic hypotension, mean arterial pressure may fall to less than 50 mm Hg before the patient exhibits signs of shock.

rise in left ventricular end-diastolic pressure (preload) and heightened resistance to left ventricular emptying (afterload) caused by ineffective pumping and increased peripheral vascular resistance. Thermodilution catheterization reveals a reduced cardiac index.

• Arterial pressure monitoring shows systolic arterial pressure less than 80 mm Hg caused by impaired ventricular ejection.

• ABG analysis may show metabolic and respiratory acidosis and hypoxia.

• Electrocardiography (ECG) demonstrates possible evidence of acute MI, ischemia, or ventricular aneurysm.

• Echocardiography determines left ventricular function and reveals valvular abnormalities.

• Serum enzyme measurements display elevated levels of creatine kinase (CK), lactate dehydrogenase (LD), aspartate aminotransferase, and alanine aminotransferase, which indicate MI or ischemia and suggest heart failure or shock. CK-MB and LD isoenzyme levels may confirm acute MI.

• Cardiac catheterization and echocardiography may reveal other conditions that can lead to pump dysfunction and failure, such as cardiac tamponade, papillary muscle infarct or rupture, ventricular septal rupture, pulmonary emboli, venous pooling, and hypovolemia.

How it's treated

Treatment aims to enhance cardiovascular status by increasing CO, improving myocardial perfusion, and decreasing cardiac workload with combinations of cardiovascular drugs and mechanical-assist techniques. These goals are accomplished by optimizing preload, decreasing afterload, increasing contractility, and optimizing heart rate.

Recommended I.V. drugs may include dopamine (a vasopressor that increases CO, blood pressure, and renal blood flow), inamrinone or dobutamine (Dobutrex) (inotropic agents that increase myocardial contractility and increase CO), and norepinephrine (when a more potent vasoconstrictor is necessary).

Nitroglycerin or nitroprusside (vasodilators) may be used with a vasopressor to further improve CO by decreasing afterload and reducing preload. However, the patient must have adequate blood pressure to support nitroprusside therapy and must be monitored closely. Diuretics may also be used to reduce preload in the patient with fluid volume overload.

And just for good measure

Additional treatment measures for cardiogenic shock may include:

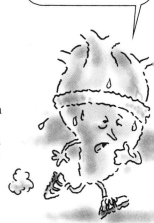

Cardiogenic shock treatment aims to decrease cardiac workload, among other things. Boy, I'd appreciate some of that right about now!

• thrombolytic therapy or coronary artery revascularization to restore coronary artery blood flow if cardiogenic shock is due to acute MI
• emergency surgery to repair papillary muscle rupture or ventricular septal defect if either is the cause of cardiogenic shock.

What to do

• Begin I.V. infusions of normal saline solution or lactated Ringer's solution, using a large-bore (14G to 18G) catheter, which allows easier administration of later blood transfusions.
• Administer oxygen by face mask or artificial airway to ensure adequate tissue oxygenation. Adjust the oxygen flow rate to a higher or lower level, as blood gas measurements indicate. Many patients will need 100% oxygen, and some will require 5 to 15 cm H_2O of positive end-expiratory or continuous positive airway pressure ventilation.
• Monitor and record the patient's blood pressure, pulse, respiratory rate, and peripheral pulses every 1 to 5 minutes until the patient stabilizes.

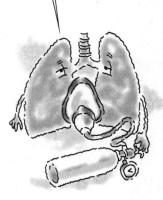

Administering oxygen by face mask ensures adequate tissue oxygenation.

Fascinating rhythm

• Monitor the patient's cardiac rhythm continuously. Systolic blood pressure less than 80 mm Hg usually results in inadequate coronary artery blood flow, cardiac ischemia, arrhythmias, and further complications of low CO. If blood pressure drops below 80 mm Hg, increase the oxygen flow rate and notify the practitioner immediately. A progressive drop in blood pressure accompanied by a thready pulse generally signals inadequate CO from reduced intravascular volume.
• Determine how much fluid to give by checking blood pressure, urine output, central venous pressure (CVP), or PAWP. (To increase accuracy, measure CVP at the level of the right atrium, using the same reference point on the chest each time.) Whenever the fluid infusion rate is increased, watch for signs of fluid overload, such as an increase in CVP.
• Keep in mind that, if the patient is hypovolemic, preload may need to be increased, which is typically accomplished with I.V. fluids. However, I.V. fluids must be given cautiously and increased gradually while hemodynamic parameters are closely monitored. In this situation, diuretics aren't given.

I'm going in

• Insert an indwelling urinary catheter if necessary to measure hourly urine output. If output is less than 30 ml/hour in adults, increase the fluid infusion rate but watch for signs of fluid overload

such as an increase in CVP. Notify the practitioner if urine output doesn't improve.
• Administer a diuretic, such as furosemide (Lasix) or bumetanide (Bumex), as ordered to decrease preload and improve stroke volume and CO.
• Monitor ABG values, CBC, and electrolyte levels. Expect to administer sodium bicarbonate by I.V. push if the patient is acidotic. Administer electrolyte replacement therapy as ordered and indicated by laboratory test results.
• During therapy, assess skin color and temperature and note changes. Cold, clammy skin may be a sign of continuing peripheral vascular constriction, indicating progressive shock.
• Prepare the patient for possible emergency cardiac catheterization to determine eligibility for percutaneous transluminal coronary angioplasty or coronary artery bypass graft in an attempt to reperfuse areas with reversible injury patterns.

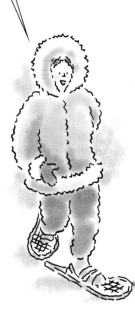

Cold, clammy skin is expected for me right now, but for a cardiogenic shock patient receiving therapy, it means the condition is progressing.

Hypovolemic shock

Hypovolemic shock most commonly results from acute blood loss—about 20% of total volume. Without sufficient blood or fluid replacement, it may cause irreversible damage to organs and systems.

What causes it

Massive volume loss may result from:
• GI bleeding, internal or external hemorrhage, or any condition that reduces circulating intravascular volume or other body fluids
• intestinal obstruction
• peritonitis
• acute pancreatitis
• ascites
• dehydration from excessive perspiration, severe diarrhea, protracted vomiting, diabetes insipidus, diuresis, or inadequate fluid intake.

How it happens

Potentially life-threatening, hypovolemic shock stems from reduced intravascular blood volume, which leads to decreased cardiac output and inadequate tissue perfusion. The subsequent tissue anoxia prompts a shift in cellular metabolism from aerobic to anaerobic pathways. This shift results in an accumulation of lactic acid, which produces metabolic acidosis.

Shock sequence

When compensatory mechanisms fail, hypovolemic shock occurs in this sequence:

intravascular fluid volume decreases

venous return diminishes, which reduces preload and decreases stroke volume

CO is reduced

MAP decreases

tissue perfusion is impaired

oxygen and nutrient delivery to cells decreases

multisystem organ failure occurs.

What to look for

The specific signs and symptoms exhibited by the patient depend on the amount of fluid loss. (See *Estimating fluid loss.*) Typically, the patient's history includes conditions that reduce blood volume, such as GI hemorrhage, trauma, or severe diarrhea and vomiting.

Estimating fluid loss

These assessment parameters indicate the severity of fluid loss.

Minimal fluid loss
Intravascular volume loss of 10% to 15% is regarded as minimal. Signs and symptoms include:
• slight tachycardia
• normal supine blood pressure
• positive postural vital signs, including a decrease in systolic blood pressure greater than or equal to 10 mm Hg or an increase in pulse rate greater than or equal to 20 beats/minute
• increased capillary refill time greater than or equal to 3 seconds

• urine output greater than or equal to 30 ml/hour
• cool, pale skin on arms and legs
• anxiety.

Moderate fluid loss
Intravascular volume loss of about 25% is regarded as moderate. Signs and symptoms include:
• rapid, thready pulse
• supine hypotension
• cool truncal skin
• urine output of 10 to 30 ml/hour
• severe thirst
• restlessness, confusion, or irritability.

Severe fluid loss
Intravascular volume loss of about 40% or more is regarded as severe. Signs and symptoms include:
• marked tachycardia
• marked hypotension
• weak or absent peripheral pulses
• cold, mottled, or cyanotic skin
• urine output less than 10 ml/hour
• unconsciousness.

Assessment findings may include:
- pale skin
- decreased sensorium
- rapid, shallow respirations
- urine output less than 25 ml/hour
- rapid, thready peripheral pulses
- cold, clammy skin
- MAP less than 60 mm Hg and a narrowing pulse pressure
- decreased CVP, right atrial pressure, PAWP, and CO.

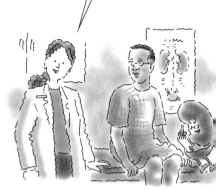

> If urine specific gravity exceeds 1.020 while urine sodium levels fall to less than 50 mEq/L, your patient may have hypovolemic shock.

What tests tell you

No single diagnostic test confirms hypovolemic shock, but these test results help support the diagnosis:
- low HCT
- decreased Hb level
- decreased RBC and platelet counts
- elevated serum potassium, sodium, LD, creatinine, and blood urea nitrogen (BUN) levels
- increased urine specific gravity (greater than 1.020) and urine osmolality
- urine sodium levels less than 50 mEq/L
- decreased urine creatinine levels
- decreased pH and PaO_2 and increased $PaCO_2$
- gastroscopy, X-rays, aspiration of gastric contents through a nasogastric tube, and tests for occult blood
- coagulation studies for coagulopathy from disseminated intravascular coagulation (DIC).

How it's treated

Emergency treatment relies on prompt, adequate fluid and blood replacement to restore intravascular volume, raise blood pressure, and maintain it above 80 mm Hg. Rapid infusion of normal saline or lactated Ringer's solution and, possibly, albumin or other plasma expanders may expand volume adequately until whole blood can be matched. If hypovolemic shock is caused by massive bleeding, lactated Ringer's solution is preferred for fluid replacement because it minimizes the risk of electrolyte imbalances.

Treatment may also include application (although controversial) of a pneumatic antishock garment, oxygen administration, control of bleeding, administration of dopamine or another inotropic drug, and surgery if appropriate.

What to do

- Assess the patient for the extent of fluid loss and begin fluid replacement as ordered. (See *Hypovolemic shock and children*.)

Ages and stages

Hypovolemic shock and children

Suspect hypovolemia in the infant or child who has a capillary refill longer than 2 seconds and accompanying history and signs of hypovolemic shock, such as tachycardia, altered level of consciousness, pale skin, lack of tears, and depressed fontanels.

Keep in mind that fluid replacement for an infant and a child is generally a crystalloid at a volume of 20 ml/kg of body weight in a fluid bolus. This bolus may be repeated for a total of three times while monitoring capillary refill as a response.

Stay on the ball

When blood pressure drops

A drop below 80 mm Hg in systolic blood pressure usually signals inadequate cardiac output from reduced intravascular volume. Such a drop usually results in inadequate coronary artery blood flow, cardiac ischemia, arrhythmias, and other complications of low cardiac output. If the patient's systolic blood pressure drops below 80 mm Hg and his pulse is thready, increase the oxygen flow rate and notify the practitioner immediately.

- Obtain type and crossmatch for blood component therapy.
- Assess the patient's ABCs.
- If the patient experiences cardiac or respiratory arrest, start CPR.
- Administer supplemental oxygen as ordered.
- Monitor the patient's oxygen saturation and ABG values for evidence of hypoxemia and anticipate the need for ET intubation and mechanical ventilation if the patient's respiratory status deteriorates.
- Place the patient in semi-Fowler's position to maximize chest expansion.
- Keep the patient as quiet and comfortable as possible to minimize oxygen demands
- Monitor the patient's vital signs, neurologic status, and cardiac rhythm continuously for such changes as cardiac arrhythmias and myocardial ischemia.

Capillary cues

- Observe the patient's skin color and check capillary refill.
- Notify the practitioner if capillary refill takes longer than 2 seconds. (See *When blood pressure drops.*)
- Monitor hemodynamic parameters—including CVP, PAWP, and CO and cardiac input—as often as every 15 minutes to evaluate the patient's status and response to treatment.
- Monitor the patient's intake and output closely.
- Insert an indwelling urinary catheter and assess urine output hourly.

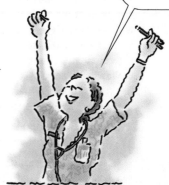

Strrretch that chest! Putting the patient in semi-Fowler's position maximizes chest expansion.

Understanding DIC

Disseminated intravascular coagulation (DIC) can occur as a complication of hypovolemic shock. As a result, accelerated clotting occurs, causing small vessel occlusion, organ necrosis, depletion of circulating clotting factors and platelets, activation of the fibrinolytic system, and consequent severe hemorrhage.

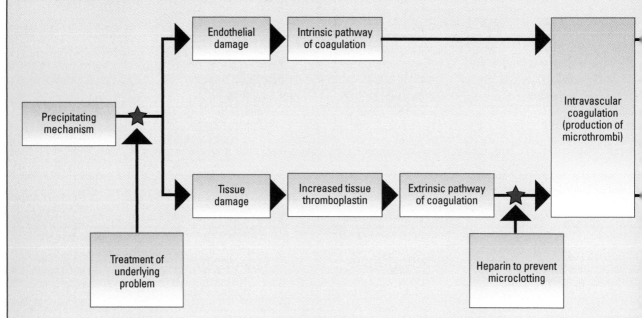

Watch for blood

• If bleeding from the GI tract is the suspected cause, check all stools, emesis, and gastric drainage for occult blood.
• If urine output falls below 30 ml/hour in an adult, expect to increase the I.V. fluid infusion rate, but watch for signs of fluid overload such as elevated CVP.
• Notify the practitioner if urine output doesn't increase.
• Administer blood component therapy as ordered; monitor serial Hb values and HCT to evaluate the effects of treatment.
• Administer dopamine or norepinephrine I.V. as ordered to increase cardiac contractility and renal perfusion.
• Watch for signs of impending coagulopathy, such as petechiae, bruising, and bleeding or oozing from gums or venipuncture sites, and report them immediately. (See *Understanding DIC.*)
• Provide emotional support and reassurance as appropriate in the wake of massive fluid losses.
• Prepare the patient for surgery as appropriate.

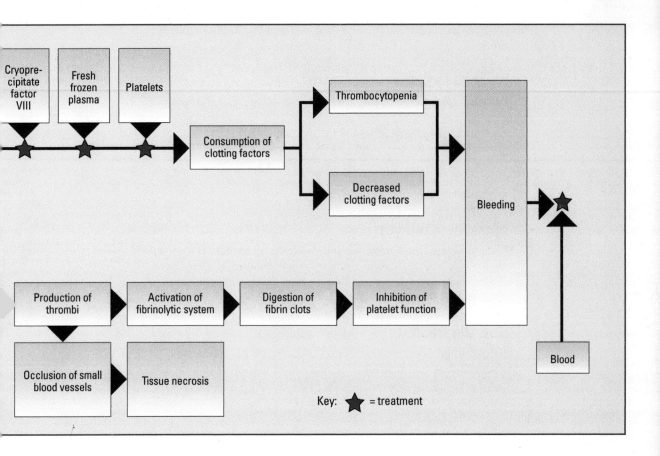

eurogenic shock

In neurogenic shock, a temporary loss of autonomic function below the level of a spinal cord injury produces cardiovascular changes. Neurogenic shock is a type of distributive shock in which vasodilation causes a state of hypovolemia. It occurs most commonly at the spinal level of T6 or above.

What causes it

It may result from spinal cord injury: spinal anesthesia, vasomotor center depression, medications, or hypoglycemia.

How it happens

A loss of sympathetic vasoconstrictor tone in the vascular smooth muscle and reduced autonomic function lead to widespread arterial and venous vasodilation. Venous return is reduced as blood pools in the venous septum, leading to a drop in CO and hypotension.

What to look for

The neurogenic shock patient will display these signs and symptoms:
- severe hypotension
- bradycardia
- slow pulse
- warm, dry, and flushed skin
- hypothermia.

What tests tell you

Tests to determine neurogenic shock should include ABG to determine the degree of cardiopulmonary compensation, ECG to determine cardiac arrhythmias, and CT scan or magnetic resonance imaging to determine the extent of spinal injury.

How it's treated

Treatment goals include assessing ABCs, treating hypothermia, administering fluid resuscitation and vasoconstrictors to increase blood pressure, and administering agents to block vagal effects that cause bradycardia, such as atropine.

What to do

- Assess the patient's LOC.
- Assess the rate, depth, and pattern of respirations, and auscultate breath sounds.
- Palpate for peripheral pulses, and auscultate the apical heart rate.
- Assess the patient's vital signs, noting hypotension and bradycardia.
- Observe the patient for warm, dry skin.
- Obtain a blood sample for ABG analysis.
- Provide supplemental oxygen and prepare the patient for ET intubation and mechanical ventilation, as necessary.
- Initiate cardiac and hemodynamic monitoring.
- Treat hypothermia with a warming blanket.
- Insert an indwelling urinary catheter.
- Initiate and administer I.V. fluid resuscitation such as normal saline solution or lactated Ringer's solution to increase intravascular volume and blood pressure.
- Administer medications such as vasopressors to increase blood pressure, blood products to increase intravascular volume, an os-

motic diuretic such as mannitol (Osmitrol), if urine output is decreased to increase renal blood flow, and atropine or transcutaneous pacing to treat symptomatic bradycardia.

Septic shock

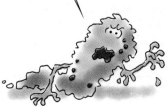

Gram-negative bacteria are the most common cause of septic shock.

Septic shock is a type of distributive shock. It can occur in any person with impaired immunity, but elderly people are at greatest risk. Low systemic vascular resistance and an elevated CO characterize septic shock. The disorder is thought to be a response to infections that release microbes or immune mediators, such as tumor necrosis factor and interleukin-1.

What causes it

Any pathogenic organism can cause septic shock. Gram-negative bacteria, such as *Escherichia coli, Klebsiella pneumoniae, Serratia, Enterobacter,* and *Pseudomonas* rank as the most common causes and account for up to 70% of all cases. Opportunistic fungi cause about 3% of cases. Rare causative organisms include mycobacteria and some viruses and protozoa.

How it happens

An immune response is triggered when bacteria release endotoxins. In response, macrophages secrete tumor necrosis factor (TNF) and interleukins. These mediators in turn increase the release of platelet-activating factor (PAF), prostaglandins, leukotrienes, thromboxane A_2, kinins, and complement.

Truth about consequences

The consequences of this immune activity are vasodilation and vasoconstriction, increased capillary permeability, reduced systemic vascular resistance, microemboli, and an elevated CO. Endotoxins also stimulate the release of histamine, further increasing capillary permeability.

Moreover, myocardial depressant factor, TNF, PAF, and other factors depress myocardial function. CO falls, resulting in multisystem organ dysfunction syndrome. (See *Understanding MODS,* pages 502 and 503.)

What to look for

The patient's history may include a disorder or treatment that causes immunosuppression, or a history of invasive tests or treatments, surgery, or trauma. At onset, the patient may have fever

Understanding MODS

Multisystem organ dysfunction syndrome (MODS) is a condition that occurs when two or more organs or organ systems can't maintain homeostasis. Intervention is necessary to support and maintain organ function. MODS isn't an illness itself; rather, it's a manifestation of another progressive, underlying condition.

MODS develops when widespread systemic inflammation, a condition known as *systemic inflammatory response syndrome* (SIRS) overtaxes a patient's compensatory mechanisms. Infection, ischemia, trauma of any sort, reperfusion injury, or multisystem injury can trigger SIRS. If allowed to progress, SIRS can lead to organ inflammation and, ultimately, MODS.

Primary or secondary

Typically, MODS is classified as *primary* or *secondary*. In *primary MODS*, organ or organ system failure is due to a direct injury (such as trauma or a primary disorder) that usually involves the lungs, such as pneumonia, aspiration, near drowning, and pulmonary embolism. The organ failure can be positively linked to the direct injury. Typically, acute respiratory distress syndrome (ARDS) develops and progresses, leading to encephalopathy and coagulopathy from hepatic involvement. As the syndrome continues, other organ systems are affected.

In *secondary MODS,* organ or organ system failure is due to sepsis. Typically, the infection source isn't associated with the lungs. The most common infection sources include intra-abdominal sepsis, extensive blood loss, pancreatitis, or major vascular injuries. With secondary MODS, ARDS develops sooner and progressive involvement of other organs and organ systems occurs more rapidly.

Regardless of the type of MODS or triggering event, the overall underlying problem is inadequate perfusion.

Assessment findings

Assessment findings associated with MODS typically reveal an acutely ill patient with signs and symptoms associated with SIRS. Early findings may include:
- fever, usually greater than 101° F (38.3° C) (early indicator)
- tachycardia
- narrowed pulse pressure
- tachypnea
- decreased pulmonary artery pressure (PAP), decreased pulmonary artery wedge pressure (PAWP), decreased central venous pressure, and increased cardiac output (CO) (due to tachycardia).

As SIRS progresses, findings reflect impaired perfusion of the tissues and organs, such as decreasing level of consciousness, respiratory depression, diminished bowel sounds, jaundice, oliguria, or anuria. PAP increases (due to pulmonary edema). PAWP increases and CO decreases with the development of heart failure.

Organ dysfunction is determined by specific criteria. For example, pulmonary organ dysfunction is identified by the development of ARDS, requiring positive end-expiratory pressure greater than 10 cm H_2O and a fraction of inspired oxygen less then 0.5. Hepatic dysfunction is evidenced by jaundice with a serum bilirubin level of 8 to 10 mg/dl. Oliguria of less than 500 ml/day or an increasing serum creatinine level indicate mild renal system dysfunction, while the need for dialysis suggests severe organ involvement. Development of disseminated intravascular coagulation typically indicates severe hematologic system dysfunction.

Understanding MODS (continued)

Treatment

Treatment focuses on supporting respiratory and circulatory function by using mechanical ventilation, supplemental oxygen, hemodynamic monitoring, and fluid infusion to expand and maintain the intravascular compartment. Renal function is closely monitored, including hourly urine output measurements and serial laboratory tests to evaluate for trends indicating acute renal failure. Dialysis may ultimately be necessary.

Numerous drugs may be used:
• antimicrobial agents to treat underlying infection
• vasopressors, such as dopamine and norepinephrine
• isotonic crystalloid solutions, such as normal saline and lactated Ringer's solutions, to expand the intravascular fluid spaces

• colloids, such as albumin, to help expand plasma volume without the added risk of causing fluid overload.

Some experimental agents are being used, such as antitumor necrosis factor, endotoxin, and anti-interleukin-1 antibodies. However, evidence supporting the effectiveness of these agents is currently unavailable.

Nursing care

Nursing care for the patient with MODS is primarily supportive. The patient is acutely ill and requires close, usually extensive monitoring. Emotional support is also crucial because mortality for a patient with MODS is directly proportional to the number of organs or organ systems affected. For example, mortality is 85% when three organs are involved; it jumps to 95% when four organs are involved and up to 99% with five-organ involvement.

and chills, although 20% of patients may be hypothermic. The patient's signs and symptoms will reflect the hyperdynamic (warm) phase of septic shock or the hypodynamic (cold) phase.

Hyper ...

The hyperdynamic phase is characterized by:
• increased CO
• peripheral vasodilation
• decreased systemic vascular resistance
• altered LOC
• rapid, shallow respirations
• decreased urine output
• rapid, full, bounding pulse.

... or hypo

The hypodynamic phase is characterized by:
• decreased CO
• peripheral vasoconstriction
• increased systemic vascular resistance
• inadequate tissue perfusion
• pale, possibly cyanotic skin color

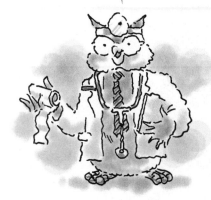

Any emergency nurse would be wise to look for these septic shock symptoms.

- mottling of extremities
- decreased LOC
- rapid, shallow respirations
- decreased or absent urine output
- absence of peripheral pulses or a rapid, weak, thready pulse
- cold, clammy skin
- hypotension, usually with a systolic pressure below 90 mm Hg or 50 to 80 mm Hg below the patient's previous level
- crackles or rhonchi if pulmonary congestion is present
- reduced or normal CVP.

What tests tell you

- Blood cultures are usually positive for the offending organism.
- CBC shows the presence or absence of anemia and leukopenia, severe or absent neutropenia, and (usually) the presence of thrombocytopenia.
- ABG studies may reveal metabolic acidosis, hypoxemia, and low $Paco_2$ that progresses to increased $Paco_2$ (indicating respiratory acidosis).
- BUN and creatinine levels are increased and creatinine clearance is decreased.
- PT, PTT, and bleeding time increase, platelets decrease, and fibrin split products increase.
- Chest X-rays reveal evidence of pneumonia (as the underlying infection) or acute respiratory distress syndrome (indicating progression of septic shock).
- ECG shows ST-segment depression and inverted T waves.
- Amylase and lipase levels may show pancreatic insufficiency.
- Hepatic enzyme levels are elevated due to liver ischemia.
- Blood glucose levels are initially elevated and then decrease.
- CT scan reveals abscesses or sources of possible infection.

How it's treated

Location and treatment of the underlying sepsis is essential to treating septic shock, including:
- removal of the source of infection, such as I.V., intra-arterial, or urinary drainage catheters
- aggressive antimicrobial therapy appropriate for the causative organism
- culture and sensitivity tests of urine and wound drainage
- surgery, if appropriate
- reduction or discontinuation of immunosuppressive drug therapy
- possible granulocyte transfusions in patients with severe neutropenia

- oxygen therapy and mechanical ventilation if necessary
- colloid or crystalloid infusions
- administration of a vasopressor such as dopamine.

What to do

- Assess the patient's ABCs; monitor cardiopulmonary status closely.
- Administer supplemental oxygen as ordered.
- Monitor the patient's oxygen saturation and ABG values for evidence of hypoxemia and anticipate the need for ET intubation and mechanical ventilation if the patient's respiratory status deteriorates.
- Place the patient in semi-Fowler's position to maximize chest expansion. Keep the patient as quiet and comfortable as possible to minimize oxygen demands.
- Monitor the patient's vital signs continuously for changes. Observe his skin color and check capillary refill. Notify the practitioner if capillary refill is longer than 2 seconds.

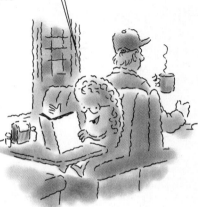

In a patient with septic shock, capillary refill shouldn't take longer than 2 seconds. I wish my "coffee-lary" refills were that quick!

Ups and downs

- Keep in mind that the patient's temperature is usually elevated in the early stages of septic shock and that he frequently experiences shaking chills. As the shock progresses, the temperature usually drops and the patient experiences diaphoresis.
- If the patient's systolic blood pressure drops below 80 mm Hg, increase the oxygen flow rate, and notify the practitioner immediately. Alert the practitioner and increase the infusion rate if the patient experiences a progressive drop in blood pressure accompanied by a thready pulse.
- Remove I.V., intra-arterial, or urinary drainage catheters and send them to the laboratory to culture for the presence of the causative organism (and prepare to reinsert or assist with reinsertion of new devices).
- Obtain blood cultures as ordered and begin antimicrobial therapy as ordered. Monitor the patient for possible adverse effects of therapy.
- Institute continuous cardiac monitoring to evaluate for possible arrhythmias, myocardial ischemia, or adverse effects of treatment.
- Monitor the patient's intake and output closely. Notify the practitioner if his urine output is less than 30 ml/hour.
- Administer I.V. fluid therapy as ordered, usually normal saline or lactated Ringer's solution. Monitor hemodynamic parameters to determine the patient's response to therapy.

Overload alert!

- Be alert for signs and symptoms of possible fluid overload, such as dyspnea, tachypnea, crackles, peripheral edema, jugular vein distention, and increased PAP.
- Administer positive inotropic agents as ordered.
- Institute infection control precautions; use strict aseptic technique for all invasive procedures.
- Monitor laboratory test results, especially coagulation studies and hepatic enzyme levels, for changes indicative of DIC and hepatic failure, respectively.
- Provide emotional support to the patient and his family.
- Prepare the patient for surgery as appropriate.

Did you know multisystem trauma is the leading cause of death for people younger than age 45?

Multisystem trauma

Trauma is a physical injury or wound that's inflicted by an external or violent act; it may be intentional or unintentional. Multisystem traumas involve injuries to more than one body area or organ, and are the leading cause of death in people younger than age 45.

I had no idea!

That's heart-wrenching!

The type of trauma determines the extent of injury:
- *blunt trauma*—leaves the body intact
- *penetrating trauma*—disrupts the body surface
- *perforating trauma*—leaves entrance and exit wounds as an object passes through the body.

A patient experiencing multisystem trauma requires immediate action and a multidisciplinary team approach. The patient may have a head injury accompanied by chest and cardiac trauma. Or, he may have experienced a spinal cord injury along with numerous fractures and contusions to other body areas.

What causes it

Trauma may be caused by weapons, automobile collision, physical confrontation, falls, or other unnatural occurrence to the body.

How it happens

Trauma typically creates wounds. Traumatic wounds include:
- *abrasion*—scraped skin, with partial loss of skin surface
- *laceration*—torn skin, causing jagged, irregular edges (severity of which depends on size, depth, and location)

• *puncture wound*—skin penetrated by a pointed object, such as a knife or glass fragment
• *traumatic amputation*—removal of part of the body (a limb or part of a limb).

What to look for

Assessment findings vary according to the type and extent of trauma. A conscious patient with multiple injuries may be able to help focus the assessment on areas that need immediate attention, such as difficulty breathing and neurologic symptoms.

Initially, the patient is assessed for life-threatening problems involving his ABCs. Monitor cardiac rhythm, initiate CPR, and administer drugs and electrical shock therapy (defibrillation and synchronized cardioversion) as appropriate for cardiac arrhythmias. After initially assessing and treating life-threatening conditions, perform a secondary assessment, including taking a history and performing a physical examination.

Out of time

During an emergency, you won't have time to obtain all of the patient's history. Focus on the most important information, including:
• signs and symptoms related to the present condition
• allergies to drugs, foods, latex, or environmental factors
• medication history, including prescription and over-the-counter medications, herbs, and supplements
• past medical history
• last meal
• events leading to the injury or condition.

When the patient's condition is stabilized, fill in the other components of the normal health history. Remember to include a history of blood transfusions and tetanus immunization if the patient has an open wound. When the patient is stable, perform a body-system examination according to your facility's policy and procedure. A thorough assessment helps systematically identify and correct problems and establishes a baseline for future comparison.

What tests tell you

The diagnostic tests performed are based on the body system affected by the trauma. For example, a patient with a blunt chest injury would require a chest X-ray to detect rib and sternal fractures, pneumothorax, flail chest, pulmonary contusion, and a lacerated or ruptured aorta. Angiography studies would also be per-

> **Memory jogger**
>
> To help remember what information to obtain during assessment of the trauma patient, use the acronym **SAMPLE.**
>
> **S**—Signs and symptoms
>
> **A**—Allergies
>
> **M**—Medications
>
> **P**—Past medical history
>
> **L**—Last meal
>
> **E**—Events leading to injury

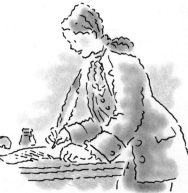

History—of the patient, that is—is always important, but in multisystem trauma emergency cases, you'll have to settle for the abridged version.

formed with suspected aortic laceration or rupture. Diagnostic tests for a patient with head trauma may include a CT scan, cervical spine X-rays, skull X-rays, or an angiogram.

Some other diagnostic tests that may be performed on the patient with multisystem trauma include:
• ABG analysis to evaluate respiratory status and determine acidotic and alkalotic states
• CBC to indicate the amount of blood loss
• coagulation studies to evaluate clotting ability
• serum electrolyte levels to indicate the presence of electrolyte imbalances.

How it's treated

Multisystem trauma care basics include:
• performing triage
• assessing and maintaining ABCs
• protecting the cervical spine
• assessing LOC
• preparing the patient for transport and possible surgery.

Six degrees of contamination

Management of traumatic wounds depends on the type of wound and degree of contamination. Treatment may include:
• controlling bleeding, usually by applying firm, direct pressure and elevating the extremity
• cleaning the wound
• administering pain medication
• administering antibiotic therapy
• undergoing surgery.

Additional treatment is based on the body system that's affected by the trauma and the extent of injury. For example, treatment of a blunt chest injury may include maintaining a patent airway, providing adequate ventilation, maintaining fluid and electrolyte balance, and inserting a chest tube for pneumothorax, hemothorax, or tension pneumothorax.

What to do

• Assess the patient's ABCs and initiate emergency measures if necessary; administer supplemental oxygen as ordered.
• Immobilize the patient's head and neck with an immobilization device, sandbags, backboard, and tape. Assist with cervical spine X-rays. Monitor vital signs and note significant changes.
• Immobilize fractures.
• Monitor the patient's oxygen saturation and cardiac rhythm for arrhythmias.

• Assess the patient's neurologic status, including LOC and pupillary and motor response.
• Obtain blood studies, including type and crossmatch.
• Insert two I.V. large-bore catheters and infuse normal saline or lactated Ringer's solution.
• Quickly and carefully assess the patient for multiple injuries.
• Assess the patient's wounds and provide wound care as appropriate. Cover open wounds and control bleeding by applying pressure and elevating extremities.
• Assess for increased abdominal distention and increased diameter of extremities.
• Administer blood products as appropriate.
• Monitor the patient for signs of hypovolemic shock.
• Provide pain medication as appropriate.
• Provide reassurance to the patient and his family.

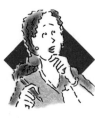

Quick quiz

1. What's the highest priority when caring for a patient with hypovolemic shock?
    A.   Assessing for dehydration
    B.   Administering I.V. fluids
    C.   Inserting a urinary catheter
    D.   Obtaining a sample for CBC

Answer: B. Hypovolemic shock is an emergency that requires rapid infusion of I.V. fluids.

2. Which sign would lead you to suspect that a patient is experiencing septic shock?
    A.   Clear, watery sputum
    B.   Severe hypertension
    C.   Hypotension
    D.   Polyuria

Answer: C. Hypotension—along with pale, possibly cyanotic skin; mottling of extremities; decreased LOC; rapid, shallow respirations; decreased or absent urine output; absence of peripheral pulses; or a rapid, weak pulse—is a sign of hypodynamic septic shock.

3. You suspect a cervical spine injury in a patient. Which action is most appropriate?

    A. Remove the cervical collar before attempting to open the airway.

    B. Use the head-tilt chin-lift maneuver to open the airway.

    C. Turn the patient on his side to prevent aspiration.

    D. Use the jaw-thrust maneuver to open the airway.

Answer: D. In a patient with a suspected cervical spine injury, the most appropriate way to open the airway is to use the jaw-thrust maneuver.

4. Which drug would you administer first to a patient with ana-phylactic shock?

    A. epinephrine

    B. diphenhydramine

    C. albuterol

    D. prednisone

Answer: A. Immediate treatment for anaphylactic shock involves the administration of epinephrine to reverse bronchoconstriction. Later, corticosteroids, such as prednisone, diphenhydramine, and albuterol, may be given.

5. Which sign would you observe in a patient experiencing in-travascular fluid volume loss of about 10%?

    A. Supine hypotension

    B. Positive postural vital signs

    C. Urine output less than 30 ml/hour

    D. Cold, mottled skin

Answer: B. An intravascular fluid volume loss of approximately 10% is classified as minimal and would be manifested by positive postural vital signs, such as a decrease in systolic blood pressure greater than 10 mm Hg or an increase in pulse rate to greater than 20 beats/minute.

Scoring

☆☆☆ If you answered all five questions correctly, way to go! Your knowledge of this chapter's information is shockingly accurate!

☆☆ If you answered three or four questions correctly, nice job! Treat yourself to a multisystem-pleasing rest before going on to the last chapter.

☆ If you answered fewer than three questions correctly, don't be shocked! Just review the material and try again.

Appendices and index

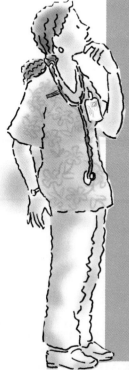

Emergency delivery

Emergency delivery refers to a situation in which the neonate's birth is imminent. It's commonly defined as labor completed within less than 3 hours, and may occur with multiparity. In such cases, rapid assessment of the mother and fetus is critical.

What causes it

Emergency delivery may result from various factors. In some situations, it results from precipitous labor in which uterine contractions are so strong and rapid that the woman delivers after only a few of them. Emergency delivery may also occur due to a lack of understanding about labor signs and symptoms. Additionally, it may be necessary when the mother or fetus exhibits distress.

What to look for

Emergency delivery due to precipitous labor may be identified from a labor graph that shows the active phase of dilation at a rate greater than 5 cm/hour in a nullipara (1 cm every 12 minutes) and greater than 10 cm/hour (1 cm every 6 minutes) in a multipara. Additionally, uterine contraction monitoring may reveal hypertonic contractions.

Vaginal examination may reveal rupture of membranes, with rapid and progressive cervical dilation. Crowning may also be evident.

What you need

- Bulb syringe
- Sterile scissors or scalpel
- Two cord clamps or sterile Kelly clamps
- Basin
- Fluid absorbent pads
- Sterile gloves
- Clean baby blankets
- Sanitary pad
- Infant stockinette hat
- Identification bands per facility policy
- Heated Isolette or warm blankets

What to do

If a patient requires emergency delivery, follow these steps.
- Explain to the patient what's happening and what to expect.

- Monitor the patient's vital signs and fetal heart rate and pattern closely, reporting any significant changes.
- Administer oxygen via face mask as ordered to ensure adequate oxygenation.
- Initiate I.V. therapy if ordered to maintain fluid balance.
- Put on appropriate attire such as a gown and gloves, adhering to standard precautions and your facility's policy.
- Assist the practitioner with delivery by applying gentle pressure with a sterile towel to the neonate's head as it crowns.
- To prevent aspiration, suction the neonate's mouth and nose immediately after the head is delivered.
- Quickly inspect the neonate's neck area for evidence of the umbilical cord; if present and loose, gently slide it over the neonate's head.
- Assist with delivering the remainder of the neonate, providing support to the head and shoulders.
- Assess for spontaneous breaths and crying; if they don't occur, gently rub the neonate's back.
- Assist with clamping the umbilical cord.
- Quickly wrap the neonate in a warmed blanket or place him under a radiant heat source such as an Isolette.
- Determine the neonate's Apgar score.
- If the neonate is stable, place him on the mother's abdomen.
- Assist with delivery of the placenta; after it's delivered, place it in a basin or plastic bag and send it with the mother to the obstetric unit.
- Document the time of delivery of the neonate and placenta. Also document the neonate's status and his Apgar score.
- Monitor maternal vital signs and vaginal bleeding. Maternal bleeding should slow significantly after the placenta's delivery.
- Assess the fundus by gently massaging it while applying moderate suprapubic pressure.
- Prepare the mother and her neonate for transfer to the obstetric unit and nursery.

Recording the Apgar score

Use this chart to determine the neonatal Apgar score at 1-minute and 5-minute intervals after birth. For each category listed, assign a score of 0 to 2, as shown. A total score of 7 to 10 indicates that the neonate is in good condition; 4 to 6, fair condition (the neonate may have moderate central nervous system depression, muscle flaccidity, cyanosis, and poor respirations); 0 to 3, danger (the neonate needs immediate resuscitation, as ordered).

Sign	Apgar score		
	0	1	2
Heart rate	Absent	Less than 100 beats/minute	More than 100 beats/minute
Respiratory effort	Absent	Slow, irregular	Good crying
Muscle tone	Flaccid	Some flexion and resistance to extension of extremities	Active motion
Reflex irritability	No response	Grimace or weak cry	Vigorous cry
Color	Pallor, cyanosis	Pink body, blue extremities	Completely pink

Glossary

abduct: move away from the midline of the body; opposite of *adduct*

adduct: move toward the midline of the body; opposite of *abduct*

advance directive: written legal document that identifies a patient's advance wishes regarding the types of health care he desires if unable to decide for himself

agonist: drug that binds to a receptor to elicit a physiologic response

alveolus: in the lung, a small saclike dilation of the terminal bronchioles

anaerobic: oxygen not required for growth

angina: pain felt in the chest region; typically associated with a heart attack

anion: ion with a negative electrical charge

anorexia: loss of appetite

antagonist: drug that binds to a receptor but doesn't produce a response or blocks the response at the receptor

anterior: front or *ventral;* the opposite of *posterior* or *dorsal*

antibody: immunoglobulin produced by the body in response to exposure to a specific foreign substance (antigen)

antigen: foreign substance that causes antibody formation when introduced into the body

anuria: urine output of less than 100 ml in 24 hours

aphasia: language disorder characterized by difficulty expressing or comprehending speech

apnea: cessation of breathing

apraxia: inability to perform coordinated movements, even though no motor deficit is present

arthrosis: joint or articulation

ascites: accumulation of fluid in the abdominal cavity

assessment: first step in the nursing process that involves data gathering

ataxia: uncoordinated actions when voluntary muscle movements are attempted

atrophy: wasting away

automaticity: ability of the heart to generate its own electrical impulse

avulsion fracture: fracture that occurs when a joint capsule, ligament, tendon, or muscle is pulled from a bone

axonal injury: diffuse brain injury that usually results from tension and shearing forces

Battle's sign: bruising immediately behind the ear that usually indicates a fracture of the posterior portion of the skull

Biot's respirations: respirations that are rapid and deep, and alternate with abrupt periods of apnea

blepharitis: inflammation of the eyelids

body mechanics: use of body positioning or movement to prevent or correct problems related to activity or immobility

borborygmi: loud sounds produced by the normal movement of air through the intestines

bradycardia: abnormally slow heart rate; usually less than 60 beats per minute

bradypnea: abnormally slow respiratory rate; usually less than 10 breaths per minute

bruit: abnormal sound heard over peripheral vessels that indicates turbulent blood flow

buccal: pertaining to the cheek

bursa: fluid-filled sac lined with synovial membrane

capillary: microscopic blood vessel that links arterioles with venules

cardiac cycle: period from the beginning of one heartbeat to the beginning of the next; includes two phases: systole and diastole

carpal: pertaining to the wrist

cartilage: connective supporting tissue occurring mainly in the joints, thorax, larynx, trachea, nose, and ear

celiac: pertaining to the abdomen

central nervous system: one of the two main divisions of the nervous system; consists of the brain and spinal cord

cognition: thinking and awareness

colloid: fluid containing starches or proteins

consciousness: state involving full awareness and ability to respond to stimuli

contralateral: on the opposite side; opposite of *ipsilateral*

coronary: pertaining to the heart or its arteries

cortex: outer part of an internal organ; the opposite of *medulla*

costal: pertaining to the ribs

crackles: intermittent, nonmusical, crackling breath sounds that are caused by collapsed or fluid-filled alveoli popping open

crepitus: noise or vibration produced by rubbing together irregular cartilage surfaces or broken ends of a bone; also the sound heard when air in subcutaneous tissue is palpated

cutaneous: pertaining to the skin

cyanosis: bluish discoloration of the skin or mucous membranes

debridement: removal of dead tissue or foreign material from a wound

dehiscence: separation of a wound's edges

deltoid: shaped like a triangle (as in the deltoid muscle)

dermis: skin layer beneath the epidermis

diaphragm: membrane that separates one part from another; the muscular partition separating the thorax and abdomen

diastole: resting portion of the cardiac cycle where the coronary arteries are filling with blood and the ventricles are relaxed

distal: far from the point of origin or attachment; the opposite of *proximal*

diuresis: formation and excretion of large amounts of urine

dorsal: pertaining to the back or posterior; the opposite of *ventral* or *anterior*

dysarthria: speech defect commonly related to a motor deficit of the tongue or speech muscles

dysphagia: difficulty swallowing

dyspnea: difficult or labored breathing

edema: accumulation of fluid in the interstitial space

empathy: process of putting oneself into the feelings of another

endocardium: interior lining of the heart

endocrine: pertaining to secretion into the blood or lymph rather than into a duct; the opposite of *exocrine*

endometrium: inner mucosal lining of the uterus

epidermis: outermost layer of the skin; lacking vessels

Erb's point: auscultatory point on the precordium at the third intercostal space to the left of the sternum

evisceration: internal organ protrusion through an opening in a wound

exocrine: pertaining to secretion; the opposite of *endocrine*

exophthalmos: abnormal protrusion of the eyeball

fistula: abnormal opening between organs or between an organ and body surface

flaccidity: decrease in muscle tone that causes muscle to become weak or flabby

fluid wave: rippling across the abdomen during percussion; indicative of the presence of ascites

fremitus: palpable vibration that results from air passing through the bronchopulmonary system and transmitting vibrations to the chest wall

gastric lavage: instillation of solution into the stomach and subsequent withdrawal to remove stomach contents

glomerulus: compact cluster; the capillaries of the kidney

hematuria: blood in the urine

hemoglobin: protein found in red blood cells that contains iron

hemoptysis: blood in the sputum

hordeolum: inflammation of the sebaceous gland of the eyelid; also called *stye*

hydrocele: accumulation of serous fluid in a saclike structure such as the testis

hyperopia: defect in vision that allows a person to see objects clearly at a distance but not at close range; also called *farsightedness*

hyperresonance: increased resonance produced by percussion

hypertonic: having a greater concentration than body fluid

hypotonic: having a lesser concentration than body fluid

hypoxemia: state in which the blood contains a lower than normal amount of oxygen

hypoxia: state in which the tissues have a decreased amount of oxygen

infarction: death of tissue due to ischemia

inferior: lower; the opposite of *superior*

infiltration: seepage or leakage of fluid into the tissues

informed consent: legal document that a patient or legal guardian signs giving permission for a procedure after the patient has demonstrated understanding of the procedure

ipsilateral: on the same side; opposite of *contralateral*

ischemia: insufficient blood supply to a part

isotonic: having the same concentration as body fluid

Korotkoff sounds: sounds heard when auscultating blood pressure denoting systolic and diastolic pressures

laceration: wound caused by tearing of the tissues

lacrimal: pertaining to tears

lateral: pertaining to the side; the opposite of *medial*

lethargy: slowed responses, sluggish speech, and slowed mental and motor processes in a person oriented to time, place, and person

living will: advance directive that states the medical care that persons would want or refuse should the person be unable to give consent or refusal

lumbar: pertaining to the area of the back between the thorax and the pelvis

maceration: tissue softening as a result of excessive moisture

manubrium: upper part of the sternum

meatus: opening or passageway

medial: pertaining to the middle; opposite of *lateral*

myocardium: thick, contractile layer of muscle cells that forms the heart wall

nephron: structural and functional unit of the kidney

neutropenia: decreased number of neutrophils

neutrophil: white blood cell that removes and destroys bacteria, cellular debris, and solid particles

Nitrazine paper: treated paper used to detect pH and determine the presence of amniotic fluid

nociceptors: nerve endings that respond to noxious stimuli

olfactory: pertaining to the sense of smell

oliguria: urine output of less than 500 ml in 24 hours

ophthalmic: pertaining to the eye

pectoral: pertaining to the chest or breast

percussion: use of tapping on a body surface with fingers

pericardium: fibroserous sac that surrounds the heart and the origin of the great vessels

peristalsis: movement through the intestines

phrenic: pertaining to the diaphragm

plantar: pertaining to the sole

pleura: thin serous membrane that encloses the lung

plexus: network of nerves, lymphatic vessels, or veins

popliteal: pertaining to the back of the knee

posterior: back or dorsal; the opposite of *anterior* or *ventral*

pronate: to turn the hand or forearm so that the palm faces down or back, or to rotate the foot so that the inner edge of the sole bears the weight of the body; opposite of *supinate*

proximal: situated nearest the center of the body; opposite of *distal*

pruritus: itching

pulse deficit: difference between the apical and radial pulse rates

pulse pressure: difference between the systolic blood pressure and diastolic blood pressure readings

purulent: pus-producing or pus-containing

range of motion: extent to which a person can move his joints or muscles

sanguinous: referring to or containing blood

serosanguineous: containing blood and serum

spasticity: sudden, involuntary increase in muscle tone or contractions

sprain: complete or incomplete tear in the supporting ligaments surrounding a joint

station: relationship of the presenting part to the ischial spines

strain: injury to the muscle or tendinous attachment

striated: marked with parallel lines, such as striated (skeletal) muscle

subcutaneous: related to the tissue layer under the dermis

sublingual: under the tongue

superior: higher; opposite of *inferior*

supinate: to turn the palm or forearm upward; the opposite of *pronate*

systole: period of ventricular contraction

tachycardia: rapid heart rate; usually more than 100 beats per minute

tachypnea: rapid respiratory rate, usually more than 20 breaths per minute

tendon: band of fibrous connective tissue that attaches a muscle to a bone

toco transducer: external mechanical device that translates one physical quantity to another, most commonly seen in capturing fetal heart rates and transmitting and recording the value onto a fetal monitor

Valsalva maneuver: forceful exhalation with a closed glottis; bearing down

ventral: pertaining to the front or *anterior*; the opposite of *dorsal* or *posterior*

ventricle: small cavity, such as one of several in the brain or one of the two lower chambers of the heart

viscera: internal organs

xiphoid: sword-shaped; the lower portion of the sternum

Selected references and Internet resources

Selected references

Bhushan, V., and Bisanzo, M. *Emergency Management of the Trauma Patient: Cases, Algorithms, Evidence*. Philadelphia: Lippincott Williams & Wilkins, 2006.

Fultz, J., and Sturt, P.A. *Mosby's Emergency Nursing Reference*, 3rd ed. St. Louis: Mosby–Year Book, Inc., 2005.

Greenberg, M.I., et al., eds. *Greenberg's Text-Atlas of Emergency Medicine*. Philadelphia: Lippincott Williams & Wilkins, 2004.

Harrison, R., and Daly, L. *Acute Medical Emergencies*, 2nd ed. London: Churchill Livingstone, 2006.

Hohenhaus, S.M. "An Informal Discussion of Emergency Nurses' Current Clinical Practice: What's New and What Works," *Journal of Emergency Nursing* 32(1): 69-70, February 2006.

Jenkins, J.L., and Braen, G.R., eds. *Manual of Emergency Medicine*, 5th ed. Philadelphia: Lippincott Williams & Wilkins, 2004.

Kothari, C.L., and Rhodes, K.V. "Missed Opportunities: Emergency Department Visits by Police-Identified Victims of Intimate Partner Violence," *Annals of Emergency Medicine* 47(2):190-99, February 2006.

Lippincott Manual of Nursing Practice Series: Alarming Signs & Symptoms. Philadelphia: Lippincott Williams & Wilkins, 2007.

Lippincott Manual of Nursing Practice Series: Diagnostic Tests. Philadelphia: Lippincott Williams & Wilkins, 2007.

Lippincott Manual of Nursing Practice Series: Pathophysiology. Philadelphia: Lippincott Williams & Wilkins, 2007.

Lomas, C. "Making a Big Event Out of Emergency Care Nursing," *Nursing Times* 102(2):60-61, January 2006.

MacKenzie, E.J., et al. "A National Evaluation of the Effect of Trauma-Center Care on Mortality," *New England Journal of Medicine* 354(4):366-78, January 2006.

McMonagle, M.P. "Images in Clinical Medicine: The Importance of Early Cervical-Spine Radiography," *New England Journal of Medicine* 354(4):e4, January 2006.

O'Shea, R.A, ed. *Principles and Practice of Trauma Nursing*. London: Churchill Livingstone, 2005.

Prentiss, K.A., et al. *Emergency Management of the Pediatric Patient: Cases, Algorithms, Evidence*. Philadelphia: Lippincott Williams & Wilkins, 2006.

Rapid Response to Everyday Emergencies: A Nurse's Guide. Philadelphia: Lippincott Williams & Wilkins, 2006.

Sheehy's Manual of Emergency Care, 6th ed. St. Louis: Mosby–Year Book, Inc., 2005.

Wellens, H.J., and Conover, M.B. *The ECG in Emergency Decision Making*, 2nd ed. St. Louis: Mosby–Year Book, Inc., 2006.

Zimmermann, P.G., and Herr, R.D. *Triage Nursing Secrets*. St. Louis: Mosby–Year Book, Inc., 2005.

Internet resources

Emergency Nurses Association:
   www.ena.org

Emergency Nursing World:
   www.enw.org

National Emergency Nurses Affiliation:
   www.nena.ca

Index

A

Abdomen, assessing, 268-273, 270i, 358
Abdominal pain, eliciting, 273, 274i
Abdominal paracentesis, 282, 283i
Abdominal reflex, assessing, 55
Abdominal sounds, 270, 271, 272t
Abdominal trauma, 292-295
Abdominal X-ray, 277
Abduction, 313, 351
Abrasions, 437-439, 506
Absence seizure, 77
Abuse, indications of, 331, 332
Accupril, 138t
acebutolol, 125t, 131t
Acetaminophen poisoning, 469t
Acetone breath odor, 457t
acetylcholine, 417
Acid-base disorders, 217, 218t
Acoustic nerve, 51
Acromioclavicular separation, 333t
Activase, 63t, 143t
Activated charcoal, 469, 470
Acute care nurse practitioners, 17-18
Acute coronary syndrome, 154-162. *See also* Angina;
    Myocardial infarction.
  causes of, 155
  diagnostic tests in, 157
  treatment of, 157, 160-161i
Acute respiratory distress, 204, 205
Acute respiratory distress syndrome, systemic inflammatory response syndrome and, 502
Adduction, 313
Adenocard, 132t
adenosine, 132t, 134
Adjuvant analgesics, 36
Adrenalin, 482
Adrenergic blockers, 124-127, 125t
Adrenergics, 121-124, 122-123t
Advance directives, 40
Advanced practice nurse, 17-18
Advocate, nurse as, 2-4, 39
Aerosol therapy, 231-232
Air transport, 21, 22
Airway, assessing, 10, 11t
Airway obstruction, 242-245, 244i
Albumin, 362
albuterol, 227t
Alcohol breath odor, 457t
Aldactone, 141t
Aldomet, 138t
Alpha-adrenergic blockers, 125t, 126
Altace, 138t
alteplase, 63t, 143t
Alu-Cap, 285t

aluminum hydroxide, 285t
aluminum hydroxide and magnesium hydroxide, 285t
Amblyopia, 406
American Nurses Association, 39
amiloride, 141t
amiodarone, 131t
amlodipine, 129t
Ammonia, ingestion of, 455
Amputation, traumatic, 326-328, 506
Analgesics, adjuvant, 36
Anaphylactic shock, 482-489, 484-485i
  causes of, 483
  epinephrine for, 488
  signs and symptoms of, 486
  treatment of, 487
Anaphylaxis. *See* Anaphylactic shock.
Anectine, 228t
Aneurysm. *See specific type.*
Aneurysm repair, 64, 145
Angina, 127
  diagnostic tests in, 157
  pain in, 100t
  signs and symptoms of, 155, 156
  treatment for, 157, 160-161i
Angiography
  in acute coronary syndrome, 157
  cerebral. *See* Cerebral angiography.
  digital subtraction, 56, 57
  fluorescein, 414-415
  in neurologic emergencies, 56-58
  pulmonary, 223-224
  renal, 366-367
Angiotensin-converting enzyme inhibitors, 138t, 139
Angiotensin II receptor antagonists, 139
Ankles
  assessing, 318, 320i
  dislocated, 334t
  fractured, 342-343t
Antacids, 285t
Anterior cord syndrome, 81t
Antianginals, 127-130, 129t
Antiarrhythmics, 130-134, 131-132t
Antibiotics, and anaphylaxis, 483
Anticoagulants, 134-136, 135t
  in neurologic emergencies, 62t
Anticonvulsants, 36, 62t
Antidiuretic hormone, 285t
Antidotes, common, 469t
Antiemetics, 285t
Antihypertensives, 136-139, 138t
Antiplatelet drugs, 62t, 134, 135t
Anturane, 135t
Anzemet, 285t
Aortic aneurysm, 162-166
  dissecting, pain in, 100t

i refers to an illustration; t refers to a table.

i refers to an illustration; t refers to a table.

i refers to an illustration; t refers to a table.

i refers to an illustration; t refers to a table.

i refers to an illustration; t refers to a table.

i refers to an illustration; t refers to a table.

i refers to an illustration; t refers to a table.

i refers to an illustration; t refers to a table.

i refers to an illustration; t refers to a table.

i refers to an illustration; t refers to a table.

Notes

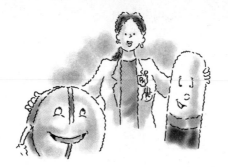

Notes

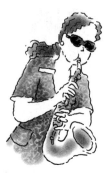

Notes

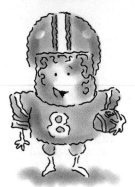

Notes

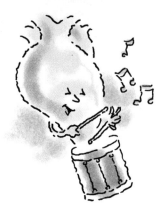